Other Books by Mark Gilberd

Natural Remedies for Animals Series
Natural Remedies for Animal First Aid
Natural Remedies for Cat Diseases
Natural Remedies for Dog Diseases
Natural Remedies for Goat Diseases
Natural Remedies for Sheep Diseases
Natural Remedies for Pig Diseases
Natural Remedies for Cow Diseases
Natural Remedies for Horse Diseases
Natural Remedies for Poultry Diseases

Lady's Companion Series
Lady's Companion to Menopause Treated Naturally
Lady's Companion to PMS Treated naturally
Lady's Companion for First Aid Treated Naturally

Pandemic Flu the Big One A Naturopaths Story
Pandemic and Disaster Diseases Treated Naturally

Pandemic and Disaster Diseases Treated Naturally

Mark Gilberd
Medical Herbalist, Homoeopath and Iridologist

Text Copyright 2013

Foreword

What are you going to do when the Hospitals are full and there are thousands of sick people outside waiting with rumors that most of the staff is sick and stocks have nearly run out? Most of the GPs are sick or closed and all the Chemists have big posters in their windows telling of the stocks that they have run out of, how are you going to treat your family, what are you going to do. This book is your last hope as there is nothing like it, as it is basically a survivors survival manual designed and set out in such a way as to teach you what you need to know at the fastest possible speed while giving you the information you need with the most important being treatment should begin at the first sign of the symptoms and should hopefully have aborted the disease before it starts or made the condition a more milder form of the disease. You will soon be sick to death at reading that same line at the beginning of lots of herbal treatment sections especially in the most nasty ones, but this is the most important point in the book, it can be too late sometimes to do anything once you learn the name of a disease, but if treatment was begun at the beginning of symptoms or before you could have a good chance. If you were using this book in a Survival situation where you were all alone you cannot afford to make mistakes and you don't want to increase your work load. Believe me, when you make mistakes in treatment it will scar you very deep and usually it takes a while to get over it. Latter on just skip the top couple of lines and get straight to the treatment.

This book gives you the edge over most especially if you have been learning from it for a while and preparing yourself. We introduce you to Herbal and Homoeopathic Medicine and go through the most nasty diseases on the planet, even the ones from the past such as Small Pox and give you the Herbal and Homoeopathic remedies for the treatments and sometimes give you the symptoms of a disease not only through the normal way but through the eyes of a Practitioner who one hundred years ago or more was having to deal with it with his back against the wall and no one to rely on but themselves, this gives you a unique perspective that few have seen. In a separate section is Herbal and Homoeopathic First Aid which focuses on injuries more on the Disaster side and gives you another perspective on using natural medicines that you can practice on yourself and family and at the same time will be adding to your knowledge. I have decided to include my novel Pandemic Flu, The Big One, A Naturopaths Story which will add life to a dry reference book and allow you to see how a paranoid lung damaged Naturopath works before and after a Pandemic using logic, the law of mechanics, a good knowledge of medicine and lots of commonsense.

Great effort has been made in the teaching part to train your mind to think like a Professional Herbalist and to give you the resources that you would need, some parts have been written in such a way that as you gain experience and read that same part again later you will get a new and different messages from it.

I have made Homoeopathy a large part of the treatment section of this book for two reasons, the first is because most Homoeopathic knowledge has been preserved over time and it is easy to reference the remedies used for let's say Cholera and Typhoid because they have been using the same remedies for hundreds of years and still are in places like India where it is on the National Health System. The second and most important reason is that a stock of Homoeopathic Medicines could easily be made to last hundreds of times longer than say a similar supply of modern or herbal medicines for the simple reasons that you use less and you can use the remedies to make more remedies.

Most teaching manuals start at the beginning and try to add knowledge upon knowledge which is how it should be done but here because time may be a luxury you do not have, you start immediately to learn how to treat the most nasty diseases on the planet, and as you read and go through each disease all their common factors slowly start to become apparent, and as you are using the same process of thinking in handling these diseases you should start becoming a little more confident, but it is only time and effort that will bring good results, but at least you are not alone anymore and you can have hope again, always remember prevention is the best way to go.

One of the main reasons for this book is that most of the Natural Remedy Treatments for the epidemics and plagues of the past are now lost in time especially in the western world and there is no quick reference such as this.

I have always wondered what would happen in a disaster so great that the drug companies collapsed along with the whole system of modern medicine. That would only leave people like me left a survivor.

Regards

Mark Gilberd

Medical Herbalist, Homoeopath and Iridologist

Willis Alonzo Dewy MD 1858 to 1938 Homoeopathic Master

Most of the Homoeopathic write ups in the diseases of this book are sourced from the Gentleman above. I am very lucky to have some of his early editions from the beginning of the 19 centaury which are now copyright expired. His work is always interesting and always very useful as he was the man on the spot as technology was changing around him, it is a pity he didn't live for ten more years to see the onset of anti-biotics. His works lives on long after his death and still is saving and giving comfort to life even today; he has surely more than paid his entrance fee to heaven and still keeps on giving which can only be said about a few people. More of interest and keeping to the title of this book during Spanish flu pandemic of 1918, which killed up to 50 million people worldwide he gathered data from homeopathic physicians treating flu patients around the country in 1918 and published his findings in the Journal of the American Institute of Homeopathy in 1920. The homeopathic physicians in the U.S. reported very low mortality rates among their patients, while flu patients treated by conventional physicians faced mortality rates of around 30 percent. Part of the reason Homoeopaths have survived pandemics for centuries is that when they get very scared they tend to make a Disease Nosode from the disease and use that to protect themselves and others and to slow down the spread. Dr Dewey was a native of Middlebury, Vermont and was born on October 25, 1858, son of Josiah Earl Dewey and Eunice Converse Carpenter and of New England ancestors of which some were patriots and soldiers of the revolution.

Dr. Dewey was educated in the high school at Middlebury in 1872, Burr and Burton Seminary, Manchester, Vermont in 1873, and the public schools of New York City, where he was a student from 1868 to 1872. He is also a graduate of Packard's Business College, New York city. He was educated in medicine at the New York Homœopathic Medical College, where he gained a degree in 1889. In 1880 he was interne at Ward's Island Homœopathic Hospital in New York City, The years 1881 and 1882 were spent in studies in Berlin, Heidelberg, Vienna, Paris and London all of which would of had large Homoeopathic communities especially Germany. From 1884 until 1888 he was professor of anatomy in Hahnemann Medical College of the

Pacific, and from 1888 until 1892 held the chair of Materia Medica in that institution and at the same time was editor of the "California Homœopath." In 1894 he filled the chair of Materia Medica in the Metropolitan Post-Graduate School of Medicine, New York City and in 1896 he was appointed to the same chair in the Homœopathic Department of the University of Michigan, with which he has since been associated.

Throughout his medical life he has been a faithful contributor to the literature of his profession and is the author of Essentials of Homœopathic Materia Medica, Essentials of Homœopathic Therapeutics, Practical Homœopathic Therapeutics and co-authored with Boericke the Boericke and Dewey's "Twelve Tissue Remedies which is a must for anyone who uses cell salts. These are but his most well-known works, there are plenty more.

Index

A Brief History Of Plagues And Epidemics
Waiting For The Big One
Some Of Our More Modern Diseases
Vaccines
Have Antibiotics Run Their Course
TB A Good Example Of Antibiotic Resistance
Treatment Of Acute Diseases

Disease Fighting Herbs

Andrographis
Astragalus
Baptisia
Boneset
Burdock
Cats Claw
Echinacea
Elecampane
Elder
Garlic
Goldenseal
Licorice
Myrrh
Plantain
Pleurisy Root
Reshi Mushroom
Shitkae Mushroom
Willow Bark
Yarrow

Herbal Actions

The Main Herbal Actions Used In Different Systems

Actions Used In The Respiratory System
Actions Used In The Digestive System
Actions Used In The Nervous System
Actions Used In The Urinary System
Actions Used In The Muscular Skeletal System
Actions Used For The Skin

Actions Used In The Reproductive System
Homoeopathic Treatment
Symptom Guide Questions
Materia Medica
Boerickes Materia Medica
Disease Nosodes
How To Make A Nosode In A Hurry
Nutritional Disease Fighting Supplements
Vitamin A
Vitamin C
Vitamin E
Selenium
Zinc
Colostrum
Fever
Rehydration Formulas
Airborne, Contact And Crowding Diseases
Influenza
Measles
Chicken Pox
Small Pox
Diphtheria
Whooping Cough
Scarlet Fever
Mumps
Meningitis
Tuberculosis
Waterborne Diseases
Rehydration Formulas
Gastroenteritis Bacterial Infections
Gastroenteritis Viral Infections
Disease Causing Organisms In Food
Shigellosis
Rota Virus
Norovirus
Cholera

Typhoid Fever
Giardia
Cryptosporidiosis
Leptospirosis
Hepatitis A

Animal And Insect Borne Diseases

Dengue
Yellow Fever
Ross River Fever
Murray Valley Encephalitis
Typhus
Plague - The Black Death

Man Made And Natural Disasters

Nuclear Weapons And Radiation
Biological And Germ Warfare
Global Warming

Surviving Natural Disasters

Tsunami
Floods
Earthquakes
Hurricanes, Typhoons And Cyclones
Volcanoes
Fires

First Aid Naturally

Tetanus
Septicemia
Gangrene

First Aid

Abscess and Boils
Bites and Stings
Bruises
Bleeding
Bones and Fractures
Burns
Cuts and Wounds - Puncture Wounds - After Surgery
Diarrhea
Dysentery

Earache
Eczema
Eye Problems
Gastritis and Gastroenteritis
Hay Fever
Hemorrhoids
Indigestion
Itching
Motion Sickness
Nose Bleed
Nausea
Ring worm
Sunburn
Sprains
Splinters
Shock
Our Two Main Wound Herbs
Calendula
Hypericum
HyperCal
Herbs Used In This Book
Glossary Of Herbal Terms
Homoeopathics Used In This Book
Pandemic Flu The Big On A Naturopaths Story (Novel).
Medical Terms

A Brief History Of Plagues And Epidemics

One of the earliest recorded plagues was in Athens in 430 BC. This was recorded by the Greek historian Thucydides. The plague killed half of the population and collapsed the state. Thucydides writes that the plague had first begun in the ports of Ethiopia and had traveled from there to Egypt, Libya and then into most of Persia.

Probably the next largest plague recorded could have been the beginning of the end of the Roman Empire. The cause is believed to have been the return of troops from a rebellion in Syria in 165 CE to Rome then a city of 2 million people. Historians believe that the plague may have been smallpox but are unsure. At the height of the plague 2000 people were dying a day and over the next 14 years the plague spread through the Roman Empire. Still worse was the plague in Rome of 251 CE that killed as many as 5000 a day and continued in the city and provinces till 266 CE.

In 542 CE the bubonic plague reached Constantinople causing untold suffering and death for 3 months until winter came and changed the disease into its worst form of contagious pneumonic plague. At its height 10,000 people a day were dying. When the crisis subsided 40% of the population was dead. For the next 6 years the disease raged across Europe killing half of the population. By 610 CE it had reached China.

After the fall of Rome and the finish of the bubonic plague we entered the dark ages for the next 900 years. The Black Plague returned again to Europe in 1340 and left about 30 million dead by the time it declined in 1351 which was about a third of the population of Europe. London alone lost 35,000 people out of a total of 60,000. In Paris 800 people died a day. Syria and Egypt lost about a third of their populations between 1347 to 1349 while China lost about two thirds of its population between 1353 and 1354. For about 50 years around this time the weather had been growing colder and stormier and crops had been failing. In 1309 the worst famine in Europe's history began and lasted for ten years. By 1325 more than one person in ten had starved to death and sickness was common.

In China in 1333 drought and famine followed the first onset of the plague then a series of floods and earthquakes happened along with the Mongol uprising. War, famine and disease followed leaving the people very vulnerable when the Black Plague returned in 1353.

Christopher Columbus discovery of the Americas in 1492 started another wave of epidemics this time going both ways. Columbus is reputed to have brought syphilis back to Portugal which from their slowly spread all through Europe. Columbus introduced smallpox, measles and most of the other European diseases to the Americas with devastating results, from 1518 to 1568 a estimated 25 million Mexican Indians died out of a total population of 28 million. Smallpox latter went on to kill most of the North American Indians. The Americas had an estimated population of 100 million before the Europeans brought their diseases and by the early 19th century the native population had been reduced to about 10 million. European arms did not conquer the Americas their microbes did.

African slaves were brought to the Americas starting from the mid-17th century bringing with them malaria and yellow fever to which both the European and Indian populations were susceptible to. Both of these diseases were later found by scientists to be caused by the mosquitoes so when the mosquitoes were killed the problem went away.

The first major cholera epidemic occurred in India in the early 1800s and from the ports of India traveled the world reaching Europe and the USA in 1832.

The Spanish Flu Pandemic went from 1918 to 1920 killing at the least 20 million people 5 million more than WW1. It is known as the Spanish flu because Spain being a neutral country in WW1 was about the only country whose media could report about the disease in the newspapers for most other countries were subject to war time censorship.

We will end with a more recent outbreak of Cholera this one in Lima Pere 1991where the cause was found to be a ship from Asian waters empting their ballast tanks into the harbor, unfortunately they had filled the tanks with cholera infected water which went on to contaminate shellfish and fish that the local population ate.

From our brief history of some of humanities biggest killers we can draw three fairly self-evident conclusions.

1. Infectious microbes can be very effective and capable travelers often adapting to problems on the way and forever evolving.
2. When infectious microbes attack a people who have never had contact with that particular species of microbes and if the microbes are of a dangerous and fatal nature there can be massive population losses.
3. If people are malnourished, poor, stressed and living in unsanitary conditions whether from famine, disaster or war they are ripe targets for infectious diseases. These will be the people with the highest death rate.

Waiting For The Big One

The nearest thing to a plague we are experiencing now is AIDS which has now been around for quite a while and yet no significant advance has been made in a cure which is very worrying but still there is hope after one man was cured in Germany but whether they can duplicate it again remains to be seen, but if they can't figure this how are they going to handle a fast moving deadly virus when their isn't really a Doctor alive who has ever dealt with a situation like this and can you make a vaccine in time when all the staff who make the vaccine are probably going down with the disease themselves along with the rest of the population. AIDS is also a good example of our three previous conclusions especially when we look at its spread through Africa, India and Asia. Our most recent scares have come from SARS (2002) and Bird Flu which is still ongoing. Let take a look at SARS first. SARS stands for Severe Acute Respiratory Syndrome and is a severe form of viral pneumonia from a cross over infection from the animal kingdom. From China SARS spread to about 24 countries till it was halted by the International Health Care Agency with only about 8000 sick resulting in 770 deaths. This was a very lucky save and hopefully it has improved the chances of stopping similar cases in the future.

Bird Flu is an ongoing problem and a possible pandemic in the making which only the future mutations of the virus will tell. So far it has a just under 50% death rate. Controlling air travel may not be a preventative for this disease as it was in SARS because it is migrating birds that are spreading the disease to local poultry populations which in turn pass the disease on to humans. It is the cross over infections from the animal kingdom that are the most dangerous for us humans as our immune systems just don't recognize them and by the time it figures something is wrong and launches its attack it may be just too late. Let's now take a look at the worst case scenario of what may be possible to happen. A chicken in Turkey has caught bird flu from a flock of migrating birds which spent the night in trees next to a pond that the chickens forage around. A child with the flu comes out to feed the chickens. The child catches bird flu from the chicken. In the Childs body the two viruses meet each other and make a new flu strain. To this newly evolved flu chickens and humans will probably have no immunities. The child gets sicker and starts to cough spreading the new flu through the family. The child's father starts to get the flu but forces himself to go to work for he is head of security at a massive multinational meeting and has to be there. At the meeting he spreads the virus to lots of people who the next day will take it back to their home countries. It is said that the Spanish Flu took four months to spread through the world and if they had the air travel that we have now experts reckon the disease could spread around the world in four days. For a more in depth and different scenario read the Pandemic Flu novel at the back.

Some Of Our More Modern Diseases

Just by reading the list below especially the causes, origins and deaths gives you a good idea of what the world is up against presently and a idea of future potentials. Bear in mind that we are just at the beginning of where the effects of climate change are going to start hitting hard, we have had it fairly easy so far our future response will tell if we really deserve this planet or not. I have left out Swine flu as this will keep on happening as long as we keep living close to pigs but have mentioned Avian flu as having the ability to fly where you please and breach boarder and quarantine creates problems. Below are some of the more well-known diseases in time line.

West Nile Disease

First Recognized - Uganda 1937 Arrived in USA 1999.
Origin - Africa and Middle East.
Host Animal - Birds but natural host is not known, kills some species of birds.
Virus Family - Flaviviruses
Number Of Cases - In the US there have been 2944 cases up to 2005.
Number Of Deaths - In the US there have been 98 deaths up to 2005.
Future Outlook - The disease is now established across the US.

This virus is interesting in that it traveled so far and then liked the environment when it got there for it is a mosquito bourn tropical disease. The virus attacks young children and the elderly and ailing. Those hospitalized complained of fevers, headaches, weakness, tremors, confusion, stiff necks and paralysis. At its worst it leads onto encephalitis which can be lethal. When this virus first arrived it started killing thousands of birds but it was the crows which suffered the worst with 90% of them dyeing in Queens (New York) which really got the investigation going. Dr McNamara a vet started the investigation and had to push the other agencies to work on the problem. It took 3 months to find the name of the virus. By 2001 the CDC had found the virus in 58 different species of animals.

Monkey Pox

First Recognized - In Monkeys 1958, Humans 1970 in Africa Traveled to USA in 2003.
Origin - Africa
Host Animal - African Squirrels
Virus Family - Pox virus
Number Of Cases - In USA 82
Number Of Deaths - In USA none but a 10% death rate in Africa.
Future Outlook - Outbreaks possible if exotic pet trade isn't controlled.

The symptoms this virus caused were feeling feverish, tired and aching all over, swollen glands, pounding head, then latter crops of pus filled sores that break open the crust and scab over. This would have scared the doctors for they would have thought it was smallpox. On investigation they found that prairie dogs were spreading the disease and tracked the disease to a pet shop that had Gambian pouched rats imported from Africa along with other rodents from Africa. The original shipment contained 800 animals. The US has now banned importation of African rodents.

Marburg Fever

First Recognized - 1967
Origin - Africa
Host Animal - Primates, reservoir is unknown but bats are suspected.
Virus Family - Filoviruses
Number Of Cases - 374
Number Of Deaths - 329
Future Outlook - Uncertain, could return but there is a vaccine successful in primates.

This virus was unknown before the outbreak. People started arriving at the hospital in Germany suffering from fever, vomiting, diarrhea, severe headache and body ache. There was no response to antibiotics. The intestinal complications were accompanied by other symptoms, a wide spread rash of bright red spots, reddening of the genitals, liver enlargement and hemorrhaging. Blood seeped out of the gastrointestinal tract, the lungs, the nose, the gums and spots where the patients had been pricked with needles. On investigation it was found 31 of the patients had handled monkey blood. The blood was from green monkeys from Uganda and apparently some of the monkeys got sick on transit.

Ebola

First Recognized - 1976
Origin - Africa
Host Animal - Primates.
Virus Family - Filoviruses
Number Of Cases - Unknowns
Number Of Deaths - Death Rate Is 50 to 90%
Future Outlook - Will keep occurring until monkey hunting stops.

Outbreaks occurred in Sudan 1976, Uganda in 2000 and Angola 2004. The disease strikes suddenly with patients complaining of terrible headaches and weakness. Within days the condition worsens to chills and high fever over 105 degrees, severe muscle and joint pains and a throat so sore it is difficult to swallow saliva let alone food. Around the 4th day the patient begins hemorrhaging from various extremities. When death comes it is from shock on account of fluid loss. The Africans wash the bodies of their dead before burial and it was found that this was one of the main ways the disease is spreading. Poor hygiene and the sharing of needles as well as handling of the patients made hospitals a spreader of Ebola. One thing to consider here is that this disease can only really be handled in a close to full bio hazard suit, imagine working in this suite on a hot summer day in Africa, you would not last long my respect goes to those who have to.

AIDS

First Recognized - Named in 1982, virus found in1985
Origin - Possibly Africa
Host Animal - Possibly monkeys
Virus Family - Belongs to a group of Retroviruses called lentivruses found in primates.
Number Cases - Tens of millions and increasing.
Number Of Deaths - Tens of millions and increasing.
Future Outlook - Bleak

The oldest known case of AIDS occurred in a man from Kinshasha near the mouth of the Congo River Africa. His blood was drawn in 1959 and later tested positive for HIV.

People with HIV are defined as having AIDS once their CD4 + T cell count goes below 200 cells per cubic millimeter of blood. AIDS refers to the end stage which can take 8 to 10 years for a HIV person to reach. AIDS is a severe impairment for the immune system and makes the person vulnerable to diseases and cancers. Most of these infections are called opportunistic because the organisms that cause them take advantage of the lowered immunity. HIV is not a single virus but a family of related virus subtypes called clades, in all there are 8 clades labeled A through to H. In addition the virus changes rapidly by mutation and never stays still long enough for a vaccine to become effective. The chance of finding a cure for AIDS looks very bleak.

Hanta Virus Pulmonary Syndrome

First Recognized - 1993
Origin - Four Corners Region USA
Host Animal - Deer Mice and other small rodents.
Virus Family - Bunya viruses
Number Of Cases - 396
Number Of Deaths - 143
Future Outlook - Possible outbreaks when rodent populations explode and invade homes

On May the 14th 1993 a 19 year old Navajo Indian long distance runner collapsed and died after difficulty breathing in a car on the way to the funeral of who was possibly another victim. The disease starts out like a cold or flu, then the lungs fill with fluid and the patient cant breath and dies. The unusual thing about the disease is that it was killing young and fit people. Later they found that the virus is shed in rodent droppings and inhaled when the soil or dust is disturbed. It can also enter the body through the eyes, broken skin or contaminated food and water.

Avian Flu

First Recognized - 1997
Origin - Southern China
Host Animal - Aquatic birds
Virus Family - Influenza Viruses
Number Of Cases - 205 by spring 2006

Number Of Deaths - 130 by spring 2006

Future Outlook - Uncertain. A pandemic is possible but not inevitable.

The reported signs and symptoms of avian influenza in humans have ranged from eye infections (conjunctivitis) to influenza-like illness symptoms e.g., fever, cough, sore throat, muscle aches to severe a respiratory illness such as pneumonia, acute respiratory distress and viral pneumonia. Sometimes it is accompanied by nausea, diarrhea, vomiting and neurologic changes. The main reason H5N1 has not caused a pandemic yet is that it does no spread from person to person. We shall have to wait and see what happens when it meets up with Swine Flu.

SARS

First Recognized - 2003

Origin - Southern China

Host Animal - Civets, possibly bats.

Virus Family - Corona viruses

Number Of Cases - 8098.

Number Of Deaths - 774

Future Outlook - The outbreak died but could happen again.

SARS was the one that nearly got away, it managed to get to about 7 countries before good policing and quarantine stopped it. The disease was very contagious being airborne along with spreading from contaminated surfaces. Some patients were found to have infected over 33 other people. The disease starts with flu like symptoms, fever, muscle aches, headaches, dry cough and a sore throat but the patient becomes short of breath from infected lungs leading then to pneumonia and for some death even after being put on respirators. The outbreak was tracked down to Civets being eaten leading to the Chinese government to kill about 10,000 of them along with raccoon dogs and badgers which were also found to be infected. SARS was the modern world's first test of tracking and treating in real time on the internet.

Middle East Respiratory Syndrome - MERS-CoV.

First Recognized - First reported in Saudi Arabia in 2012.

Origin - So far, all the cases have been linked to four countries in or near the Arabian Peninsula.

Host Animal - MERS-CoV is more closely related to the bat coronaviruses

HKU4 and HKU5
Virus Family - Coronavirus called MERS-CoV
Number Of Cases -
Number Of Deaths - Over a hundred and rising
Future Outlook - Uncertain

(MERS) is viral respiratory illness caused by a coronavirus first reported on 24 September 2012. MERS-CoV is the sixth new type of coronavirus like SARS but still distinct from it. Most people who have been confirmed to have the MERS-CoV infection developed a severe acute respiratory illness. They had fever, cough, and shortness of breath. About half of these people died.

This virus has spread from ill people to others through close contact. However, the virus has not shown to spread in a sustained way in communities. The situation is still evolving.

Vaccines

The best way to fight diseases is to prevent people from getting them in the first place. After town planning and hygiene vaccination is the main preventative. Being a Natural Practitioner I know the cases for and against vaccination and know vaccination is more about numbers rather than an individual being protected immediately after their shot but in this book I have to be for it because of the extreme conditions I am writing about, as an example let's take a look at a worst case scenario. Ebola is treated in a near full biohazard suit as contact with the patient spreads the disease. Imagine Ebola has now mutated and is now an airborne infection. You now have a fatal disease which can only be treated in quarantine situations running havoc and there is no cure and the death process is like something out of a horror movie. There is only one hope, vaccinate the population before they come into contact with the disease and do it fast. That is of course if they can make a vaccine in time, in a worse case example as this a vaccine may be the only hope so for this reason alone let us hope that vaccine technology makes the leap into Vaccines made of genetic material which hopefully will provide all the benefits of the existing vaccines but with less risk.

Let's take a quick look at how they make some of our vaccines now. In the first stage the target microbe has to be cultured in vast quantities, once enough have been grown they are killed, changed or weakened so that they cannot cause a infection. Each batch is then tested to make sure it is effective against the intended microbe and is strong enough and does not have any contaminates. Then the vaccine is sent off for government testing. Upon its return it is then put into one dose bottles or syringes.

Active immunity against a specific disease is given by injecting a person with weakened poisons or proteins of an infectious organism which stimulates the immune system and programs it for defense should the person latter come into contact with the disease. A vaccine creates a immune response which causes the production of antibodies and memory cells without making us sick most of the time.

Vaccines can give protection to the following diseases - Smallpox, anthrax, chickenpox, hepatitis A and B, mumps, rubella, diphtheria, polio, rabies, tetanus, yellow fever, cholera and many other diseases.

Vaccines are mainly used to prevent large outbreaks in communities as well as to give individual protection. One of the main reasons for mass vaccination is to cut down the numbers of susceptible people in a community making it harder for a disease to spread. This has actually succeeded in wiping out the disease smallpox and polio is the one they next hope to end. The main problem with vaccinations is that it is not always easy to make a vaccine that is safe and effective especially when you are dealing with viruses like the flu or AIDS which keep on mutating and changing their shapes all the time.

The future of vaccines lies in embracing the new technology of genetics. Vaccines made of genetic material either DNA or RNA should provide all the benefits of existing vaccines without the risk of infection and hopefully any allergic response. They should be able to activate the immune system, be inexpensive, stable and easy to store. The problem with today's technology is that it can take 3 to 6 months to make a vaccine if they can at all and that is a far to slow response to a raging pandemic. The problems of bringing in the new technology are the usual ones, it costs a lot of money in an area where there is not much profit to be made and they are scared of the media and law suits if anything goes wrong.

Have Antibiotics Run Their Course

Bacteria have been on this planet far longer than we have and they have also survived all the disasters that have wiped out our past species such as the dinosaurs so you can say that they are the ultimate survivor. Part of their survival mechanism is their ability to multiply rapidly and adapt to new circumstances. Some bacteria if the conditions are right are capable of dividing every 20 minutes, by doubling the number of bacteria at this rate you can start with a single bacterium at 6 in the morning and have a quarter of a million by noon. Six hours latter you could theoretically be up to well over 68 billion. Add to this equation that every new lot would have their weak ones, strong ones and mutant ones, now shuffle the deck and see what happens, I suppose we should call this evolution, but look at the speed that it is taking place.

Let's look at some of the common bacteria that infect us.

Cocci Bacteria - These are shaped like round balls and cause the diseases - pneumonia, tonsillitis, bacterial heart disease, meningitis, some blood poisonings and various skin diseases.

Bacilli bacteria - These a rod shaped looking like a pill capsule and cause the diseases - TB, whooping cough, tetanus, typhoid, diphtheria,

salmonellas, legionnaires disease and botulism.
Spirochetes - These are shaped like a spiral and cause the diseases - syphilis, leptospirosis, and lymes disease.

Let's look at some of the ways antibiotics fight these bacteria.

1. The penicillin family of antibiotics work by stopping the microbes from making new cell wall materials, as the walls become weak they cannot be mended and the microbes eventually burst open and die.
2. Sulfa Drugs prevent microbes from reproducing, if no more microbes are produced then the body's natural defenses can deal with the problem.
3. Streptomycin's prevent proteins being made inside the microbes which stop the microbes from functioning properly and eventually kills them.

Antibiotics usually come from nature mostly from the fungi family but there are lots of others for our example we will use the fungi family. Fungi and bacteria share a lot of the same likes such as warm damp places to live and colonize. No doubt back in time when our planet was young there was once a nice warm damp rock on which one side there were mold spreading happily and then along came some bacteria who thought this is a nice place I think I will stay and colonize. The mold was not happy at all about this and finally come up with the first antibiotic and reclaimed its home. This is also the beginning of antibiotic resistance for a few bacteria survived the mold attack and on their little cold damp rock while they were recovering started to make new plans. That's a cute little story but it is probably very close to the truth.

In 1928 Alexandra Flemming went away from the lab for a few days leaving cultures and microbes to grow while he was gone. When he returned and studied his cultures he found to his surprise that a colony of microbes had begun to grow and then died. Strangely a patch of mold was growing in the same dish. Flemming isolated the new chemical from the mold and called it penicillin. Starting from the middle of WW2 the Growth Industry of Medical Antibiotics began and Doctors started writing scripts to the masses who took the pills but usually stopped taking them as soon as they started feeling better, little did they know that they were only killing off the susceptible bacteria and leaving those with a partial resistance to survive, change and fight another day. Today the Doctors should insist that we take the whole course of antibiotics, so there is no chance of survivors.

The early scientists had a suspicion that drug resistance would become a problem in the future but the problem arrived sooner and bigger than any could believe. Latter a new and terrifying truth was discovered. What was discovered was that antibiotic resistance could be handed to neighboring bacteria that happened to be living nearby even if it was a different species of bacteria. The learning and evolution of one species can be simply handed over to another. The mechanism involves plasmids which are small loops of DNA that sit inside bacteria and are separate from the main chromosomes. There is a mechanical exchange by the bacteria coming next to each other and then joining themselves by a small tube which allows the plasmid to travel to the other bacteria.

Bacteria have now evolved further by developing Transposons. Transposons are even smaller pieces of DNA then the plasmids and they are able to jump from one piece of genetic material to another, they can jump from the plasmid to the chromosome or vice versa. These can easily transfer resistance genes within a bacterial cell or from one cell to another. This is an even faster and more efficient way of spreading resistance genes among the populations of bacteria. Spontaneous mutations, plasmids and transposons are the main methods bacteria employ to survive in the presence of antibiotics.

Another large cause of antibiotic resistance is the use of antibiotics in animal feeds. Farm animals are given large amounts of antibiotics as growth enhancers and to treat specific infections. The bacteria on and inside these animals tend to be multi resistant and they can pass this on especially to the people who work closely with them. The speed at which bacterial resistance is now developing is much faster than the pace at which drug companies can produce new antibiotics and some have even given up trying. I doubt if we will ever be able to get out of the mess we have created with farmers with no knowledge or training in antibiotics able to buy and use them at will and markets in Africa and other countries selling them to anyone with money along with Doctors prescribing them to shut up complaining and insistent mums even when they know it is of no use, its time these truths were brought out to the general public for they are not fools because if the experts won't do anything who else will.

Below is an anonymous quote from a WHO report on Infectious Disease in 2000

2000 BC - Here eat this root
1000 AD - That root is heathen. Here say this pray.
1850 AD - That prayer is superstition. Here drink this potion.
1920 AD - That potion is snake oil. Here swallow this pill.
1945 AD - That pill is ineffective. Here take this penicillin.
1955 AD - Oops bug mutated. Here take this Tetracycline.
1960 - 1999 AD - 39 more oops. Here take this more powerful antibiotic.
2000 AD - The bugs have won. Here eat this root.

TB Is A Good Example Of Antibiotic Resistance And Our Past Coming Back To Haunt Us

TB is caused by the bacteria Mycobacterium Tuberculosis which spreads through airborne droplets sprayed out when a infected person coughs. The bacteria can remain in the air for up to 2 hours. The symptoms are cough, weight loss, night sweats, fever, chest pains and the coughing up of blood. TB has largely been forgotten about by the major industrialized countries and is often thought of as something that happened in the past. In the early 1800s it was a major cause of death by eating away at the body tissues such as the lungs until they no longer worked. In 1882 Robert Koch identified the TB bacteria thus proving TB was a infectious disease which started measures to be taken by the authorities to prevent the spread. The next main step in the fight against TB was in 1908 when the BCG vaccination was developed giving children immunity to the disease.

By the 1950s effective antibiotics had been found that treated and cured most cases. Across Europe and the US it seemed that they had won the battle against TB. Recently there has been a massive worldwide resurgence of TB starting in the early 1990s infecting 8 million people and killing about 2 million annually. Additionally the disease is also implicated in the death of another 1 million HIV infected people. TB now kills more people then AIDS and Malaria combined.

MDR - TB refers to TB that is resistant to 2 or more of the primary drugs used to treat it. TB treatment can extend for months or even years and can cost up to $250,000 per person. It is now feared that up to a third of the world's population is infected with TB. In Eastern Europe in 1997 the region reported 67.6 TB cases per 1000 people. Russia saw a 300% rise in TB cases between 1992 and 1996 and in 1998 alone saw 250,000 new cases of infection with 10 to 20% of them being the new MDR -TB. WHO has identified eight hot spots of MDR-TB they are Russia, Central Africa, India, Pakistan, Thailand, The Philippines, Indonesia and South Africa. In Sub Saharan Africa about 1.5 million TB cases are reported annually while Asia reports 3 million annually.

Presently they have started putting the three main TB drugs Isoniazid, Rifamoin and Pyrazinamide into one new pill called Rifater and toughened up the treatment regime for example in South Africa and many other places now if you have MDR-TB you must get someone to sign a document that they will witness you taking the medicine and ensure you run the whole course before they will give you the medicine. This situation can only get worse.

Treatment Of Acute Diseases With Herbal And Homoeopathic Medicines

My Personal Survival Story

The best way to treat acute disease is to prevent it from happening. We usually get warning that something is wrong, when you get that I think I am coming down with something feeling that's the time to start treatment. The following story is how I found a way to do just that. In the year 2000 after heaps of lung abuse I hit the side of a MDF particle board dust silo while wheeling a big bin out from under it and half buried me in what dropped down on me. About midnight I didn't feel well and coughed and my mouth tasted of iron. I got up went to the bathroom coughed again and spat in the wash bowl and it was mostly blood. I quickly drove to hospital; it felt like my lungs were filling up with blood. It was the fasted admission I have ever had I just got to the counter at the hospital pulled out my hanky coughed into it and made a mess of it and they just grabbed me and took me out the back. To cut a long story short after a scary 24 hours I became a death reject with a great fear of coughing and much damaged lungs. After Workcare weaseled out (its only registered as a carcinogen in Europe, it doesn't kill Australians) and the Hospital got rid of me a week later after managing to pass the lung function test (if you can walk and feed yourself we've got no room for you in a Queensland Hospital) I was left on my own to somehow survive in a world full of flu and cold germs that might make me cough but I was determined to survive even if I had to hang myself upside down to let the blood drain out.

The first 2 years were the worst but I developed a good system and didn't get anything for about 3 years. This is what I did. At the first hint that I might be coming down with something I would start taking Vitamin C in 1000 mg doses every hour and start on the Garlic Oil capsules as they are anti-viral, antibiotic, anti-fungal and lots more but the main important reason is that they exit the body via the lungs which concentrates their actions just where I want, sometimes when I was really scared I used to take up to 36 capsules a day so I would be nearly sweating garlic. Echinacea was the next main one that I would take in tincture form so as to stimulate the bone marrow to make an army of more white blood cells as well as to take care of anything wandering around the blood stream. My other main weapon was Tea Tree Oil which I used with water as a gargle especially when you feel the dry pain beginning in the top of your throat in the nasal passage area that usually precedes a cold. What you do is gargle and try to wash a bit of gargle into this area without choking yourself. The whole idea is that if you take out the scouting parties the main force won't arrive. Some of these doses were extreme for example the Vitamin C dose would have been on the border of making the bowels loose while the Garlic dose would be close and probably past the dose you would use for worming purposes but I live and didn't cough for three years. Unfortunately it took about another 5 years after that to get the voice box working properly.

Now let's look at giving treatment immediately instead of waiting to find out what the disease is called and maybe then finding out that it is too late which generally happens in the case of males. And even if we fail to stop the disease it will most likely run a milder course because it is now weaker from our efforts.

Disease Fighting Herbs

These are the herbs you need to learn in case one day you have to fight a really strong acute disease. Use Homoeopathic Aconite 30C first in any severe disease that comes on fast as this remedy can sometimes abort the condition, and while this remedy is working you can get your Herbs ready. In respiratory diseases always use the Tea Tree Oil gargle as soon as you feel pain and dryness in the nasopharynx area and try to wash some gargle in their without choking yourself (usually 3 to 6 drops of oil to a wine glass of water. Echinacea and Garlic are our main herbs and most of the time we start with them at the beginning of a disease especially if we don't know what it is. Always try to focus on the cause as well as the end results so if you think the cause is bacterial then focus on antibacterial Herbs, if it's a virus focus on antiviral Herbs etc, you will soon be given a list of these herbs.

When learning herbs focus and think in the Actions of the Herbs and never use more than 5 herbs mixed together. First learn the Actions and what the different Actions mean and can do as well as learning the herbs below. After this we shall go through the Body Systems and the Actions needed for them. I want you to learn to think in Actions for example this person has dysentery so I need to use Astringent Herbs or this person has a cough but is not bringing anything up so I need Expectorant Herbs. Don't suppress nature by giving them something to just stop the cough and leave all the rubbish in the chest, work with nature and help get rid of the rubbish in other words help the body to help its self. This is the way you must train your mind, I need that Action for this condition and I need to add to it the Actions of this and that as well instead of thinking that Herb worked well last time so I will use it again. Think holistically try to see the whole picture of what that disease is doing to that patient and make a tailor made herbal formula to that individual using no more than 5 Herbs with one of those Herbs in the formula not only helping the patient but also for pushing the formula into the body (Licorice or Ginger). Keep reading the above paragraph over and over again for it's what you have to achieve to work correctly, train your mind to the above and over time things will fall into place also there is a vast amount of information in that paragraph and over time as you keep reading it you should find something new. We will start with the disease fighting herbs, note that I put the Actions first so at a glance you can see what the herb can do and we end with the dosage and any warnings. Most of these herbs are the first herb that you need at the onset of a severe disease. With herbs like Echinacea you can use them let's say a month before winter to build up the immune system to protect you from colds and flu's or maybe a month before you go into hospital so as to save you from a nasty hospital bug. Garlic is another good preventative which kills lots of bugs and unfortunately relationships as well but to prevent this you can use Kyolic which is an aged Garlic that does not smell.

Disease Fighting Herbs

Andrographis

Actions - Anti Viral, antibacterial, anti-inflammatory, bitter, immune stimulant.

An herb used extensively in India and China. Used in a wide variety of conditions including fever, gastrointestinal diseases like dysentery, hepatitis, stomach ulcers and colitis, respiratory diseases (influenza), allergies, venomous snake and scorpion bites. Andrographis is frequently used for preventing and treating the common cold and flu. Some people claim it stopped the 1919 flu epidemic in India, although this has not been proven. Andrographis has become popular in the treatment of colds, with research showing that it can reduce the severity of cold symptoms and also help to prevent colds. Try not to take for more than two weeks.

Astragalus

Actions - Immuno-modulator, anti-viral, adaptogen, hypotensive, immune stimulant, adrenal tonic, diuretic, vasodilator, blood tonic.

Stimulates the natural production of interferon (helps to stop viruses replicating) and intensifies the white cell destruction of germs in other words it is an immune booster. A good tonic for strengthening the resistance to disease. Is very useful for people in a state of chronic debility and fatigue by restoring the immune function and giving them energy especially in those with cancer undergoing chemo or people with Ross River Fever this is why the herb is known as an Adaptogen because it helps people adapt and have the energy to cope with changes. Use as a lung tonic to help expel toxins and pus in flu's, colds and sinusitis. Increases stamina and can accelerate wound healing.

Uses - Boosting immune system, disease preventative, fatigue, healing wounds, good for use in those with chronic diseases that cause immune problems such as AIDS.

Baptisia (Wild Indigo)

Actions - Anti microbial, anti-viral, astringent, laxative, anti-catarrhal, febrifuge

Useful in the treatment of infections and catarrh in the ear, nose and throat such as tonsillitis, laryngitis, sinusitis and generally for any infection of the respiratory tract. Systemically use for enlarged and inflamed lymph glands throughout the lymphatic system, helps to reduce fevers, stimulates the immune system, use as a mouthwash to heal mouth ulcers and gingivitis.

Uses - Boils, diphtheria, infected eczema applied topically, fatigue, gangrene, glandular fever, scarlet fever, toxemia, typhoid, typhus.

Warning - Large doses are emetic (causes vomiting) and can be purgative.

Dose - 1 to 2mls of the tincture three times a day

Boneset (Eupatorium perfoliatum)

Actions - Diaphoretic, immune stimulant, bitter, laxative, tonic, anti-spasmodic, carminative, astringent.

Boneset is one the best remedies for the relief of the associated symptoms that accompany influenza. Influenza with deep aching, and congestion of the respiratory mucosa (British Herbal Medicine Association, 1983). It will speedily relieve the aches and pains as well as aid the body in dealing with any fever that is present. Boneset may also be used to help clear the upper respiratory tract of mucous congestion. In influenza it relieves the pain in the limbs and back. Its popular name "boneset" is derived from its well-known property of relieving the deep seated pains in the limbs which accompany this disorder, and colds and rheumatism. It was used by nearly every Eclectic physician in the treatment of fevers and flu and for the common cold "especially when accompanied by deep-seated, aching pain". The most well documented use of E. perfoliatum by Eclectic physicians was during the 1918-19 influenza epidemics, highlighted by two practitioner reports of over 1,000 treated cases with only five fatalities. Rudolf Weiss (1988) lists boneset alongside other tonics such as Echinacea spp. for treating acute viral infections and enhancing overall immune resistance. A classic indication is fevers with "dry skin, not followed by perspiration, with deep seated aching pain and great thirst" (Harper-Shove, 1952).

Combinations - In the treatment of influenza it may be combined with Yarrow, Elder Flowers, Cayenne or Ginger. With Pleurisy Root and Elecampane in bronchial conditions.

Preparations & Dosage - Infusion: pour a cup of boiling water onto 1-2 teaspoonful's of the dried herb and leave to infuse for 10-15 minutes. This should be drunk as hot as possible. During fevers or the 'flu it should be drunk every half hour. Tincture: take 2-4 ml of the tincture three times a day.

Burdock Root

Actions - Alterative, diuretic, bitter, antibacterial, antifungal, anti-tumor.

The sliced and bruised roots are one of the finest blood cleansers known to herbalists. The bruised leaves applied externally are a remedy for ring worm and scabies. Soothing to the kidneys and an excellent diuretic. Aids in the elimination of uric acid so it is good for rheumatic conditions and gout, by improving the function of the elimination organs (liver, kidneys, bowels) many health conditions can be improved, valuable remedy for skin conditions,

Uses - Remedy for all blood disorders, rheumatism, skin parasites, skin conditions resulting in dry scaly skin, psoriasis, eczema, dandruff, chicken pox, aids digestion and appetite, aids kidney function and helps with cystitis, speeds up the healing of wounds and ulcers.
Dose - 2 to 4mls of tincture 3 times a day.

Cats Claw

Actions - Anti oxidant, immune stimulant, anti-inflammatory, anti-fungal, anti-rheumatic, anti-viral, anti-tumor, anti-microbial.
To alleviate allergic sinus type conditions, boost the immune system, asthma, bursitis, Candida, immune deficiency disorders, chronic inflammatory diseases, auto immune conditions.
Human Dose - 30 to 75ml per week
Cautions - Don't use during pregnancy.

Echinacea

Actions - Immune stimulant, anti-microbial, anti-inflammatory, alterative. One of our most important remedies for treating acute and recurring infections. It is an infection fighter active against strep bacteria (abscesses and boils), a blood cleanser, (blood poisons, snake bites, poisonous insects and bacterial disease toxins) and a glandular and lymphatic system cleanser. Use it particularly for respiratory infections and for any disease above the waist. Boosts the white blood cells by stimulating the bone marrow to increase their production. Generally boosts the whole immune system
Uses - All infections especially those ones that cause septic conditions of the blood such as Typhoid and Diphtheria, depressed immune function, inflammatory conditions, allergies, effective against both bacteria and viruses. Mostly to fight acute diseases in their first stages.
Warning - Do not use continually as you may burn out the immune system, month on month off if you want to use it long term.

Elecampane

Actions - Expectorant, antitussive, anti-bacterial, antifungal, alterative,

diaphoretic, stomachic, demulcent, astringent, carminative, digestive tonic.
This herb is meant to be named after Helen of Troy and is a very ancient herb used for thousands of years especially by the Romans. Specific for irritating bronchial coughs, lots of catarrh, has a soothing and anti-bacterial action. Mainly used for treating chronic coughs, bronchitis and asthma especially in the young. It is also used for digestive problems. Elecampane also contains Alantolactone which helps to expel intestinal parasites such as pin worms. An external wash can help deter Scabies.

Uses - Bronchitis, emphysema, pneumonia, chest colds, whooping cough, coughs, emphysema, asthma and digestive problems. In the past was used for TB and Diphtheria

Dose - 1 to 2mls 3 times a day.

Elder

Actions - Diaphoretic, alterative, antispasmodic, diuretic, anti-catarrhal, expectorant.

Used for the treatment of all gastric, hepatic, and pulmonary ailments, all fevers, skin disorders especially scabies and ring worm, externally as an insecticide.

Leaves - Externally emollient and vulnerary (bruises, sprains and wounds). Internally used as a purgative, expectorant, diuretic and diaphoretic. Topically the lotion makes an anti-inflammatory wash, salve, eyewash and gargle for sore throats.

Flowers - Diaphoretic and anti-catarrhal. Use for colds and flu.

Berries - Diaphoretic and anti-catarrhal. The uses are similar to the flowers but the berries are used for rheumatism. The berries have been used as a nutrient rich tonic given after birth to help build the blood.

Uses - Colds, chills, fevers, respiratory infections, flu, gout, measles.

Dose - Really depends on which part of the plant you are using the leaves, flowers or berries. The tincture made of flowers is 2 to 4mls 3 times daily.

Garlic

Actions - Immune stimulant, anti-bacterial, anti-viral, anti-protozoan, anti-septic, anti-oxidant, diaphoretic, cholagogue, hypotensive, antispasmodic, vermifuge and many more.

The plant is rich in volatile oil and sulphur and because of its remarkable penetrating, disinfecting and mucous expelling powers garlic is a valuable basic remedy for the treatment of all ailments in which the cleansing of the blood stream and expulsion of mucous accumulations is required. Garlic is extremely effective in dissolving and cleansing cholesterol from the blood stream, it stimulates the digestive tract, kills worms, parasites and harmful bacteria, normalizes blood pressure, reduces fever, gas and cramps. Garlic is very high in sulphur so think of it as working as a Sulphur antibiotic but without the complications. Recent research has shown that Garlic can slow the growth or kill more than 60 species of fungi and more than 20 of bacteria. The oil in Garlic contains the active substance responsible for its antibiotic and antimicrobial actions which is a sulphur compound called allicin. When eaten the oil enters the digestive system and is absorbed into the blood stream, it is later excreted via the lungs hence the Garlic breath. For this reason Garlic is best used for infections of the digestive and respiratory system.

Uses- All infections, coughs, colds, flu, bronchitis, all fevers, pulmonary conditions, gastric and skin complaints, rheumatism, all worms and also liver fluke, mange.

Externally you can use garlic for ring worm and ear ache, to disinfect wounds, sores, and parasitical infections.

Goldenseal

Actions - Astringent, anti-catarrhal, cholagogue, anti-inflammatory, antibiotic, antiviral, alterative, bitter, laxative, tonic especially for the Digestive System, oxytocic.

Effective anti-catarrhal for drying up mucous membranes, has a activity against Staf, Strep, Chlamydia, Diphtheria, Protozoa, Coccidiosis, E Coli, Salmonella, Cholera and Candida. It is a liver cleanser and antiseptic and is used for internal bleeding and bowel diseases. It lowers blood sugar and is a natural insulin.

Uses - Cholera, catarrh, dysentery, gastritis, Giardia, hepatitis, jaundice, TB, Malaria, Thrush

Warnings - Avoid during pregnancy, long term use kills friendly bacteria in the intestines and reduces the assimilation of the B Vitamins, avoid in high blood pressure, for short term use only.

Licorice

Actions - Anti bacterial, anti-viral, expectorant, demulcent, anti-inflammatory, adrenal tonic, anti-spasmodic, mild laxative, nutritive.

Licorice improves macrophage activity and increases the production of interferon. Licorice extract also has broad spectrum anti-microbial effects along with being an antioxidant protecting the tissues especially those of the liver from free radical damage. The root part is used, licorice is one of our best demulcents especially for sore throats and painful and inflamed airways where it hurts to cough and is also good for gastric ulcers as it coats and soothes them giving them protection and reducing the inflammation, it is also nutritive and slightly laxative, It contains the building blocks of hormones, has a marked effect on the endocrine system and the glands of the body, catarrh, bronchitis, coughs, gastric and peptic ulcers, abdominal colic.

Uses - Treatment of cough, inflamed throat, pneumonia, pleurisy, TB, all catarrhal conditions, gallstones, chronic constipation, arthritis, fatigue, female infertility, pains of colic, stress, easing gastric ulcers, inhibits the herpes simplex virus.

Dose - 1 to 3mls of the tincture 3 times a day.

Caution - Do not use with high blood pressure. Long term use can also raise the blood pressure.

Myrrh

Actions - Anti microbial, astringent, carminative, anti-catarrhal, expectorant, vulnerary, antiseptic, antifungal, alterative.

Stimulates production of white blood cells and also has a good anti-microbial action so this is a good herb for immune boosting and fighting diseases. Good for use in respiratory infections, boils and abscesses and viral infections

Uses - Viruses, coughs, asthma, infections of the mouth, mouth ulcers, gingivitis, sinusitis, laryngitis.

Externally - Healing and antiseptic to wounds and abrasions.

Dose - 1 to 4mls 3 times a day.

Cautions - Use only in small amounts for short periods. Large amounts can speed heartbeat.

Plantain

Actions - Expectorant, demulcent, astringent, antibacterial, diuretic, alterative, anti-inflammatory, antispasmodic, decongestant.

Plantain clears heat and removes excess fluid from the body while at the same time soothing inflammation and irritated tissues. The whole plant yields soothing mucilage similar to linseed, gentle expectorant while soothing sore and inflamed membranes, coughs, bronchitis etc. Its astringency aids in diarrhea and cystitis where there is bleeding. Is good for using in the treatment of stomach ulcers and has been used for blood poisoning. The plant is high in chlorophyll and good for use on wounds.

Uses - Treatment of bronchitis, laryngitis, enteritis, TB, dysentery, urinary infections hemorrhages, internal obstructions and ulcers, fevers.

Externally - Wounds, sores, boils piles, ulcers and all bites, eye disorders.

Dose - 2 to 3mls of tincture 3 times a day.

Pleurisy Root

Actions - Diaphoretic, expectorant, anti-spasmodic, carminative, anti-inflammatory.

This herb was originally named for its ability to reduce the pain and inflammation of the disease pleurisy which is a very painful condition. Pleurisy Root is effective against respiratory infections where it reduces inflammations and assists expectoration and is best adapted to the acute stage. It can be used in the treatment of bronchitis and other chest conditions. The addition of diaphoretic and anti-spasmodic powers will show why it is so highly valued in the treatment of pleurisy and pneumonia. It can also be used in influenza.

Preparations & Dosage - Infusion: pour a cup of boiling water onto 1/2-1 teaspoonful of the herb and let infuse for 10-15 minutes. This should be drunk three times a day. Tincture: take 1-2 ml of the tincture three times a day.

Reshi Mushroom

Actions - Immune stimulant, antibacterial, anti-tumor, adaptogen, rejuvenative, anti-inflammatory.

As an immune stimulant it helps to activate the phagocytosis of macrophages and may increase interferon. Aids in the prevention of illness as well as in recovery. Helps normalize blood pressure reduces cholesterol and can inhibit histamine release (anti-inflammatory). Inhibits the inflammation associated with allergies, bronchitis, conjunctivitis and rheumatism. Good for treating chronic hepatitis. Good for over overcoming fatigue, anxiety and stress while improving stamina at the same time.

Uses - Good as an all-round immune booster and restorative tonic. Works well with its fellow mushroom Shitake as they tend to complement each other's actions and together they can be used to attack acute viral diseases. In chronic disease use 1/10 of the recommended dose.

Shitake Mushroom

Actions - Immune stimulant, antiviral, rejuvinative, aphrodisiac.

Animal studies have shown an antiviral and anti-tumor activity as well as the stimulation of killer T cells. Shitake enhances the stem cells in the bone marrow to create more B and T cells. Lowers blood pressure by helping the body get rid of excessive salt and can be used in AIDs like diseases. Stimulates the production of interferon and provides significant protection against type A Viruses which causes epidemic influenza.

Uses - Good as an all-round immune booster and restorative tonic. Works well with its fellow mushroom Reshi as they tend to complement each other's actions and together they can be used to attack acute viral diseases. In chronic disease use 1/10 of the recommended dose.

Willow Bark (White Willow)

Actions - Febrifuge, bitter tonic, astringent, antiseptic, analgesic, anti-inflammatory, anti-rheumatic.

Willow Bark can be thought of as caveman's Aspirin as it was developed from this. It is a refrigerant herb valuable in fevers and pain relief but can take a while to get into the system so think of looking for results especially in pain in about a day's time.

Uses - Treatment of all fevers, debility, enteritis, colic, pleurisy, rheumatism, sciatica and urinary infections as the excretion of salicylic acid in urine soothes an inflamed tract.

Externally - Rickets and cramp.

Dose - 2 teaspoonful's of powdered bark twice daily. Externally - Use the same brew as a massage in pain effected areas.

Yarrow

Actions - Diaphoretic, astringent, diuretic, antiseptic, hypotensive.

It is a famed wound herb for staunching excess bleeding and derives its name from the Greek Warrior Achilles who healed his wounds and those of his soldiers with yarrow blossoms.

The herb is one of the best diaphoretics known to herbalists opening the skin pores and inducing lavish perspiration, use for fevers, as a urinary antiseptic it can be used for cystitis, specific in thrombotic conditions associated with high blood pressure.

Uses - Treatment of all fevers, pneumonia, pleurisy, inflamed throat, hemorrhages, uterine hemorrhages, dysentery, hysteria, epilepsy, rheumatism, colic.

Externally - Wounds, skin eruptions, abscess, earache.

Dose - 2 to 4mls 3 times a day.

The Main Herbal Actions Used In Different Body Systems

Now we are going to go through the body systems and give you the Actions that are commonly used within that Body System starting with the Respiratory System we are also going to give you 2 or 3 of the major herbs used for that system in detail for you to learn. As mentioned before you never use more than 5 herbs in a formula and one of those herbs is used to push the formula into the body as well as to work in harmony with the rest of the formula. The main one for this we shall use is Licorice which works by spreading the formula over the small intestines which allows for better absorption because it is now covering a larger surface area. Other herbs you use for forcing a formula into the system are the hot herbs such as Ginger and Cayenne. The hot herbs work because they are hot and this increases the blood supply around the areas where they are and thus enhances their absorption into the body. We are going to mainly use Licorice for 2 reason the first being that it tastes nice so it makes the formula more palatable especially to children the second reason is that it has a strong Action on enhancing the immune system. Have a read of the herb and you will see why I want you to use it in most of your formulas.

Licorice

Actions - Anti bacterial, anti-viral, expectorant, demulcent, anti-inflammatory, adrenal tonic, anti-spasmodic, mild laxative, nutritive.

Licorice improves macrophage activity and increases the production of interferon. Licorice extract also has broad spectrum anti-microbial effects along with being an antioxidant protecting the tissues especially those of the liver from free radical damage. The root part is used , licorice is one of our best demulcents especially for sore throats and painful and inflamed airways where it hurts to cough and is also good for gastric ulcers as it coats and soothes them giving them protection and reducing the inflammation, it is also nutritive and slightly laxative, It contains the building blocks of hormones, has a marked effect on the endocrine system and the glands of the body, catarrh, bronchitis, coughs, gastric and peptic ulcers, abdominal colic. Can be used for treating inflammatory and allergic conditions.

Uses - Treatment of cough, inflamed throat, pneumonia, pleurisy, TB, all catarrhal conditions, gallstones, chronic constipation, arthritis, fatigue, female infertility, pains of colic, stress, easing gastric ulcers, inhibits the herpes simplex virus.

Human Dose - 1 to 3mls of the tincture 3 times a day.

Caution - Do not use with high blood pressure. Long term use can also raise the blood pressure.

You really need to get an Anatomy book that also gives you a good write up on how the different body systems work so you have a good reference to work with and learn from for you will need a basic understanding of how most things work to get the most out of the following information.

Actions Used In The Respiratory System

There are many problems that can affect the respiratory system from coughs to colds leading to bronchitis and maybe then to pneumonia. The infections are many and varied form a sore throat to pleurisy. Then you have people who have an existing chronic lung disease or conditions such as Asthma or like me damage from an industrial accident and lung abuse. Below are the Actions to think of when dealing with the Respiratory System. Consider also if the condition is affecting another system. Is this just one part of a disease condition? Is there diarrhea, is there any unusual behavior, is there fever, what is the temperature, is the patient anxious, what's the breathing like, are the lungs full of mucous, etc, etc, learn to be very observant and always listen to what the patient says.

Respiratory Herbs - Angelica, Cat Mint, Coltsfoot, Comfrey, Elder, Elecampane, Eyebright, Fenugreek, Fennel, Garlic Golden Rod, Hyssop, Horehound, Horse Radish, Licorice, Mullein, Myrrh, Plantain, Sage and Thyme.

Some Good Respiratory Herbs

Elecampane

Actions - Expectorant, antitussive, anti-bacterial, antifungal, alterative, diaphoretic, stomachic, demulcent, astringent, carminative, digestive tonic.

This herb is meant to be named after Helen of Troy and is a very ancient herb used for thousands of years especially by the Romans. Specific for irritating bronchial coughs, lots of catarrh, has a soothing and anti-bacterial action. Mainly used for treating chronic coughs, bronchitis and asthma especially in the young. . It is also used for digestive problems. Elecampane contains Alantolactone which helps to expel intestinal parasites such as pin worms. An external wash can help deter Scabies.

Uses - Bronchitis, emphysema, pneumonia, chest colds, whooping cough, coughs, emphysema, asthma and digestive problems. In the past was used for TB and Diphtheria

Human Dose - 1 to 2mls 3 times a day.

Elder

Actions - Diaphoretic, alterative, antispasmodic, diuretic, anti-catarrhal, expectorant.

Used for the treatment of all gastric, hepatic, and pulmonary ailments, all fevers, skin disorders especially scabies and ring worm, externally as a insecticide.

Leaves - Externally emollient and vulnerary (bruises, sprains and wounds). Internally used as a purgative, expectorant, diuretic and Diaphoretic. Topically the lotion makes a anti-inflammatory wash, salve, eyewash and gargle for sore throats.

Flowers - Diaphoretic and Anti catarrhal. Use for colds and flu.

Berries - Diaphoretic and Anti catarrhal. The uses are similar to the flowers but the berries are used for rheumatism. The berries have been used as a nutrient rich tonic given after birth to help build the blood.

Uses - Colds, chills, fevers, respiratory infections, flu, gout, measles.

Dose - Really depends on which part of the plant you are using the leaves, flowers or berries. The tincture made of flowers is 2 to 4mls 3 times daily.

Plantain

Actions - Expectorant, demulcent, astringent, antibacterial, diuretic, alterative, anti-inflammatory, antispasmodic, decongestant.

Plantain clears heat and removes excess fluid from the body while at the same time soothing inflammation and irritated tissues. The whole plant yields soothing mucilage similar to linseed, gentle expectorant while soothing sore and inflamed membranes, coughs, bronchitis etc. Its astringency aids in diarrhea and cystitis where there is bleeding. Is good for using in the treatment of stomach ulcers and has been used for blood poisoning. The plant is high in chlorophyll and good for use on wounds.

Uses - Treatment of bronchitis, laryngitis, enteritis, TB, dysentery, urinary infections hemorrhages, internal obstructions and ulcers, fevers.

Externally - Wounds, sores, boils, piles, ulcers and all bites, eye disorders.

Dose - 2 to 3mls of tincture 3 times a day.

Actions For The Respiratory System

Anti-biotic - Chaparral, Echinacea, Elecampane, Garlic, Myrrh.

Anti-catarrhal - Helps the body to remove excess catarrhal build ups.

Herbs - Cayenne, Coltsfoot, Cranesbill, Echinacea, Elder, Eyebright, Garlic, Golden Rod, Hyssop, Marshmallow, Mullein, Myrrh, Peppermint, Sage, Thyme, Yarrow.

Anti-inflammatory - Helps the body to combat inflammations. Herbs mentioned under demulcents will often act in this way especially when they coat sore throats and pipe lines and other inflamed areas that lead to pain.

Herbs - Angelica, Comfrey, Cranesbill, Eyebright, Feverfew, Ginger, Golden Rod, Ladys Mantle, Licorice, Marshmallow.

Anti-microbial - Helps the body destroy or resist pathogenic micro-organisms.

Herbs - Aniseed, Echinacea, Garlic, Myrrh, Peppermint, Plantain, Rosemary, Sage, Thyme.

Antispasmodic - Prevents or eases spasms and cramps.

Herbs - Aniseed, Angelica, Coltsfoot, Fennel, Horehound, Hyssop, Mullein, Rosemary, Sage, Skullcap, Thyme

Astringent - Contracts tissue which in turn reduces discharges, these herbs contain tannins which also have a slight anti-bacterial action. (Bacteria don't like to be contracted)

Herbs - Agrimony, Angelica, Comfrey, Elecampane, Eyebright, Golden Rod, Marshmallow, Mullein, Myrrh, Plantain, Sage, Rosemary, Shepherds Purse, Thyme.

Demulcent - Soothes and protects irritated or inflamed internal tissues.
Herbs - Coltsfoot, Comfrey, Fenugreek, Licorice, Marshmallow, Mullein, Oats, Plantain.

Diaphoretic - Aids the skin in the elimination of toxins and produces sweat thus reducing the temperature of fevers by evaporation.
Herbs - Angelica, Cayenne, Elder, Elecampane, Fennel, Garlic, Ginger, Golden Rod, Hyssop, Peppermint, Thyme, Yarrow.

Expectorant - Supports the body in the removal of excess mucous from the respiratory system and helps in the control of coughs.
Herbs -Angelica, Aniseed, Coltsfoot, Comfrey, Elder, Elecampane, Fennel, Fenugreek, Garlic, Hyssop, Horehound, Licorice, Marshmallow, Mullein, Myrrh, Plantain, Sweet Violets, Thyme.

Febrifuge - Helps the body to bring down fevers.
Herbs - Cayenne, Elder Flowers, Hyssop, Penny Royal, Peppermint, Plantain, Raspberry, Sage, Thyme, Vervain.

Immune Booster - Astragalus, Echinacea, Reshi, Shitake.

Pectoral - Has a general strengthening and healing effect on the respiratory system.
Herbs - Aniseed, Coltsfoot, Comfrey, Elder, Garlic, Hyssop, Licorice, Mullein, Horehound.

Actions Used In The Digestive System

The Digestive System is a large system composed of many separate parts that are usually doing more than one job especially the liver and pancreas. You must learn the basics of how this works and the process of food moving from one end to another. In dealing with problems of the digestive system its always best to start with a purge so as to clean the system and bowels out. This is very important especially when you do not know what you are dealing with because you are purging out hopefully most of the toxins that are causing the condition. After the purge fast the patient for 24 hours and see what happens. Below is a list of Actions that are used for the digestive system read through them and become familiar with them for in Herbal Medicine you always think in Actions needed not the Herb needed this way the mind stays on the big picture.

Digestive Herbs - Agrimony, Aniseed, Burdock, Calendula, Catmint,

Centaury, Chamomile, Cranesbill, Devils Claw, Dandelion, Fennel, Fenugreek, Feverfew, Garlic, Gentian, Hops, Horseradish, Licorice, Marshmallow, Meadowsweet, Milk Thistle, Pau D'Arco, Pennyroyal, Peppermint, Raspberry, Slippery Elm, Vervain, Wild Yam, Yarrow, Yellow Dock

Centaury

Actions - Bitter, aromatic, mild nervine, gastric stimulant, cholagogue, febrifuge, vermifuge.

This is a very bitter herb that enhances most of the digestive secretions and is good for stimulating the appetite and improving digestion. If being used as a bitter tonic take 10 minutes before a meal. Use whenever a gastric stimulant is required especially in cases of anorexia and liver weakness. This is a good herb for use in the young. This herb also promotes circulation and has a tonic effect on the blood vessels.

Uses - For digestive ailments, jaundice, bloating, indigestion, malaria, as a vermifuge, use externally for lice, wounds and warts. In the past it was also used as a birth remedy.

Dose - 1 to 2 mls of tincture 3 times daily, best 20 minutes before meals.

Meadowsweet

Actions - Anti-inflammatory, anti-rheumatic, analgesic, antacid, anti-emetic, stomachic, astringent, diaphoretic, sedative.

A important fever and diarrhea herb, acts to protect and soothe the mucous membranes of the digestive tract reducing excess acidity and easing nausea, heart burn, hyperacidity, gastritis, peptic ulcers. This herb is a good acid balancer and is good for correcting over acid systems. Meadowsweet is the forerunner of aspirin as this is the first herb it was synthesized from in 1835 but as this herb contains its own buffering agents it is gentle on the stomach.

Uses - Fevers, arthritis, gout, diarrhea and the above mentioned.

Dose - 1 to 4mls 3 times daily.

Caution - Avoid if sensitive to salicylates.

Milk Thistle

Actions - Cholagogue, galactagogue, demulcent, anti-oxidant, bitter tonic. This herb is said to rejuvenate the liver and helps to protect it from toxins and chemicals. For problems like hepatitis it is used alone at first as it drains the liver probably by its action of stimulating the gallbladder to release bile (which is the waste product of the liver). Used to increase milk production in mothers and for gallbladder problems.

Uses - Liver problems, gallbladder problems, hepatitis, alcohol abuse, chemo therapy nausea, drug abuse, to increase milk production.

Dose - 1 to 2mls 3 times daily.

Actions For The Digestive System

Anti-emetic - Can reduce a feeling of nausea and can help to relieve or prevent vomiting.
Herbs - Cayenne, Cloves, Dill, Fennel, Lavender, Meadowsweet, Peppermint.

Anti-inflammatory - Helps the body to combat inflammations, there will always be pain, heat and maybe fever when these are called for. Herbs mentioned under demulcents will often act in this way especially when they are applied to coat for example an inflamed intestine or any other inflamed organ.(Slippery Elm).
Herbs - Cranesbill, Chamomile, Eyebright, Feverfew, Ginger, Golden Rod, Ladys Mantle, Licorice, Marshmallow, Meadowsweet, Marigold, Pau D' Arco, Witch Hazel, Wormwood.

Anti-microbial - Helps the body destroy or resist pathogenic micro-organisms.
Herbs - Aniseed, Cayenne, Echinacea, Garlic, Gentian, Marigold, Myrrh, Peppermint, Rosemary, Rue, Sage, Thyme, Wormwood.

Antispasmodic - Prevents or eases spasms and cramps especially of the intestines.
Herbs - Aniseed, Angelica, Chamomile, Fennel, Rosemary, Rue, Sage, Skullcap, St johns Wort, Thyme, Valerian, Vervain.

Anthelmintic - Destroys or expels worms from the digestive system.
Herbs - Garlic, Tansy, Wormwood, Thyme, Rue.

Aperient - Mild laxative.

Herbs - Burdock, Dandelion.

Astringent - Contracts tissue which in turn reduces discharges, these herbs contain tannins. In the digestive system they can be used to stop diarrhea and in the treatment of ulcers. Most astringents also have an anti-bacterial action.

Herbs - Agrimony, Bear Berry, Cranesbill, Comfrey, Eyebright, Golden Rod, Hops, Ladys Mantle, Marigold, Marshmallow, Meadowsweet, Nettles, Raspberry, Sage, Rosemary, Slippery Elm, Shepherds Purse, St Johns Wort, Slippery Elm, Thyme, Witch Hazel, Yarrow.

Bitter - Herbs that taste bitter act as stimulating tonics for the digestive system.

Herbs - Burdock, Centaury, Feverfew, Gentian, Hops, Horehound, Rue, Tansy, Wormwood.

Carminative - Stimulates peristalsis of the digestive system and relaxes the stomach and helps remove gas and wind from the system. These herbs are usually rich in volatile oils.

Herbs - Aniseed, Angelica, Cayenne, Chamomile, Fennel, Garlic, Ginger, Golden Rod, Hyssop, Horseradish, Juniper, Parsley, Peppermint, Penny Royal, Sage, Rosemary, Tansy, Thyme, Valerian, Wormwood.

Cholagogue - Stimulates the release of bile from the gallbladder which can relieve gallbladder problems, bile is also the body's natural laxative so cholagogues have a laxative effect as well.

Herbs - Agrimony, Blue Flag, Dandelion, Fumitory, Gentian, Marigold, Milk Thistle, Yellow Dock.

Demulcent - Soothes and protects irritated or inflamed internal tissues.

Herbs - Bear Berry, Corn Silk, Coltsfoot, Comfrey, Fenugreek, Licorice, Marshmallow, Milk Thistle, Mullein, Oats, Plantain, Slippery Elm.

Diaphoretic - Aids the skin in the elimination of toxins and produces sweat thus reducing the temperature of fevers.

Herbs - Angelica, Black Cohosh, Cayenne, Chamomile, Elder, Elecampane, Fennel, Garlic, Ginger, Golden Rod, Guaiacum, Hyssop, Lime Blossom, Peppermint, Sarsaparilla, Thyme, Vervain, Yarrow.

Hepatic - Tones and strengthens the liver, may increase the flow of bile.

Herbs - Agrimony, Blue Flag, Dandelion, Fennel, Fumitory, Gentian, Horseradish, Hyssop, Motherwort, Milk Thistle, Vervain, Wormwood, Yarrow.

Laxative - Promotes the evacuation of the bowels.
Herbs - Burdock, Dandelion., Fumitory, Horseradish, Licorice,
Parasiticide - Kills parasites and insects.
Herbs - Aniseed, Rosemary,
Sialagogue - Stimulates the secretion of saliva.
Herbs - Blue flag, Cayenne, Gentian, Ginger.
Vermifuge - An agent that causes the expulsion of intestinal worms, see anthelmintics.

Actions Used In The Nervous System

The nervous system touches and joins every part of the body to the brain and when there is something wrong with this system it can have a devastating effect on other parts and produce the worst pains imaginable. One of the most important herbs in this system is Hypericum also known as St Johns Wort. This herb is anti-viral (specific to shingles virus), probably antibacterial as well, anti-inflammatory, a sedative and one of our main first aid remedies for wounds which helps relieve pain and can kill the tetanus bacteria, this is only mentioning a part of its uses, always consider this herb when there are problems with this system especially if you don't know what the problem is. Another good herb for rebuilding this system is Oats which is a Nervine tonic also think of Valerian which is our main Tranquilliser but also a good tonic for this system. A lot of the herbs mentioned below are used in other systems as well so when you want the action of a Nervine to use in another system try to match the herb to one used in that system as well.
Nervous System Herbs - Brahimi, Chamomile, Cramp bark, Damiana, Gotu Kola, Hypericum, Hops, Hyssop, Linden Flowers, Mistletoe, Passion Flower, Skullcap, Valerian, Vervain

Chamomile

Actions - Antispasmodic, nervine, sedative, carminative, anti-inflammatory, analgesic, antiseptic, allergies.
An excellent gentle sedative with a relaxing action that is good for easing anxiety and helping with sleep. Helps to restore the nervous system. In the digestive system it can be used for indigestion especially when there is

colicky pains and is ideal for colitis and IBS type problems. For females Chamomile is good for amenorrhea, spasmodic dysmenorrhea, premenstrual irritability and menopausal tensions. This herb is also a good source of calcium and magnesium which are the nervous systems favorite minerals.

Uses - Anxiety, colic, diverticula's, flatulence, gastritis, indigestion, insomnia, irritable, nervousness, restlessness, stress, ulcers.

Doses - Tincture 2 to 4mls 3 times daily, for teas just the one teabag.

Skullcap

Actions - Nerve tonic, sedative, antispasmodic, stress, anxiety, PMS, antidepressive, alterative, bitter tonic, cerebral tonic.

Skullcap has a wide range of use mostly focusing on the nerves. It relaxes states of nervous tension while at the same time renewing and revivifying the central nervous system. It has a specific use in the treatment of seizure, epilepsy and hysterical states. It may be used in all exhausted or depressed conditions. Good for easing Pre Menstrual Tension and painful menstruation.

Uses - Alcoholism, arthritis, delirium, convulsions, drug withdrawal, epilepsy, headache, hypertension, nerve pain, panic attacks, Parkinson's disease, restlessness, tremors.

Doses - Tincture 2 to 4mls 3 times a day, 1 to 2 teaspoonfuls of dried herb in tea 3 times a day.

Actions For The Nervous System

Antispasmodic - Prevents or eases spasms and cramps.
Herbs - Aniseed, Angelica, Black Cohosh, Chamomile, Fennel, Horehound, Hyssop, Lime Blossom, Mistletoe, Motherwort, Rosemary, Rue, Sage, Skullcap, St johns Wort, Thyme, Valerian, Vervain.

Antidepressive - Damiana, Rosemary, Skullcap, St Johns Wort, Valerian, Vervain.

Analgesic - Herbs that reduce pain.
Herbs - Chamomile, Dong Quai, Hops, Ladys Mantle, Passion Flower, St Johns Wort, Skullcap, Valerian, Wild Yam, Withania.

Nervine - Has a beneficial effect on the nervous system, acts like a tonic to

this system.
Herbs - Black Cohosh, Chamomile, Hops, Lime Blossoms, Mistletoe, Motherwort, Oats, Peppermint, Rosemary, Skullcap, St Johns Wort, Tansy, Thyme, Valerian, Vervain, Wormwood.

Sedative - Calms the nervous system and reduces stress and nervousness throughout the body.
Herbs - Black Cohosh, Chamomile, Hops, Hyssop, Motherwort, Skullcap, St Johns Wort, Valerian, Vervain.

Actions Used In The Urinary System

Most infections get to the kidneys via the blood for the kidneys are the main filter of the blood removing wastes and water. Other infections can start off as cystitis and travel up the ureters from the bladder and infect the kidneys that way so you must consider both ways. Always ask yourself is the infection traveling from the kidney down or the bladder up? Urinary antiseptics are good for this system whether for treating infection or preventing it as in cases of stones scraping the sides as they go down leaving a wound ripe for infection. Also think of Cranberry for this system as it coats the pipes and stops bacteria getting a foot hold literally.

Urinary System Herbs - Agrimony, Bearberry, Buchu, Celery Seed, Cornsilk, Couch grass, Chaparral, Gravel Root, Damiana, Golden Rod, Horsetail, Marshmallow, Parsley, Plantain, Sarsaparilla, Saw Palmetto, Shepherds Purse, Tribulas, Yarrow.

Buchu

Actions - Diuretic, urinary antiseptic, digestive tonic, carminative, kidney tonic.

Used in any infection of the genito-urinary system such as cystitis, urethritis and prostatitis. Especially useful in painful and burning urination. Good kidney tonic. Used to treat blood in the urine, stones and chronic urinary infections especially if started by colon bacteria. Helps in incontinence associated with prostatitis. Aids in the elimination of stone debris and uric acid from the kidneys. Soothes and strengthens the urinary system.

Uses - Bladder stones, flatulence, gonorrheal, gout, incontinence, kidney inflammation, kidney stones, prostatitis, urethritis, urinary infections.

Dose - 2 to 4mls 3 times a day.

Corn Silk
Actions - Diuretic, demulcent, tonic, antiseptic, antilithic.
A soothing diuretic that is helpful in any irritation of the membranes of the urinary system. Used as a urinary demulcent along with other herbs. Combined with other herbs in the treatment of cystitis, urethritis and prostatitis. Cleanses and soothes the urinary system.
Uses - Bed wetting, cystitis, gout, hypertension, kidney stones, prostatitis, urinary infections.
Dose - 3 to 6mls 3 times a day.

Actions For The Urinary System
Anti-inflammatory - Helps the body to combat inflammations.
Herbs - Cats Claw, Chaparral , Cleavers, Cranesbill, Eyebright, Ginger, Golden Rod, Guaiacum, Licorice, Marshmallow, Pau D' Arco.
Anti-lithic - Prevent the formation of stones or gravel in the urinary system and helps the body to remove them.
Herbs - Bearberry, Corn Silk, Chaparral , Gravel Root, Horsetail.
Anti-microbial - Helps the body destroy or resist pathogenic micro-organisms.
Herbs - Echinacea, Garlic, Juniper, Myrrh,
Astringent - Contracts tissue which in turn reduces discharges and bleeding, these herbs contain tannins.
Herbs - Agrimony, Cranesbill, Chaparral, Golden Rod, Horsetail, Shepherds Purse.
Cystitis - Agrimony, Bearberry, Buchu, Celery Seed, Corn Silk, Gravel Root, Golden Rod, Horsetail, Plantain,
Demulcent - Soothes and protects irritated or inflamed internal tissues.
Herbs - Bearberry, Corn Silk, Licorice, Marshmallow, Plantain, Slippery Elm.
Diuretic - Increases the secretion and elimination of urine.
Herbs - Agrimony Angelica, Bear Berry, Blue Flag, Burdock, Buchu, Broom, Coltsfoot, Chaparral, Corn Silk, Dandelion Leaves, Elder, Fumitory, Golden

Rod, Guaiacum, Gravel Root, Hawthorn, Horseradish, Horsetail, Juniper, Lime Blossom, Nettles, Pau D' Arco, Penny Royal, Plantain, Parsley, Shepherds Purse, Sarsaparilla, Yarrow.

Urinary Antiseptics - These herbs have a antiseptic action as they pass through the system.

Herbs - Angelica, Bearberry, Buchu, Corn Silk, Golden Rod, Shepherds Purse, Yarrow.

Actions Used In The Muscular Skeletal System

For bruising think about Arnica in a lotion and use the Homoeopathic dose internally, for broken bones think about Comfrey as its old name is knit bone. For arthritis and rheumatism use your Anti Rheumatics, Anti Inflammatories, and Analgesics but also think of Celery Seed as this is called the acid remover and another herb to think of is Meadowsweet as this herb is called the acid balancer along with having a Anti-inflammatory Action. It is usually the high acid in the system that irritates the joints and starts the inflammation so these 2 herbs could remove the cause for the condition, also consider diet as a diet high in protein will create a lot of acid waste. For blood borne bacterial infections think of the Alteratives (blood cleansers) and Anti Bacterials especially our main ones Garlic and Echinacea. If there is damage to the joints use a nutritional supplement with these 3 together - Glucosamine Sulphate, Chondroitin and MSM as these together will help rebuild the joints. Never forget about using ice packs straight away on sprains and strains the old freezer bag of peas is good as it takes shape to the limb. Hot and cold treatment can be of great benefit if done soon after a sprain this involves putting the foot in a bucket of really hot water and then putting it in a bucket of really cold water this acts like a pump to the blood and gets it circulating in the damaged area instead of the swelling slowing blood circulation and starting a full on attack of the inflammatory process which will slow down the healing.

Muscular Skeletal System Herbs - Black Cohosh, Burdock, Chickweed, Cats Claw, Celery, Dandelion, Devils Claw, Feverfew, Meadowsweet, Sarsaparilla, Willow bark.

Celery Seed

Actions - Anti rheumatic, diuretic, carminative, sedative, alterative, hypotensive, anti-inflammatory, urinary antiseptic.

The main use for this herb is in the treatment of rheumatism, arthritis and gout. Celery seed can help soothe the nerves and relieve pain and also aids the body in the removal of uric acid. Celery seed mixed with food aids in the digestion of protein.

Uses - Arthritis, hyperacidity, pain, hypertension, digestion, kidney stones, urinary tract infections

Dose - 2 to 4mls of tincture 3 times daily.

Caution - Not to be used with kidney diseases or during pregnancy.

Guaiacum

Actions - Anti rheumatic, anti-inflammatory, anti-spasmodic, laxative, diaphoretic, diuretic, alterative, peripheral circulatory stimulant.

Specific for rheumatic complaints with lots of inflammation, aids in the treatment of gout and can be used here as a preventative. Care must be taken with this herb especially in allergic conditions. Can be used topically on swelling, arthritic joints and herpes.

Uses - Arthritis, gout, rheumatism, syphilis,

Dose - 1 to 4mls 3 times a day.

Actions For The Muscular Skeletal System

Alterative - Herbs that gradually restore proper function to the body, they increase health and vitality. They were once known as the blood cleansers.

Herbs - Black Cohosh, Blue Flag, Burdock, Chaparral, Echinacea, Garlic, Nettles, Pau D'Arco, Sarsaparilla, Yellow Dock.

Analgesic - Herbs that reduce pain.

Herbs - Black Cohosh, Chamomile, Hops, Meadowsweet, Pau D'Arco, Peppermint, Skullcap, St Johns Wort, Valerian.

Antispasmodic - Prevents or eases spasms and cramps.

Herbs - Angelica, Black Cohosh, Chamomile, Skullcap, St Johns Wort, Valerian.

Anti-inflammatory - Helps the body to combat inflammations.

Herbs - Cats Claw, Devils Claw, Chaparral, Feverfew, Ginger, Guaiacum, Licorice, Meadowsweet, Pau D' Arco, Sarsaparilla, St Johns Wort, Willow Bark.

Anti-Rheumatic - Angelica, Burdock, Black Cohosh, Chaparral, Cats Claw, Celery Seed, Dandelion, Garlic, Guaiacum, Nettles, Willow Bark, Yellow Dock.

Rubefacient - Causes a gentle local irritation to the skin which stimulates the capillaries to open increasing the blood flow.

Herbs - Cayenne, Garlic, Ginger, Horseradish, Nettles, Peppermint Oil, Rosemary Oil, Rue.

Actions For The Skin

For the long drawn out chronic diseases of the skin use the Alteratives especially the ones with a strong affinity to the skin such as Sarsaparilla, Burdock, Cleavers and Nettles. The blood cleansers need time to do their work so always consider using them for 3 months as this is the life cycle of the red blood cells so you would of cleaned most of the blood after using them for this time.

Good Skin Herbs - Burdock, Calendula, Chickweed, Cats Claw, Dandelion, Gotu kola, Nettles, Red Clover, Sarsaparilla, Pau D; Arco

Calendula

Actions - Anti-inflammatory, astringent, vulnerary, anti-fungal, cholagogue, emmenagogue.

The flowers are tonic and a good heart medicine they possess restorative powers over the arteries and veins, also used for liver problems, vomiting and internal ulcers. Calendula is one of the best first aid remedies out, it is said no pus will form where Calendula is and it has done its job well form the amputation wards of the American Civil War to the present. Calendula is good for stopping bleeding and can seal wounds up to a certain extent so you have to be very careful that wounds are well cleaned so as to not seal up any rubbish.

Uses - Cuts, grazes, infected sores, fungal infections, any skin inflammations, regulates the oil production of the skin so is good for acne, to stop bleeding, bruises and sprains, skin ulcers and minor burns and scolds, healing, soothing, anti-microbial. Use as a lotion to clean wounds, one of our main germicides for wounds and if Hypericum is added to the lotion you may prevent tetanus as well.

Dose - Use internally as a cholagogue, for Candida, gallbladder problems, ulcers, indigestion, painful periods, delayed menstruation - Dose 1 to 4 mls of tincture 3 times daily. Use externally as a lotion (1 to 20) or a cream.

Caution - Calendula closes wounds rapidly so make sure they are very clean and no foreign bodies remain.

Chickweed

Actions - Healing, alterative, anti-bacterial, anti-inflammatory, astringent, demulcent, emollient, nutritive, febrifuge.

Rich in copper, highly tonic food for the digestive system and a remedy for all stomach ailments, allergies, colon problems, constipation, piles, rheumatism, skin problems, eczema, psoriasis, itching, irritation, cuts and wounds. Chickweed is soothing and helps to dissolve mucous, warts and cysts in the body. It is a herb that was traditionally given to strengthen the frail.

Uses - One of the main uses of this herb is for itching skin conditions whether from insect bites or eczema like conditions. Has wound healing and demulcent properties, eczema, throat ulcers, burns, mouth sores, ulcers.

Dose - Usually given in infusions or used as a lotion or cream.

Actions For The Skin

Alterative - Herbs that gradually restore proper function to the body, they increase health and vitality. They were once known as the blood cleansers.

Herbs - Black Cohosh, Blue Flag, Burdock, Cleavers, Chaparral, Echinacea, Fumitory, Garlic, Nettles, Pau D'Arco, Sarsaparilla, Sweet Violets, Yellow Dock.

Anti-biotic - Echinacea, Garlic, Myrrh, Pau D' Arco, Tea Tree Oil

Anti-fungal - Marigold, Cats Claw, Pau D' Arco, Myrrh, Sweet Violets.

Anti-inflammatory - Helps the body to combat inflammations. Herbs mentioned under demulcents, emollients and vulneraries will often act in this way especially when they are applied externally.

Herbs - Arnica, Blue Flag, Cats Claw, Chaparral, Chickweed, Cleavers, Cranesbill, Chamomile, Eyebright, Ginger, Golden Rod, Guaiacum, Licorice, Marshmallow, Marigold, Pau D' Arco, St Johns Wort, Sweet Violets, Witch Hazel.

Astringent - Contracts tissue which in turn reduces discharges, these herbs contain tannins.
Herbs - Agrimony, Bear Berry, Cranesbill, Chaparral, Chickweed, Comfrey, Eyebright, Golden Rod, Hops, Horsetail, Ladys Mantle, Marigold, Marshmallow, Meadowsweet, Myrrh, Nettles, Raspberry, Sage, Rosemary, Slippery Elm, Shepherds Purse, St Johns Wort, Slippery Elm, Thyme, Witch Hazel, Yarrow.
Emollient - Soothing to the skin. Acts externally the way demulcents do internally.
Herbs - Chickweed, Coltsfoot, Comfrey, Fenugreek, Licorice, Marshmallow, Mullein, Plantain, Slippery Elm.
Parasiticide - Kills parasites and insects.
Herbs - Aniseed, Rosemary,
Vulnerary - Applied externally and aid the body in the healing of wounds and cuts
Herbs - Arnica, Burdock, Chickweed, Comfrey, Cranesbill, Elder, Fenugreek, Garlic, Horsetail, Hyssop, Marigolds, Marshmallow, Mullein, Myrrh, Plantain, Shepherds Purse, Slippery Elm, St Johns Wort, Thyme, Witch Hazel, Yarrow.

Actions For The Reproductive System

Below are some of the actions to consider for this system. In the Astringents the herbs underlined are the best to use to stop bleeding. Use the Alteratives for Chronic diseases of this system and maybe add some of the Emmenagogues to them after reading up on the individual herbs and adding the one that works in the direction you want.
Reproductive System Herbs - Black Cohosh, Damiana, Dong Quai, Fenugreek, Feverfew, Hops, Ladys Mantle, Motherwort, Pennyroyal, Raspberry, Saw Palmetto, Shepherds Purse, Skullcap, Squaw Vine, Tribulus, Vitex, Wild Yam, Yarrow

Black Cohosh

Actions - Emmenagogue, anti-spasmodic, nervine, alterative, sedative, tonic, anti-inflammatory, circulatory stimulant. vasodilator.
Black Cohosh has a normalizing action on the balance of female sex

hormones and may be safely used to regain normal hormonal activity that should give relief to Menopause and PMS symptoms. This would be the herb to use if your patient also suffered from rheumatism or arthritis. Has hormone balancing properties, encourages oestrogen production, use for painful or delayed menstruation, ovarian cramps or cramping pain in the womb, used to regain normal hormone activity, good for hot flashes, rheumatoid and osteoarthritis, muscular and neuralgic pains with a good example being sciatica. Black Cohosh may also lower blood pressure, lower cholesterol, help with insomnia and help with tinnitus.

Uses - Amenorrhea, arthritis, debility, depression, hypertension, hysteria, labor inducement, moodiness, snake bites and TB.

Doses - For tincture is 2 to 4mls 3 times a day, One and a half teaspoonfuls for tea 3 times a day.

Cautions - Best taken with meals so as to avoid any chance of upsetting tummy. Allow up to 8 weeks to see benefits in menopausal problems and even then the full benefit of the herb may not be reached till 6 month's time. Antibiotics can reduce the effect of this herb. This herb can interfere with hormonal medications eg The Pill. Contra indicated in pregnancy.

Saw Palmetto

Actions - Diuretic, urinary antiseptic, endocrine agent, nutritive, sedative. This herb tones and strengthens the male reproductive system. It is the specific in cases of enlarged prostrate and is of value for infections of the urinary tract. It is considered a reproductive tonic for men and women.

Uses - Enlarged prostrate, cystitis, infertility, convalescence, impotence, wasting diseases.

Dose - 1 to 2mls of tincture 3 times daily.

Actions For The Reproductive System

Alterative - Herbs that gradually restore proper function to the body, they increase health and vitality. They were once known as the blood cleansers.
Herbs - Black Cohosh, Dong Quai, Damiana, Skullcap.
Adaptogen - Helps the body overcome its problems and work to the best of its ability. Good convalescent herbs.
Herbs - Panax Ginseng Siberian Ginseng .Schizandra, Withania.

Anti-biotic - Chaparral, Echinacea, Garlic, Myrrh, Pau D' Arco, Reshi.

Antidepressive - Damiana, Rosemary, Skullcap, St Johns Wort, Valerian.

Anti-fungal - Marigold, Cats Claw, Pau D' Arco, Myrrh, Sweet Violets.

Anti-inflammatory - Helps the body to combat inflammations. Herbs mentioned under demulcents, emollients and vulneraries will often act in this way especially when they are applied externally.
Herbs - Cranesbill, Chamomile, Eyebright, Feverfew, Ginger, Golden Rod, Ladys Mantle, Licorice, Marshmallow, Meadowsweet, Marigold, Pau D' Arco, St Johns Wort, Witch Hazel.

Anti-Tumor - Burdock, Cleavers, Reshi, Shitake, Sweet Violets.

Antispasmodic - Prevents or eases spasms and cramps.
Herbs - Aniseed, Angelica, Black Cohosh, Chamomile, Fennel, Hyssop, Motherwort, Rosemary, Rue, Sage, Skullcap, St Johns Wort, Thyme, Valerian, Vervain.

Astringent - Contracts tissue which in turn reduces discharges, these herbs contain tannins.
Herbs - Agrimony, <u>Cranesbill</u>, Eyebright, Golden Rod, <u>Ladys Mantle</u>, <u>Marigold</u>, Raspberry, <u>Shepherds Purse</u>, St Johns Wort, <u>Witch Hazel.</u>

Emmenagogue - Stimulates and normalizes the menstrual flow, tonics for the female reproductive system.
Herbs - Black Cohosh, Chamomile, Fenugreek, Gentian, Ginger, Juniper, Ladys Mantle, Marigold, Motherwort, Parsley, Penny Royal, Peppermint, Parsley, Raspberry, Sage, Rosemary, Rue, Shepherds Purse, St Johns Wort, Tansy, Thyme, Valerian, Vervain, Wormwood, Yarrow.

Galactagogue - Helps increase the flow of milk in females.
Herbs - Aniseed, Fennel, Fenugreek, Milk Thistle, Raspberry, Vervain.

Hormone Precursors - Provide the building blocks for hormones.
Herbs - Black Cohosh, Blue Cohosh, Licorice, Fenugreek, Ginseng, Sarsparillia, Wild Yam, Withania

Sedative - Calms the nervous system and reduces stress and nervousness throughout the body.
Herbs - Black cohosh, chamomile, cramp bark, hops, motherwort, passion flower, skullcap, St Johns Wort, schizandra, valerian, vervain.

Urinary Antiseptic - Angelica, damiana, shepherds purse, yarrow.

Homeopathic Treatment

Homeopathy has been around now for hundreds of years and unlike most other forms of medicine its rules have not changed and will not for they are based on an essential truth. The main rule is Like cures Like or if we break down the word Homeopathy homo means the same and pathy means disease. As Homoeopathy is a very hard science to learn and as it kind of sits or balances on the border of hard science and metaphysics I will not try to explain to you what it is here as it would probably take a whole book to do this but I will say this, in the UK and a lot of countries in Europe it is on and paid for by the National Health System and anything that can get a politician to open their purse must work.

It is said that Homeopathy sits on a three legged stool. What this means is that if a remedy has at least three symptoms in the same strength as the symptoms you are trying to match then that remedy is a potential cure for your condition or if not cure it will offer the condition relief. The more symptoms you can match to the remedy the better the remedy will work for the rule is likes cure likes not vaguely similar cures. To make the remedies as closer a match as we can we ask lots of questions like the ones below and after we gather all the answers we have what is called a good Symptom Picture which we then try to match as accurately as we can to a Remedy. Most Homeopathic Materia Medicas (remedy references) are set out to answer the questions listed below with the mind symptoms being the most important. Questions on time, position and temperature are good for making a choice between two very close remedies. The best Materia Medica for the lay person is Boerickes and you should be able to view this on a few Homeopathic websites.

Symptom Guide Questions

1/. Was there a sudden onset of the condition, at what time?
2/. What time of the day does the patient feel either better or worse?
3/. What is the effect of motion? jarring? walking? running?
4/. What is the effect of drinking fluids? Warm and or cold drinks?
5/. Is the patient thirsty or not at all? Sips or gulps?
6/. Is the onset from exertion? Overeating? Weather changes? Emotions?
7/. Mental emotional state of patient?
8/. Better warm room? Warm air?

9/. Better cool room? Cool open air?
10/. Are the respirations upper chest movements or in the abdomen?
11/. Respirations - dry or wet?
12/. Expectoration - watery or stringy mucous, easy or difficult.
13/. Is there coughing
14/. Position - better or worse from sitting? standing? lying? Lying on which side?
15/. Along with the condition is there fever? Gas? Belching? Wind?

Modality - The questions above are covering what the Homoeopaths call modalities which basically mean are covering a condition that makes the patient better or worse. I will list the other main Modalities below. The Modalities help us to distinguish which remedy is right for the case especially when we have a group that look as though they may all work which is what I am giving you und the disease heading. Using modalities forces you to think what really is going on, is this the nature of the beast or the nature of the disease.

Time - Better or Worse morning, night, weekly, monthly, seasonally etc.

Motion - Better or Worse first movement, rest, exertion, walking, stretching, rising up etc

Temperature - Better or Worse heat, cold, cold air blowing, sudden change etc.

Body Activity - Better or Worse eating, drinking, urinating, defecating, sleep, coughing etc

Weather - - Better or Worse, damp, sunny, foggy, storms, sudden changes etc.

Senses - Better or Worse - touch, pressure, noise, light, odors etc.

Position - Better or Worse lying, standing, sitting, stretched out, doubled up, right side etc.

Mind - Excitement, anger, fear, stress, better busy, nervous all the time etc.

Now read through all the remedies in the Marteria Medica below (Homoeopathic Remedy Reference) and you will notice that most of them have Mind or mental symptoms kind of describing the personalities or moods a good example is Nux Vomica, I think we all know a nasty type of individual that this remedy would be suited to and meaning as though the individual is suited to this remedy then the remedy would have a curative action on them but don't expect it to change the nature of the beast. One of the main rules of Homeopathy is the closer the match of the remedy the higher the Potency you use but if you are not used to Homoeopathy just use the 30C potency and remember what I said about the 3 legged stool. Potency is a measure of strength and depth of action.

Remember as mentioned before Homoeopathy sits on a three legged stool. What this means is that if a remedy has at least three symptoms in the same strength as your symptoms then that remedy is a potential cure.

Note - The best prescribing guide for the layman is **Boerickes Materia Medica With Repertory.**

Another good guide is **The Complete Book Of Homeopathy by Dr Michael Weiner.**

I always buy my books on Homeopathy from India as they are quarter the price and there is always a wide selection. Put B. Jain Publishers into the google search engine go to their web site and check out these books and I am sure you will be pleased with what you find.

Materia Medica

Note - All Homeopathic Remedies are given in Potency and not in material Form.

Aconite

Characteristics - Aconite is best used in the first stages of a illness, especially when fear and anxiety are present. Symptoms appear suddenly, without warning and they may be caused by exposure to cold winds or draughts or by a severe fright. Symptoms are a marked restlessness, animal displays extreme anxiety or fear, high fever with a burning skin, extreme sweating and a burning thirst, a hoarse dry painful cough, bright light noises stress and cold worsen the symptoms, rest and quiet relieves the symptoms. The pains of Aconite are unbearable, sharp, shooting, burning pains, tingling and numbness. A remedy for fevers and inflammatory states, use at the first sign of all fevers, shivering with cold sweats, difficult breathing, animal shows desire for large quantities of water, symptoms worse at midnight, symptoms improve in the open air.

Mind - Great fear, anxiety, restlessness, extreme sensitivity to pain, worry, foreboding.

Better - In open air, warmth, rest.

Worse - In the evening and night, particularly before midnight, lying on affected side.

Allium Cepa

Characteristics - Increased secretions from the eyes and nose, like those of the common cold. Frequent sneezing with watery discharge which burns the nose and upper lip, but the eye discharge is bland and doesn't burn (the opposite of Euphrasia). Tickling in the throat with incessant cough (feels as if larynx is split) holds throat when coughing. Being in cool open air relieves the symptoms, eyelids are swollen and red, abdominal tympany with wind, this remedy is indicated in the early stages of most catarrhal conditions, mild forms of cat flu can be cut short if given early.

Better - Cold room (except cough), open air.

Worse - Evening, warm room, odors.

Antimonium Tartaricum - Ant Tart

Characteristics - Is characterized by a loose rattling unproductive cough such as is often herd in cats. Respiration can be very difficult with much gasping. There is usually thirst for little and often. Symptoms are worse in the evening, lying down and in cold damp weather or a warm room. Confined largely to respiratory diseases, abundant bronchial secretions, great rattling of mucous with little expectoration, drowsiness, debility and sweat.

Mind - Drowsy and despondent, fear of being alone, child will not be touched without whining.

Better - Sitting erect, from burping and expectoration.

Worse - Evenings, lying down, damp cold weather.

Apis

Characteristics - Apis is used for various types of swelling and inflammation such as that from animal bites and bites and stings from insects, it is also used for measles, mumps, sore throats, sore red eyes and fever. Apis is a quick acting remedy for inflammations especially those ones with edema and lots of swelling which is its main use. Acute nephritis with scanty and burning urine there may be some blood in the urine. . Symptoms are swelling with edema which makes the effected parts look shiny, red and puffy, the swollen parts feel soggy and waterlogged, a fever that develops rapidly but without thirst, extreme restlessness and fidgeting, an irritable nature and perhaps jealous, cool air and cold compresses relieve the symptoms. Pains are burning and stinging, arthritis with swelling, animals seek cold surface to lie on, swollen eyelids, may be swollen ears, may be blood in the urine, in the horse and cow there may be edema in the lower limbs while in dogs abdominal dropsy is seen. Symptoms get worse from heat and improve in the open air and from cold bathing.

Mind - Apathy, indifference, awkward.

Better - By cold, (room, air or application)

Worse - From warmth, pressure, late in the afternoon, from sleeping.

Arnica

Characteristics - Bruises and similar injuries where the skin is unbroken and there is mental or emotional shock. Symptoms are any type of bruising or similar injury caused by crushing, squeezing or wrenching, muscles strains which feel sore and bruised, shock after accidents, there is a fear of being touched because of the pain, good for the soreness after birth and medical operations.

Arnica can be used in potency and also as a cream. The cream must not be used on broken skin or wounds. Animal shrinks away when you try to touch it, symptoms improve when lying down.

Mind - Fears touch or approach, whole body oversensitive.

Better - Lying down or with head low.

Worse - Least touch, motion, damp and cold.

Arsenic Album

Characteristics - Burning pains relieved by heat, anxious, restless, weak and chilly with an air of fear and hopelessness. Anxiety or restlessness are often present where this remedy is indicated. Discharge from eyes and nose are watery and acrid causing ulceration in those regions. The mouth is usually dry and the patient is usually thirsty. Dramatic vomiting and diarrhea often simultaneously indicate its use if the modalities agree. The patient may have wheezing respiration and allergic asthmatic conditions can respond well. The skin can be dry, scaly and scruffy. Symptoms are worse for cold and wet better for warmth. Tries to find relief in motion but immediately feels weak with movement. Restless, feels cold, complains of general weakness, discharges burn the skin.

Mind - Fear with despair and restlessness.

Better - Warmth, open air, relieved by sweat, hot drinks, lying down (but restless).

Worse - Cold air, after midnight eg 1 to 3am. Wet damp weather and near sea shore.

Belladonna

Characteristics - This is one of the great fever remedies, conditions requiring its use usually being of violent and sudden onset. Heat, redness, pain and swelling characterize its symptoms. It is one of the main remedies used in convulsions. Pupils are usually dilated which is a keynote for this remedy. Acute ear inflammation where there is heat, pain and swelling respond well. The mouth is usually dry and there is great thirst. With Belladonna always think BIRDS. B for burning, I for irritability, R for redness, D for delirium and S for spasms.

Mind - Hallucinations, delirium, rages, bites, strikes, desire to escape.

Better - For quiet, dark, rest with slight warmth.

Worse - For noise, touch or jarring motion.

Bellis Perennis

Characteristics - Trauma to abdomen and pelvic organs especially after surgery and child birth if arnica does not give relief. Injuries to the nerves with intense soreness, back ache from hard physical work such as gardening, pain is bruised sore and aching, better cold presses, worse touch, after getting wet.

The animal is unwilling to move and when made to do so evinces pain,

muscular stiffness is prominent.
Worse - Left side and cold wind.

Bryonia

Characteristics - This remedy shows both diarrhea and constipation symptoms, the latter usually in chronic conditions. The mouth is often dry and there is great thirst. The tongue is often coated yellow. It is of great help in many cases of rheumatism or arthritis where the symptoms agree. There is often respiratory signs with a hoarse hacking cough. All symptoms are worse for movement and better for rest.

Mind - Irritable, delirium.

Better - Lying on the painful side, pressure, rest and cold things.

Worse - Warmth, motion, morning, eating and touch.

Calendula

Characteristics - The part used is the Flowers and it is used for wounds and skin irritations, it is healing, soothing, anti-inflammatory, astringent, anti-fungal and anti-microbial.

Use as a lotion for cuts, grazes, infected sores, fungal infections, any skin inflammations, regulates the oil production of the skin so is good for acne, to stop bleeding, for bruises and sprains, skin ulcers and minor burns and scolds.

Note - The tincture of this is used as a lotion diluted at 1 to 10.

Cantharis

Characteristics - Important first aid remedy for minor burns and for other pains that feel burning and fiery, also has a healing effect on the bladder, urethra and other parts of the urinary tract where burning pain is the key symptom, burns and scalds especially where blistering and inflammation occur, sunburn, insect bites that feel hot and burn, cystitis. Pains are violent burning, cutting, stabbing or smarting, rawness, use when the animal appears distressed when passing urine, or tries to pass and cannot. Better from warmth rest and rubbing.

Mind - Furious delirium, acute mania generally of a sexual type, crying, barking.

Better - From rubbing

Worse - From touch or approach, from urinating, from drinking cold water.

Carbo Vegetabilis

Characteristics - Patient exhibits mental and physical sluggishness and symptoms come on slowly, generalized weakness of all functions especially digestion, overweight, torpid, lazy, complaints of coldness, pains usually described as burning, pressing pains, wishes to be fanned, digestive problems such as belching often accompany any illness.

Mind - Aversion to darkness, sudden loss of memory.

Better - Being fanned, passing gas, rest.

Worse - Morning and evening, exertion, cold, tight clothes at abdomen.

Causticum

Characteristics - Burns and burning pains such as cystitis also used for dry coughs, burns to the skin especially with marked inflammation and blistering, coughs, laryngitis and hoarseness from straining and over using voice, cystitis especially with involuntary passing of urine when coughing, chronic cystitis, exposure to cold dry air may make symptoms worse.

Mind - Least thing makes it cry, sad, hopeless. Ailments from long lasting grief.

Better - In damp wet weather, warmth.

Worse - Cold winds.

Euphrasia

Characteristics - Affects the mucous membranes of the eyes, nose and chest producing copious watery secretions, eye secretions cause smarting of the skin while the nose discharge is bland. Used for conjunctivitis, eye strain generally but especially from computers, eyes that feel sore and inflamed and look red, hay fever symptoms including a tickly throat, sneezing, a runny nose, and itchy red watering eyes. Sunlight wind and warmth worsen the symptoms. Use for Dogs who have had their head out of the window for too long, symptoms better in dim light or darkness, in all species a tendency to diarrhea occurs.

Better - In the dark

Worse - From light, indoors, in the evening.

Hypericum

Characteristics - Used for bruises and other injuries especially to nerve rich areas like the fingers, lips, ears, eyes, tail bone, good for the pain of puncture wounds of any cause eg animal or insect. Helps with the pains after operations especially amputations. Pains are violent shooting pains along a nerve path, burning, tingling and numbness. Worse from shock and touch and better from rubbing, horse fly bites, symptoms worse cold better warmth.

Mind - Anxiety, melancholy, effects of shock.

Better - Bending head backward.

Worse - Cold, dampness and touch.

Ipecac

Characteristics - Indicated for complaints of persistent nausea not relieved by vomiting, ailments caused by eating rich or indigestible type of foods such as ice-cream, sweets etc., useful to stop bleeding if blood is bright red.

Mind - Easily irritated, child cries or screams continuously, wanting something but not sure what they desire, holds everything in contempt.

Worse - Warm, moist weather, lying down.

Kali Bichromicum

Characteristics - Has a affinity for the mucous membranes of the body, tough stringy viscid secretions sometimes forming thick yellow green mucous, sinus infections, suited for fleshy fat light complexioned people, general weakness.

Better - Heat

Worse - Cold, beer, morning, undressing.

Kali Carbonicum

Characteristics - Has a affinity for the mucous membranes digestive and respiratory, very tired, anemic, flabby tissues which may be swollen, sweat, backache, weakness, many conditions have a aggravation at 2am to 4am, often stays immobile when ill.

Mind - Very irritable, hypersensitive to pain, despondent.

Better - During the day, sitting down, bending forward, warmth.

Worse - Cold weather, between 2am and 4am.

Lachesis

Characteristics - Many symptoms tend to be left sided, cannot bear tight clothing, symptoms worse on awakening, symptoms relieved with onset of the menstrual flow. Short dry cough, feels relief after coughing up watery phlegm, feeling of constriction in throat and chest, better bending forward.

Mind - Overly talkative, impatient, sad, jealous, no desire to mix with world.

Better - Release of pressure, eating fruit, cold, discharges.

Worse - Pressure, touch, after sleep, heat, hot weather.

Ledum

Characteristics - Has a action on the capillaries and is useful for cleaning up bruises especially around the eyes, mainly used for puncture wounds made by sharp points such as nails and wood splinters and insect bites and stings especially ones that don't heal properly and look blue and puffy. Wounds that feel cold to the touch, septic conditions, sprains, pains are throbbing, tearing ,prickling, they shoot upwards, stiff and sore. Better cold, cold bathing. This remedy was used in the past along with hypericum to ward off tetanus especially in deep wounds

Better - From cold.

Worse - At night and from heat.

Lycopodium

Characteristics - Exerts most of its effects on the digestive organs, liver, kidneys and respiratory systems. The patient dislikes being left alone and appears apprehensive. The nose is often blocked and there may be blisters on the tongue. Eating a little food always satisfies the appetite but appetite is very marked. The belly is usually bloated. The stool appears hard and small and is expelled only with difficulty accompanied by ineffectual straining. Urination is also a slow process and the urine has a red sediment. Symptoms are worse for heat generally and better for cold.

Mind - Melancholy, afraid to be alone, apprehensive.

Better - By motion, on getting cold.

Worse - From heat.

Natrum Sulphuricum

Characteristics - A good liver remedy, emotional and mental difficulties arising after head injury, useful in problems associated with rainy weather and dampness, patient feels every change from dry to wet weather, may remove excess water and fluid retention from the body.

Mind - Lively music saddens, melancholy, inability to think, dislikes to speak or be spoken to.

Better - Dry weather and environments, pressure, change of position.

Worse - Damp weather, damp basements, lying on left side.

Nux Vom

Characteristics - The remedy for overindulgence, adapted especially to thin irritable energetic people who attend with great detail to tasks, quarrelsome, nervous, intelligent, hypochondriacal, oversensitive to noise music and light, craves stimulants.

Primarily used in the digestive sphere, its greatest reputation is in helping disturbances following overeating of unsuitable foods. Feces is usually hard but diarrhea can follow overeating. There is abdominal discomfort, flatulence, irritability and sensitivity to noise. Symptoms are generally worse for noise and better after rest or for damp weather.

Mind - Very irritable, sensitive to all impressions, malicious, disposed to reproach others.

Better - Wet weather, lying down, uninterrupted nap.

Worse - Overeating, mental over exertion, sensory stimulation ie sound, sight, touch etc.

Phosphorus

Characteristics - Irritated and inflamed mucous and serous membranes are the key feature of this remedy. Is a very sudden remedy with suddenness of symptoms. The patient is sensitive to loud and sudden noises (eg thunder fireworks etc). Degenerative processes and bone destruction respond well to Phosphorus. Food is suddenly vomited back up when it has been warmed in the stomach, gums can be ulcerated and bloody. Hepatitis, jaundice, pancreatic disease and nephritis come into its sphere. Urine may be bloody. A very painful cough is also a symptom. Wounds that perpetually bleed may also be helped. The patient is usually in poor body condition. Symptoms are worse for touch, exertion, in the evening and during thunder storm. Better for cold and sleep.

Mind - Low spirits, restless, fidgety.

Better - In the dark, lying on the right side, from the cold, sleep.

Worse - Touch, from exertion and in the evening.

Pulsatilla

Characteristics - Often indicated for those with mild, gentle, timid yielding dispositions who are easily moved to laughter and tears, The Pulsatilla person wants to be held and loved, moods changeable and fickle, the patient is chilly but desires strolling in cold air, symptoms are erratic and change frequently, pains are wandering, pains that grow gradually in intensity, fever without thirst despite dry mouth, bland yellow discharges.

Mind - Weeps easily, timid, fears to be alone - dark - ghosts, likes sympathy and fuss, highly emotional, easily discouraged, sensitive.

Better - Open air, cold applications, consolation relieves symptoms.

Worse - Evening before midnight, warmth, after eating fat rich food.

Rhus Tox

Characteristics - Is the most famous of the rheumatic remedies. The skin and muscular skeletal system are its main spheres. Small red papules in the skin and sometimes vesicles are typical lesions with much scratching. In all cases of damage to muscles think of Rhus and the symptoms of arthritis which are worse after rest particularly if this follows strenuous exertion. The symptoms improve with limbering up, The worst pains are seen as the animal arises from its bed.

Mind - Listless, sad, extreme restlessness, great apprehension at night.

Better - Warmth, walking, from stretching out limbs.

Worse - During sleep, cold wet rainy weather and at night.

Ruta

Characteristics - Has effects on the joints, tendons, cartilages, and the periosteum which is a fine membrane that covers bones and gives it that shiny look, it is also used for eye strain where the vision goes dim.

Used for painful bruises affecting the bones, dislocations, strains to the tendons or joints, aching with restlessness, pains are gnawing, digging, burning, bruised, sore as if beaten, bones as if broken, pain deep in the bones, rheumatism.

Better - From lying and warmth.

Worse - From over exertion, touch, cold wet weather.

Silica

Characteristics - Fits the shy chilly patient who is reluctant to enter the room, chronic inflammatory conditions such as sinus, helps in the removal of foreign bodies such as splinters and seeds, ripens abscesses, ailments attended with pus formation. Use silica and be prepared to use it for a while sometimes up to 3 weeks.

Mind - Faint hearted, anxious, yielding.

Better - Warmth, wet or humid weather.

Worse - Morning, from lying down, cold.

Staphysagria

Characteristics - Suits sensitive people who suppress their feelings and suffer in silence or who boil over with indignation, remedy for cuts and wounds especially those that are from medical procedures and have the mentioned feelings. Nervous states of animals. The pains are stinging, stitching, smarting, squeezing, as if stabbed by a knife. Worse from touch, emotions and suppressed anger.

Better - Warmth, rest at night.

Worse - Touch on affected parts, loss of fluids.

Symphytum

Characteristics - Causes bone to grow and promotes fast healing should be given for all fractures. Used for injuries to the hard parts of the body while arnica is for the soft parts. Also used for eye injuries caused from blows.

Caution - do not use if a pin has been placed in the bone as the pin has to be removed latter.

Tarentula Cubensis

Characteristics - For abscesses, boils, carbuncles, swellings of any kind but especially on the back of the neck where the skin turns black, red/blue or purple with great pain. Deep septic conditions with hardening of the effected part, condition comes on fast, pains are burning, stinging, throbbing, pricking like a needle.

Worse - Night.

Urtica Urens

Characteristics - Can be used for burns and also for cystitis where the urine burns the skin and there is difficulty passing urine. Symptoms are stinging pains, swellings particularly blistery swellings, itching.

Worse - Cool moist air, touch.

Boerickes Materia Medica

Boerickes Materia Medica is the best one for use by the lay person, once you have mastered it you can move on to the many others. To make the remedies as closer a match we can we ask lots of questions like the ones we have just read and after we gather all the answers we have what is called a good Symptom Picture which we then try to match as accurately as we can to a Remedy. Homoeopathic Repertories are used for matching symptoms to remedies but in this book you get the specific for each disease so try to match them as best as you can. Below is a example page out of Boerickes Materia Medica 1927 which is found easily on the internet as it is well out of the 70 year copyright period but it is still a very valuable reference to have and Boericke can be very proud of his work as it still is saving lives long after he is gone. All Materia Medicas are laid out in the same format, my layout concentrates more on the mind as we have matched the symptoms with the disease but still you should try to do it properly all I am trying to do is to make you able to work fast in emergencies.

ARSENICUM ALBUM
Arsenious Acid-Arsenic Trioxide

A profoundly acting remedy on every organ and tissue. Its clear-cut characteristic symptoms and correspondence to many severe types of disease make its homeopathic employment constant and certain. Its general symptoms often alone lead to its successful application. Among these the all-prevailing debility, exhaustion, and *restlessness*, with *nightly aggravation*, are most important. *Great exhaustion after the slightest exertion*. This, with the peculiar irritability of fiber, gives the characteristic *irritable weakness*. *Burning pains*. Unquenchable thirst. Burning relieved by heat. *Seaside complaints* (*Nat mur; Aqua Marina*). Injurious effects of fruits, especially more watery ones. Gives quiet and ease to the last moments of life when given in high potency. *Fear fright and worry*. Green discharges. Infantile Kala-azar (Dr. Neatby).

Ars should be thought of in ailments from alcoholism, *ptomaine poisoning*, stings, dissecting wounds, chewing tobacco; ill effects from decayed food or animal matter; odor of discharges is *putrid*; in complaints that return annually. Anæmia and chlorosis. Degenerative changes. Gradual loss of weight from impaired nutrition. Reduces the refractive index of blood serum (also *China* and *Ferr phos*). Maintains the system under the stress of malignancy regardless of location. Malarial cachexia. *Septic infections and low vitality.*

Mind - *Great anguish and restlessness. Changes place continually. Fears*, of death, of being left alone. Great fear, with cold sweat. Thinks it useless to take medicine. Suicidal. Hallucinations of smell and sight. Despair drives him from place to place. Miserly, malicious, selfish, lacks courage. General sensibility increased (*Hep*). Sensitive to disorder and confusion.

Head - Headaches relieves by cold, other symptoms worse. Periodical burning pains, with *restlessness*; with cold skin. Hemicrania, with icy feeling of scalp and great weakness. Sensitive head in open air. Delirium tremens; cursing and raving; vicious. Head is in constant motion. Scalp *itches* intolerably; circular patches of bare spots; rough, dirty, sensitive, and covered with dry scales; nightly burning and itching; dandruff. Scalp very sensitive; cannot brush hair.

Eyes - *Burning in eyes, with acrid lachrymation.* Lids red, ulcerated, scabby, scaly, granulated. Œdema *around* eyes. External inflammation, with extreme painfulness; *burning, hot,* and excoriating lachrymation. Corneal ulceration. *Intense photophobia*; better external warmth. Ciliary neuralgia, with fine burning pain.

Ears - Skin within, raw and burning. *Thin, excoriating, offensive* otorrhœa. Roaring in ears, during a paroxysm of pain.

Nose - *Thin, watery, excoriating* discharge. Nose feels *stopped up*. Sneezing *without* relief. Hay-fever and coryza; worse in open air; better indoors. *Burning* and bleeding. Acne of nose. Lupus.

Face - Swollen, pale, yellow, *cachectic*, sunken, cold, and covered with sweat (*Acetic acid*). Expression of agony. Tearing *needle-like* pains; burning. Lips black, livid. Angry, circumscribed flush of cheeks.

Mouth - Unhealthy, easily-bleeding gums. Ulceration of mouth with dryness and burning heat. Epithelioma of lips. Tongue dry, clean, and red; stitching and burning pain in tongue, ulcerated with blue color. Bloody saliva. Neuralgia of teeth; feel long and very sore; worse after midnight; better warmth. Metallic taste. *Gulping up of burning water.*

Throat - Swollen, œdematous, constricted, *burning*, unable to swallow. Diphtheritic membrane, looks dry and wrinkled.

Stomach - *Cannot bear the sight or smell of food.* Great thirst; drinks much, but *little at a time*. Nausea, retching, vomiting, after eating or drinking. Anxiety in pit of stomach. *Burning pain*. Craves acids and coffee. Heartburn; gulping up of acid and bitter substances which seem to excoriate the throat. Long-lasting eructations. Vomiting of blood, bile, green mucus, or brown-black mixed with blood. Stomach extremely irritable; seems raw, as if torn. Gastralgia from slightest food or drink. Dyspepsia from vinegar, acids, ice-cream, ice-water, tobacco. Terrible fear and dyspnœa, with gastralgia; also faintness, icy coldness, great exhaustion. Malignant symptoms. Everything swallowed seems to lodge in the œsophagus, which seems as if closed and nothing would pass. *Ill effects of vegetable diet, melons, and watery fruits generally*. Craves milk.

Abdomen - Gnawing, burning pains like coals of fire; relieved by heat. *Liver and spleen enlarged and painful*. Ascites and anasarca. Abdomen swollen and painful. Pain as from a wound in abdomen on coughing.

Rectum - Painful, spasmodic protrusion of rectum. Tenesmus. *Burning* pain and pressure in rectum and anus.

Stool - *Small, offensive, dark, with much prostration. Worse at night, and after eating and drinking*; from chilling stomach, alcoholic abuse, spoiled meat. Dysentery dark, bloody, very offensive. Cholera, with intense agony, prostration, and burning thirst. Body cold as ice (*Verat*). Hæmorrhoids burn like fire; relieved by heat. Skin excoriated about anus.

Urine - Scanty, burning, involuntary. Bladder as if paralysed. *Albuminous*. Epithelial cells; cylindrical clots of fibrin and globules of pus and blood. After urinating, feeling of weakness in abdomen. Bright's disease. Diabetes.

Female - Menses too profuse and too soon. Burning in ovarian region. Leucorrhœa, acrid, burning, offensive, thin. Pain as from red-hot wires; worse least exertion; causes great fatigue; better in warm room. *Menorrhagia*. Stitching pain in pelvis extending down the thigh.

Respiratory - Unable to lie down; fears suffocation. Air-passages constricted. Asthma worse midnight. Burning in chest. Suffocative catarrh. Cough worse after midnight; worse lying on back. Expectoration *scanty, frothy. Darting pain through upper third of right lung*. Wheezing respiration. Hæmoptysis with pain between shoulders; burning heat all over. Cough dry, as from sulphur fumes; *after drinking*.

Heart - Palpitation, pain, dyspnœa, faintness. Irritable heart in smokers and tobacco-chewers. *Pulse more rapid in morning (Sulph)*. Dilatation. Cyanosis. Fatty degeneration. Angina pectoris, with pain in neck and occiput.

Back - Weakness in small of back. Drawing in of shoulders. Pain and burning in back (*Oxal ac*).

Extremities - Trembling, twitching, spasms, weakness, heaviness, uneasiness. Cramps in calves. Swelling of feet. Sciatica. Burning pains. Peripheral neuritis. Diabetic gangrene. Ulcers on heel (*Cepa; Lamium*). Paralysis of lower limbs with atrophy.

Skin - Itching, burning, swellings; œdema, eruption, papular, *dry, rough, scaly; worse cold* and scratching. Malignant pustules. Ulcers with offensive discharge. Anthrax. Poisoned wounds. Urticaria, with burning and restlessness. *Psoriasis*. Scirrhus. Icy coldness of body. Epithelioma of the skin. Gangrenous inflammations.

Sleep - Disturbed, anxious, restless. Must have head raised by pillows. Suffocative fits during sleep. Sleeps with hands over head. Dreams are full of care and fear. Drowsy, sleeping sickness.

Fever - High temperature. *Periodicity marked with adynamia*. Septic fevers. *Intermittent. Paroxysms incomplete, with marked exhaustion. Hay-fever*. Cold sweats. Typhoid, not too early; often after Rhus. Complete exhaustion. Delirium; worse after midnight. Great restlessness. Great heat about 3 am.

Modalities - *Worse*, wet weather, after midnight; from cold, cold drinks, or food. Seashore. Right side. *Better* from heat; from head elevated; warm drinks.

Complementary: *Rhus; Carbo; Phos. Thuja; Secale*. Antidotal to lead poison.

Antidotes: *Opium; Carbo; China; Hepar; Nux*. Chemical Antidotes: Charcoal; Hydrated Peroxide of Iron; Lime Water.

Compare: *Arsenic stibatum* 3x (Chest inflammations of children, restlessness with thirst and prostration, loose mucous cough, oppression, hurried respiration, crepitant rales). *Cenchris contortrix; Iod; Phosph; China; Verat alb; Carbo; Kali phos. Epilobium* (intractable diarrhœa of typhoid). *Hoang Nan. Atoxyl*. Sodium arseniate 3x, sleeping sickness; commencing optic atrophy. *Levico Water*--(containing Ars, Iron and Copper of South Tyrol). Chronic and dyscratic skin diseases, chorea minor and spasms in scrofulous and anæmic children. Favors assimilation and increases nutrition. Debility and skin diseases, especially after the use of higher potencies where progress seems suspended. Dose. Ten drops in wine glass of warm water 3 times a day after meals (Burnett). *Sarcolatic acid* (influenza with violent vomiting).

Dose - Third to thirtieth potency. The very highest potencies often yield brilliant results.

Low attenuations in gastric, intestinal, and kidney diseases; higher in neuralgias, nervous diseases, and skin. But if only surface conditions call for it, give the lowest potencies, 2x to 3x trit. Repeated doses advisable.

Disease Nosodes

This section on Nosodes is the most important in the book as if you are caught in a fast moving Pandemic a Disease Nosode could save you and yours lives. There is no Doctor alive now who has experience in a fast full on Pandemic with the Spanish Flu being the last one. Nosodes were made and used for hundreds of years by Pandemic Hardened Veterans bear this in mind as well as this. If they came up with a vaccine for a fast moving Pandemic earlier then their usual six months would they still have healthy staff to make it? Would the power still be on anyway with most of the power workers sick? Would the transport infrastructure still be working?

Nosodes are remedies made from disease material mainly from the tissues, discharges, exudates, excretions, suppurations or secretions of an infected being. Simply stated a Nosode is a homeopathic remedy prepared from a pathological specimen. Rabies Nosode, for example starts with the saliva of a rabid dog and is then potentized.

Nosodes have many uses and are widely used in homeopathic practice to help limit cases of infectious diseases and to help during the recovery phase of a disease especially the ones that linger and drag on. There are Nosodes for most infectious diseases of animals and humans the use of Nosodes in this way is referred to as isopathy rather than Homoeopathy. They are often used in farm situations, to limit the spread and the effects of infectious diseases. This has especially been used as a vital component of mastitis control on many farms, both organic and conventional as they can limit their use of antibiotics and the hold back time of milk. One documented event about Nosodes dates back to Napoleon marching his Legions through Europe and spreading Typhoid in their wake, the towns that had the best cure rates were the ones where the local Homoeopaths used a Nosode of the disease.

Nosodes can be used in the prevention of infectious diseases in the manner similar to vaccination but they work by a completely different mechanism then from the raising of antibodies that vaccines work by. As yet it is not actually known how they work but they have survived hundreds of years ridicule by producing results and will carry on doing so.

The best known study into Nosodes was done by Dr. Christopher Day of England involving 'kennel cough' in a boarding kennel. At the time he was called in, there were 40 dogs in the kennel with 35 that had kennel cough. About half had been vaccinated for this malady. He gave a Nosode to all the animals that were there and all the dogs that came in through the rest of the summer, which was another 214 dogs. He successfully reduced the incidence of kennel cough from over 90% to less than 2%.

Nosodes used for the prevention of diseases are usually given in the 30C potency. A good dosing regime is one dose given night and morning for 3 days followed by one per month for the next 6 months. This generally provides a good level of protection after the first week. Nosodes can have homeopathic therapeutic properties in their own right. Such Nosodes are found in the Homoeopathic Materia Medica and have undergone a proper 'proving'. Examples are Bacillinum, Carcinosinum, Medorrhinum, Psorinum and Tuberculinum.

How To Make A Nosode In A Hurry

This is not the right way of making a Homoeopathic preparation but it is an effective way when you have an emergency situation and have to react fast.

1/. Get a sample of the pathogen you need from the patient, for example, Pus from a wound or papular eruption,, sputum coughed up from the lungs or any other disease product, it can even be the scrapings from a stubborn ringworm infection that won't go away. Sometimes the more sources of the same disease combined e.g. sputum and pus from an eruption the better the result.

2/. Find a clean 600ml jar and sterilize it by putting it in the oven at a high temperature for a while as you would for sterilizing preserving jars. After the jar is sterilized place your disease products in and fill with sterilized water or distilled water which is cheap and easy to buy from an auto shop as they use it in batteries. Shake the jar for a while until you are sure the mixture is dissolved.

3/. Empty the jar, there will always be a residue from whatever sticks to the sides and you will see the drops gather again at the bottom of the jar after it is upright.

4/. Fill the jar again with distilled water, this time at about 500mls. This will become our first potency. Get a book and put it on a table and sit down and get comfortable. We are going to gently bang the jar against the book for 100 percussions. Homoeopathic remedies are energy medicines; we are imprinting our disease products onto the universal medium, water.

5/. Repeat steps 3 and 4 again for 27 times bringing our remedy close to a normal 30C homoeopathic potency, now you can see why I told you to sit down and get comfortable.

6/. On the 29 time use half and half water and vodka. We still have one more to go after this but we are going to save most of this as a stock to make more if needed. This is very important especially in cases of epidemics where you can give your friends and others some of this and they only have to percuss a part of this 100 times to get the needed nosode for medicating others and themselves.

7/. Make the last potency again in half water and half vodka. This is our last potency to make for we are as close as we can get to the 30C potency by doing it this way. The dose will be 10 drops under the tongue 3 times a day as a preventative or 5 drops every 30 minutes at the beginning of an acute infection. Take the normal precautions used with Homoeopathic Potencies i.e. no coffee or anything strong half an hour before or after the remedy.

Nutritional Disease Fighting Supplements
Vitamin A

Increases resistance to infections and enhances phagocyte and antibody production. Maintains the tissue that makes up the skin and mucous membranes this is very important especially in respiratory and digestive diseases as both these systems have massive mucous membranes so in diseases of these systems consider put the dose up a bit.
Dose - 5000 to 10000 IU daily or 5000 twice daily for maximum assimilation.
Food Sources - Apricots, carrots, fish liver oils, green leafy veges, liver, egg yolk.

Vitamin C

Vitamin C is the most critical supplement for the natural treatment of any disease especially those of the Respiratory System as it is the primary antioxidant in the lungs and a powerful antihistamine without side effects. Low vitamin C dramatically increases histamine levels which put you at greater risk for allergic reactions, rhinitis, and asthma attacks. 1000mg of C for three days reduces blood histamine to normal levels. Vit C reduces the severity of allergic responses but be aware that your body gobbles up C during prolonged colds, asthma or allergy attacks and if it is not replaced the attacks may get worse and worse. Vitamin C is needed by the immune system and is necessary for healing and the prevention of infections along with being a potent antioxidant with anti-bacterial and antiviral actions. Humans do not manufacture Vitamin C and neither is it stored by the body so the diet is the only source. Vitamin C is easily depleted in the body especially by smoking (25mg per cigarette), stress, pollution and alcohol.

High doses of vitamin C have shown itself to act against bacteria and viral activity (especially retroviruses) in general as well as to protect tissue against inflammatory damage caused by them. During Active infection a high dosage is recommended for those strong and fit who don't get kidney stones. Take the dose up to bowel tolerance then reduce a bit for others try to get at least 3000mg into the system spread through the day. Magnesium Ascorbate is considered by many to be a better form for the body to use.

One of the studies performed by Dr Linus Pauling showed a concentration of 1mg of Vitamin C per decilitre of growth medium prevented the growth of TB bacteria and in another of his experiments he showed that higher dosages can neutralize the toxins associated with diphtheria, tetanus and staphylococcus. High levels of vitamin C increase the killing ability of the white blood cells, helps increase the interferon levels and antibody levels in the blood stream along with boosting the activity of the thymus gland. From reading the above you should be realizing what a great tool vitamin C is for the treatment of some of our more nasty types of diseases such as Typhoid. As Typhoid has a long period before the real nasty symptoms come on using our other herbs and vitamin C we could abort the disease in the beginning just from the big boost we gave to the immune system, if this failed the patient would hopefully run a milder form of the disease because we had depleted the bacterial population, so there would be less bacteria putting toxins in the blood poisoning the system and even the toxins would to a certain extent be neutralized by the vitamin C.

Food Sources - Black currants, broccoli, citrus fruit, guava, parsley, pineapple, rosehips and strawberries.

Vitamin E

The production of antibodies is increased when vitamin E is supplemented especially when it is accompanied with Selenium as a deficiency of these two can lead to a decline in T and B cells. These two supplements work together in strengthening the walls of cells hopefully slowing down the invaders attempting to break in the cell. Vitamin E also reduces the allergic response and is one of the main blood borne antioxidants. Vitamin E can inhibit excessive arachidonic acid production and is involved in the production of some of the pituitary and adrenal hormones and is needed in the body for healing.

Dose - 200iu is recommended as a maintenance dose for healthy people so this could be safely doubled for the sick.

Food sources - Wheat germ oil and all cold pressed oils from vegetable sources, sesame seeds, sunflower and pumpkin seeds, hazel nuts, walnuts, peanuts, sprouted seeds, spinach, Brussels sprouts, brown rice, asparagus, celery, peas, avocado.

Caution - No one taking anticoagulant drugs for thrombosis or other similar conditions should take Vitamin E.

Selenium

Selenium is a potent anti-oxidant which Australian soils are deficient in. Helps in the detoxification of chemicals and maintenance of cellular membranes. Selenium is needed for utilization of essential fatty acids and regulation of prostaglandin synthesis. New research has found that healthy individuals taking 200 micrograms daily for 8 weeks had a 100% increase in their lymphocyte activity. Other people say it has a anti-viral effect and reduces viral replication along with boosting the immune system by increasing immune cells.

Food Sources - Garlic, brewer's yeast, kelp and eggs, brazil nuts, mushrooms, tuna, sunflower seeds, kidneys and whole grain cereals.

Dose - Take in very low doses and do not exceed 100mcg a day.

Zinc

Most people these days are deficient in zinc which is required by the immune system for optimum function and healing. Nearly 100 important enzymes depend upon a adequate supply of zinc and many of them are involved with the immune system. Normal levels of zinc in the blood stream inhibit the release of histamine from mast cells. Zinc is also a potent antioxidant.

Food sources - One of the richest sources of zinc are oysters, other sources are liver, meat, seeds, green leafy vegetables, rose hip tea, brewer's yeast, wheat germ, pumpkin seeds, egg yolk and whole grains.

Dose - 40 to 50mg per day.

Colostrum

Colostrum is a special form of milk produced by mammals during late pregnancy, soon before birth and is very rich in nutrients such as protein, vitamins, as well as antibodies for use by the infant.

Newborns do not yet have their own immune system, and this first milk of antibodies will help to protect the baby in the months to come. Colostrum has been used through the ages, Ayurvedic physicians in India have used it as a treatment for thousands of years and for those that knew, it was the main anti biotic of the Middle Ages and many a cow was deprived of its first milk. Colostrum contains Immunoglobulins G which counteracts bacteria and toxins in the blood and lymphatic system; immunoglobulin M which seeks out and attaches itself to viruses in the circulatory system; immunoglobulins D and E which remove foreign substances from the bloodstream. Other ingredients are Lactoferrin which helps deprive bacteria of iron, growth factors, leukocytes and enzymes. More recent clinical studies have demonstrated that it is effective in preventing intestinal infections by first keeping the bacteria from attaching themselves to the intestinal wall, and secondly by killing the bacteria themselves. Colostrum has proved to be capable of killing Campylobacter, Helicobacter pylori, Listeria, Salmonella, Shigellosis, and five types of streptococci. This is a very important supplement especially in digestive problems or those of lowered immunity. Most Health Shops sell Bovine Colostrum.

Caution - Allergic reactions in persons who are known to be allergic to cow's milk

Fever

Normal body temperature is considered to be 98.4 degrees (37C) but can range between 96 to 99 degrees (35.6 to 37.2C). Onset of a fever can be gradual or sudden and the temperature can remain fairly normal during the day time but rise dramatically at night.

Fever is one of the bodies main defense mechanisms as the extra heat speeds up the chemical reactions in the body and hinders the germs as they do not like excessive heat, so fever is the body's way of taking the battle to the invader. As the temperature raises so will the pulse and respiration and as the temperature goes down so will they.

In herbal medicine we support the fever because it has a job to do, the idea is to keep the fever out of the danger areas, in other words not to high but not too low. Herbalists treat fevers with herbs that are called Diaphoretics. Diaphoretics are herbs that cause the body to sweat, they mimic the action of fevers and rid the body of toxins and can reduce the fever in a short time. We use the Actions of Febrifuges when the body temperature gets into the danger areas and needs to be brought down a good example would be Dengue Fever. Take the temperature frequently so you know which way it is going. Drink plenty of fluids. If the temperature is very high one should begin sponging, this should be done with just warm water and should not be overdone. Start sponging only the forehead and face and observe the effect on the temp. If the temp drops below 102 the sponging can be stopped. If more extensive sponging is required the extremities and the torso can be moistened. Do not attempt to drop the temp back to normal as this will merely suppress the fever and likely chill the patient.

Normal Temp	**37 C**	**98.6 F**
Oral Ranges	36 to 37.5	96.8 to 99.5
Rectally	0.5 Higher	1 F higher
Axillary	0.5 Lower	1 F Lower

The number is followed by the method taken.

1/. Low grade fever is from 37.5 to 38.2 C or 99.5 to 101 F

2/. High grade fever is from 38.2 C and above or 101 F and above.

Fevers can rise dramatically at night. As the temperature rises so will the pulse and breathing rate with the amount of urine passed reduced and concentrated due to the sweating. Other symptoms such as lassitude, feelings of hot and cold, shivering, aches and pains in the back and limbs are common. If the temperature rises above 103 (39.4 C) delirium may occur which may lead to convulsions and finally coma if no attempt is made to reduce the temperature. Convulsions are fairly common in children between the ages of 1 and 3 but are rare after the age of 5.

Treatment - Keep fever out of the danger areas, not to high not to low, give diaphoretics to reduce heat and cause sweating for the removal of toxins eg Peppermint and Ginger tea hot and at frequent intervals to promote sweating. After the temperature has returned to normal the teas may be taken cold for their tonic properties. The teas can be taken every one or two hours hot in about 60mls doses until perspiration has taken place. A lot of this depends on the patient if they want a bit more give it to them.

Patients with dry fevers ie no sweating usually feel agitated, restless and distressed and may be in some danger. High dry fevers should be treated with herbs that relax and Moisten e.g Yarrow, Chamomile, Elder, **Boneset, Pleurisy root.**

Foe sluggish fever use stimulants - *Ginger, Cayenne, Horse Radish*.

Herbal Treatment

Peppermint tea - diaphoretic, is cooling.

Ginger - diaphoretic, circulatory stimulant, these two actions make ginger good for a fever that has chills.

Chamomile has a good all round action but the herbs above are the main and easy to get ones for fever though you could mix them all together.

Herbal Actions for Fevers

Diaphoretics - Aids the skin in the elimination of toxins and produces sweat thus reducing the temperature of fevers.

Herbs - Angelica, Boneset, Catnip, Cayenne, Elder Flower, Ginger, Hyssop, Lemongrass, Lemon balm, Penny Royal, Peppermint, Pleurisy Root, Yarrow.

Febrifuge - Helps the body to bring down fevers.

Herbs - Angelica, Boneset ,Cayenne, Elder Flowers, Hyssop, Lobelia,

Marigold, Penny Royal, Peppermint, Plantain, Peruvian Bark, Raspberry, Sage, Thyme, Vervain.

Rehydration Formulas

Dehydration and severe diarrheal diseases particularly in epidemics are massive killers in the third world especially among children. The death rate is dramatically reduced now due to the use of Oral Rehydration Solution (ORS) packed into millions of sachets and sent around the world by WHO.

Many diseases can dehydrate you not only from diarrhea but also from the fever and vomiting alone so great care must always be paid to dehydration in any disease. In the western world hospitals they don't use ORS but use the IV drips instead but if there is a massive pandemic then we all have to look after ourselves so let's get used to the idea of making and using Oral Rehydration Solutions now and of always keeping an eye open for the possibility of Dehydration in any condition. Remember when you make your own ORS that ingesting plain water does not help restore the salt content of the body. But ingesting water with too much salt will draw fluids from the body, and make the dehydration worse.

Sugar is also added to the ORS solutions for two reasons. First because sugar helps with the transport of fluids across the cellular membranes in the bowel and second because sugar also provides needed calories to keep the strength up but as with salt too much sugar can be detrimental, it can promote diarrhea and make the loss of fluids worse.

Symptoms of dehydration can be weakness, headache, and fainting, dryness of the mouth, decreased saliva, lack or very decreased urine that is dark in color and highly concentrated, sunken eyes, loss of the elasticity of the skin, low blood pressure especially upon sitting up or rising from the sitting to the standing position and a fast pulse when laying or sitting up.

Formulas

1/. The simplest formula is 3 Tablespoons of sugar and 1 teaspoon of salt dissolved in 1 quart (946 mls) of potable water.

2/. An alternative simple formula is 8 teaspoons of sugar and 1 teaspoon of salt dissolved in 1 quart (946 mls) of potable water. This basic formula has been used effectively for more than 30 years by WHO.

3/. A slightly more complicated formula may be used to replace lost potassium, and to help control diarrhea. This formula is from Dr. Steven J. Greenwald and is designed specifically to help people who were being threatened with extreme diarrhea.

ORAL REHYDRATION FLUID FORMULA
1/4 teaspoon Salt (common table salt - sodium chloride)
1/4 teaspoon Salt Substitute or "Lite Salt" (potassium chloride)
1/4 teaspoon Baking Soda
2 ½ tablespoons Sugar
Combine these ingredients and dissolve them in 1000 ml (1 liter) of sterile water.

Chemists will be able to help with any problem here.

Airborne, Contact And Crowding Diseases

It is interesting some of the nasty diseases nature has created and is in the process of creating. One of the worst is the Plague, who would of even dreamed that a bite from a flea would of caused a disease that would turn airborne and be so fast acting that it could at worst kill you in 12 to 24 hours. Today the odds are again going against us with Climate Change Disasters popping up all over the place, Civil Wars causing mass migrations, famines and Refugee Camps, Disease Vectors are also changing because of the heat and we have had Swine Flu traveling around the world which no doubt has a date with Bird Flu especially when it crosses the main bird migration paths and no doubt when they have got together they will meet up with our yearly changed Human Influenza and then Death might really of hit the Jackpot. The potential is always out there after all it's really a numbers game and we humans are not really doing anything to put the odds in our favor. In this section we will also look at the Crowding Diseases especially the ones associated with Refugee Camps such as Measles and Meningitis caused by *Neisseria meningitidis* which is transmitted from person to person, particularly in situations of crowding along with Acute Respiratory Infections which are a major cause of morbidity and mortality among displaced populations especially in children aged less than 5 years. We shall start with Human Influenza so you have a fair idea how to treat it Homoeopathically and with Herbal medicine so if you ever have to treat a Animal Crossover Flu the treatment would be similar and you would only have to add Herbs that correspond with the new Herbal Actions that you require caused by the altered or different symptoms from the Animal side. If some time in the future the worst happens always keep an eye on what the Homoeopaths are doing for we are the great survivors who have suffered ridicule and disease for hundreds of years and if we get really scared we would probably make a Nosode Potency of the disease product and survive that way along with all our usual treatment. But remember the most important thing is to treat the symptoms immediately and to try to prevent them from happening in the first place, a simple thing such as gargling with a few drops of Tea Tree Oil mixed with water as soon as you feel that dry pain starting in the nasopharynx area could save your life or buy you the extra time needed to save your life. If you wait to learn the name of the disease you have got it could be too late.

Influenza

Cause - Influenza refers to a illness caused by the influenza viruses, Influenza viruses are classified as types A, B, or C by their nucleoproteins and matrix proteins. Influenza C virus infection does not cause the typical Influenza illness. Influenza viruses may be spread by airborne droplets, person-to-person contact, or contact with contaminated items. Airborne spread appears to be the most important mechanism.

Disease Process - Hemagglutinin (HA) is a glycoprotein on the influenza surface that allows the virus to fuse with the host membrane. Neuraminidase (NA), another surface glycoprotein, promotes viral dispersion from the infected cell. Relatively minor mutations in HA and NA of influenza A and B result in the frequent emergence of new viral strains. The result is decreased protection by antibodies generated to the previous strain. A major change in NA or HA occurs in influenza A at infrequent intervals (10 to 40 years during the last century); as a result, the population has no immunity to the new virus, and pandemic influenza may occur. Influenza produces widespread sporadic illness yearly during fall and winter in temperate climates. Pandemics caused by new influenza A serotypes may cause a particularly severe disease as the body has no immunities to it. Influenza B viruses typically produce mild disease but can cause epidemics with moderate or severe disease, usually occurring in 3 to 5 year cycles. Although most influenza epidemics result from a single serotype, other viruses may appear simultaneously, with one virus predominating in one location and another virus predominating elsewhere. Seasonal epidemics often occur in 2 waves with the first appearing in schoolchildren and their household contacts (generally younger people) and the second mostly in housebound or institutionalized people, particularly the elderly.

Diagnosis - Diagnosis is usually clinical and depends on local epidemiologic patterns. Definitive diagnosis requires cell cultures of nasopharyngeal swabs or aspirate or acute and convalescent antibody samples. This testing takes several days or more and is useful for establishing the presence of influenza in the community and detecting antigenic changes.

Prevention - High-risk patients, their caregivers and household contacts along with health care practitioners should receive annual influenza vaccination.

Symptoms - Influenza is a viral respiratory infection causing fever, coryza, cough, headache, and malaise. The incubation period ranges from 1 to 4 days with an average of about 48 hours. In mild cases many symptoms are like those of a common cold, mild conjunctivitis may also occur. Typical influenza in adults is characterized by the sudden onset of chills, fever, prostration, cough, and generalized aches and pains especially in the back and legs. Headache is prominent, often with photophobia. Respiratory symptoms may be mild at first, with scratchy sore throat, nonproductive cough, and sometimes coryza. Later, lower respiratory tract illness becomes dominant; cough can be persistent, raspy, and productive. Children may have prominent nausea, vomiting, or abdominal pain. After 2 to 3 days acute symptoms rapidly subside although the fever may last up to 5 days. Cough, weakness, sweating, and fatigue may persist for several days or occasionally for weeks.

Pneumonia is suspected by a worsening cough, purulent or bloody sputum, dyspnea, and rales. Secondary bacterial pneumonia is suggested by persistence or recurrence of fever, cough, and other respiratory symptoms in the second week.

Encephalitis and myocarditis develop infrequently usually during convalescence. They occur more frequently after influenza A pandemics.

Prognosis - Most patients recover fully, although full recovery often takes 1 or 2 weeks. However, influenza and influenza-related pneumonia are important causes of death in high-risk patients, young children, the elderly, and those with chronic disease. Death is possible during epidemics, particularly among high-risk patients at the extremes of age, or have cardiopulmonary insufficiency, or are in late pregnancy.

Treatment - Antiviral treatments include the neuraminidase inhibitors zanamivir and oseltamivir, which are effective for both influenza A and B, and amantadine and rimantadine, which are effective only against influenza A.

Herbal Treatment

Follow the directions given in The Acute Treatment Of Disease. If this has been done hopefully this will now be a milder form of the disease. A good basic formula for the flu is Boneset, Elder and Peppermint. They all cover the fever side of the condition with Boneset covering the aches and pains, Elder the symptoms in general and Peppermint the pain and any nausea and digestive problems. Add to this Licorice to push the formula into the body and you have an Antiviral and Expectorant Action as well. Keep on using the Garlic Oil that you were using as a preventative as it has a Antiviral Action and will help in the prevention of any secondary bacterial infections. Other herbs to consider are Ginger, Golden Rod, Golden Seal, Hyssop, Lemon Balm, Lemongrass, Pleurisy Root, Shitake, and Yarrow. The first settlers of Australia used to use a drop of Eucalyptus Oil on a sugar cube taken internally for the treatment of flu. Eucalyptus has a Antiviral and Bronchodilator Action.

Homoeopathic Treatment

Gelsemium 6C to 30C - This remedy corresponds to the commencement of the trouble, when the patient is weak, tired and aches throughout the body. It removes speedily the intense aching and muscular soreness. There is constant chilliness and the patient hugs the fire; the fever is less acute than that of Aconite, and the cough is hard and painful. There are paroxysms of sneezing with excoriating discharge, and great torpor and apathy. An extensive experience with this remedy in the great Epidemic of 1918 proved its usefulness. Simple cases were speedily cured. Those that were complicated with initial treatments by Aspirin were only those which had dangerous complications. Aconite will sometimes prove the better remedy for children, but the drug will never be a prominent one in influenza. Still it may be prescribed when indicated; it will, perhaps, soothe and moderate the subsequent attack, but its action is not quick here as in simple fevers, as we have to do with a blood affection. Baptisia. The gastro-intestinal form of grippe may need this remedy, especially when there are present putrid diarrhea stools. Clarke considers this remedy the nearest specific for the disease; he prefers the 30th potency. Hughes also praises it, but uses it in the 1x and 2x dilutions, which seem to have more extensive testimony as to their efficacy.

Eupatorium Perfoliatum 6C to 30C - This remedy has much soreness and aching of the entire body; hoarseness and cough, with great soreness of the larynx and upper respiratory tract. Coryza with thirst and drinking causes vomiting. The cough is a very shattering one, hurts the head and chest, and as in Drosera, the patient holds the chest with the hands. The breakbone pains are characteristic of the remedy. Add to these symptoms acute bilious derangements, and it is all the more indicated. Many physicians rely on this remedy in la grippe almost exclusively in the early stages.

Sabadilla 6C to 30C - Sneezing is the great keynote of this remedy. Sneezing and lachrymation on going into the open air. The throat is swollen and the pain is worse on empty swallowing; the sneezing is excessive, shaking the whole body. Shudderings , with gooseflesh chills creeping upwards, are also prominent symptoms. Frontal headache, dryness of mouth, without thirst and cough, worse on lying down, are additional symptoms. It suits well many cases of the catarrhal form of grippe; other remedies having sneezing are Cyclamen and Euphorbia.

Arsenicum 6C to 30C - This remedy corresponds to the trial form of influenza. It covers more phases of grippe than perhaps any other remedy. Hughes believes that it will cut short an attack, especially when there is a copious flow, prostration and paroxysmal coryza. Its periodicity makes it suitable to epidemics, and it suits the early symptoms when the affection is in the upper portion of the respiratory tract. The burning dryness and copious watery excoriating secretion and the involvement of the conjunctiva are unmistakable indications. Langour and prostration are prominent symptoms. Arsenicum iodide. Chills, flushes of heat and severe fluent coryza, discharge irritating and corrosive, sneezing and prostration. It corresponds to true influenza and is highly recommended by Hale. Sanguinaria nitrate is especially valuable when the trachea and larynx are affected. Phytolacca. Specific when the throat is inflamed and spotty, with great hardness and tenderness of the glands.

Dulcumara 6C to 30C - This is one of our best remedies in the acute form; the eyes are suffused, the throat is sore and the cough hurts because of the muscular soreness. If brought on by damp, cold changes in the weather, so much the surer is Dulcamara indicated. Bryonia. The trouble here is largely bronchial and going down. Phosphorus may be indicated, especially when the trouble moves towards the chest. It is a very useful remedy for the debility following la grippe, as it is usually of the pure nervous type. It is the great post-influenza "tonic."

Rhus Tox 6C to 30C - Influenza, with severe aching in all the bones, sneezing and coughing. The cough is worse evenings and is caused by a tickling behind the upper part of the sternum. Especially is it useful in cases brought on by exposure to dampness. There is much prostration and depression, and the patient may have some symptoms which are suspicious as pointing towards typhoid fever, such as burning tongue, stupor and delirium. Aching pains, nightly restlessness are keynotes symptoms. Causticum, like both Rhus and Eupatorium, has a tired, sore, bruised sensation all over the body and soreness in the chest when coughing, but it has in addition involuntary urination when coughing.

Allum Cepa 6C to 30C - Profuse catarrhal coryza; the nose runs freely, there is sneezing, irritability cough, the face is swollen and looks inflamed. Camphora. This remedy is often sufficient at the outset to cut short an attack, or at least modify the severity.

Sticta 6C to 30 - Nasal catarrh; headache, thirst, nightly expectoration, great watering of eyes, running at nose, hoarseness of voice, frontal headache and depression of whole system. Tuberculous subjects attacked by grippe. "There is no better remedy," says Dr. Fornias, "for the incessant wearing, racking cough of this class of patients." Tuberculinum is an excellent prevention of recurring attacks of la grippe in those who have annual attacks. NOTE: Those who were guided during the great Epidemic by the indications given in the previous edition of this work have amply verified all of them, so little change appears.

Measles

Cause - Measles is caused by a paramyxovirus. It is extremely contagious probably the most contagious of the fevers and is spread mainly by secretions from the nose, throat, and mouth during the early eruptive stage or by airborne droplets. The disease is contagious from several days before until several days after the rash appears. Lifelong immunity is conferred by infection. Measles is most common in children. It is characterized by fever, cough, coryza, conjunctivitis and a maculopapular rash. Worldwide, measles infects about 30 to 40 million annually, causing about 800,000 deaths, primarily in children.

Diagnosis - Typical measles may be suspected in an exposed patient who has coryza, conjunctivitis, photophobia, and cough but usually is confirmed only after the rash appears. Diagnosis is usually clinical, by identifying Koplik's spots or the rash. Drug rashes often resemble the measles rash but can usually be distinguished by the absence of other symptoms.

Prevention - Vaccine provides long-lasting immunity. The vaccine produces a mild non-infectious infection. Fever greater than 38° C occurs 5 to 12 days after inoculation in less than 5% of vaccines and can be followed by a rash. In the past there was a 3 week quarantine period for those who had come into contact with the disease.

Symptoms - Measles begins after a 7 to 14 day incubation period usually starting with coryza, sneezing and a thin nasal discharge, hacking cough, moderate fever commonly about 102 degrees which rises to its maximum at the onset of the rash, furred tongue and conjunctivitis often with photophobia. Latter the face becomes puffy and the eye symptoms become worse. The rash appears 3 to 5 days after symptom onset, usually 1 to 2 days after Koplik's spots appear (minute white spots surrounded by a red areolae on buccal mucous membrane most commonly at level of lower second molar or milk molars) in the mouth. The rash begins earliest on the temples, on forehead at the margin of the hair and behind the ears. The rash spreads rapidly in some cases a few hours over the face, trunk and finally the limbs. In the early stage the rash begins as small brownish macules that disappear under pressure, latter they become papular and fuse. Within 24 to 48 hours, the lesions have spread to the trunk and extremities, including the palms and soles, as they begin to fade on the face. Petechiae or ecchymoses may occur with severe rashes. During the severest part of the disease the temperature may exceed 104 degrees, with conjunctivitis, photophobia, a hacking cough, extensive rash, prostration, and mild itching. In 3 to 5 days, the fever falls, the patient feels more comfortable, and the rash fades rapidly, leaving a coppery brown discoloration followed by desquamation.

Bacterial complications include pneumonia, otitis media, and encephalitis and can sometimes be shown by the fever resuming again. Encephalitis occurs in about 1 in a 1000 cases, usually 2 days to 1 week after onset of the rash often beginning with high fever, headache, seizures, and coma. Encephalitis may resolve in about 1 week or may persist longer, causing morbidity or death.

Prognosis - Mortality is low in western countries but much higher in the developing world. Poor nutrition and vitamin A deficiency may predispose to mortality. Vitamin A supplementation is recommended in populations at risk. In the past TB used to be a common sequel.

Treatment - Treatment is supportive, including for encephalitis. Vitamin A reduces mortality in malnourished children but is not needed in others. Cod Liver Oil was given in the past for deficiencies of Vitamin A. Keep in bed in a darkened room so as to help with the photophobia till temperature is normal and take special care of the cough.

Herbal Treatment

Follow the directions given in The Acute Treatment Of Disease. If this has been done hopefully there will be no complications. In this disease try to treat all the symptoms as best as you can and keep an eye out for unexpected changes as we do not want any complications. For the fever think of Diaphoretic herbs such as Catnip, Yarrow and Linden. Alleviation of itching can be achieved by the use of the Anti-pruritic herbs with Chickweed being one of the best in a cream or lotion. Eyebright is the herb to think of for the eye problems and its strong Astringent Action will help with the watery eyes and runny nose. A compress of Chamomile and Eyebright Lotion 1 to 10 parts water over the eyes will help also. Other herbs to think of are Pasque Flower, Lemon Balm, Lemongrass and Golden Seal can help with the itching and burning skin, Pleurisy Root, Peppermint, Valerian when they are restless or can't sleep, Grindelia, Elder, Catnip and Calendula as a lotion to the spots so as to prevent any secondary infections, you could even mix it with Chickweed so as to relieve the itching.

Homoeopathic Treatment

Also think of Apis and Pulsatillia.

Acconite 6C to 30C - Aconite is one of the first remedies for measles; that is, while the case is presumed to be one of measles, and a hard croupy cough are present. Ferrum phosphoricum in many respects is similar to Aconite, and will take its place where restlessness and anxiety are wanting. It is somewhat questionable whether Aconite will ever be strictly indicated in any disease depending on a poisoned or infected condition of the blood, since in its pathogenesis it does not show any evidence of such condition; however, it may be indicated in the catarrhal irritation, sneezing, etc., before the case can be fully determined to be measles. In catarrhal conditions Aconite ceases to be of use after exudation has taken place, and so in measles; it would cease to be of use after it modified the fever, and the eruption appears and the disease is diagnosed as measles. Ferrum phosphoricum will perhaps be the better remedy if there be chest involvement together with the catarrhal symptoms.

Gelssemium 6C to 30C - Gelsemium is, on the whole, a more useful remedy in commencing measles than Aconite; that is, it is oftener indicated; there is much chilliness, the fever is a prominent symptoms, the child is dumpish, apathetic, does not want to be disturbed; there is watery coryza which excoriates the upper lip and nose, and there is harsh, barking, croupy cough, with chest soreness and hoarseness. Gelsemium, too, has an action on the skin and may be continued with benefit after the eruption has appeared; there is an itching and redness of the skin, and a decidedly measly eruption produced by it. It has some aching in the limbs, and may be compared with Dulcamara, but seldom be mistaken for that remedy. Gelsemium has more coryza, Dulcamara more aching. Both may be useful in an undeveloped eruption; Gelsemium when there is pain at the base of the brain, high fever and passive brain symptoms; Dulcamara when occurring from damp, cool air, rainy weather or sudden changes. Belladonna may be indicated in measles when sore throat is present and the cerebral excitement indicating that remedy, together with moisture and heat; but it corresponds more closely to scarlet fever.

Euphrasia 6C to 30C - When the catarrhal symptoms greatly predominate Euphrasia may be used. Acrid tears stream out of the eyes, with a red and swollen conjunctiva. The cough is dry and very hoarse, and there is an intense throbbing headache which is relieved on the appearance of the eruption. The excoriating discharge from the eyes will distinguish from Allium cepa. The photophobia of Euphrasia is worse in artificial light , and a brightness of the eyes despite the catarrhal condition is characteristic.

Pulsatillia 6C to 30C - A little later in the disease Pulsatilla symptoms may make their appearance. The fever has subsided or entirely disappeared. There is coryza and profuse lachrymation. The cough is still dry at night, but loosens a little in the daytime. The child sits up to cough. There is much predisposition to earache and sometimes sickness at the stomach. Where there is catarrh of the digestive canal and diarrhoea Pulsatilla will be found useful. The eyes agglutinate and the discharge is purulent. Kali bichromicum is so similar to Pulsatilla in many respects that it may be mentioned here, as the two remedies seem to differ in intensity only. Kali bichromicum has pustules developing on the cornea. The throat is swollen and there is catarrhal deafness. It produces an eruption which closely resembles measles. It comes in very well after Pulsatilla when the patient develops more intense symptoms. Measles associated with ear symptoms and swollen glands especially call for Kali bichromicum, and it is one of our best remedies for laryngeal affections, with a hoarse, dry, croupy cough. Dr. Jousset recommends Viola odorata for the cough. Sulphur is a great measles remedy. It is useful where the skin is dusky and the rash does not come out, or is purplish when it does appear.

Arsnicum 6C to 30C - In measles which do not run a favourable course, in malignant type or black or haemorrhagic measles we have two or three important remedies. The first of these is Arsenicum. There will be sinking of strength, diarrhoea, delirium, restlessness and debility, petechiae and general typhoid symptoms. The stools are particularly offensive and exhausting. Arsenicum may save the patient in these conditions. Dr. Gaudy, of Brussels, considers Arsenicum almost specific in measles. He says that its action is little short a marvellous. It is prophylactic and curative, and one of the best remedies to remove all sequelae of the disease. It corresponds to the insidious phenomena of severe epidemics of measles. Crotalus may also be indicated in the form known as black measles. Also Baptisia, with its foetor and prostration, may prove useful. Lachesis is the fourth remedy for these conditions. The individual symptom of each remedy will differentiate them, but all four should be studied carefully in these low conditions of measles.

Stramonium 6C to 30C - When the eruption does not come out properly, or when it disappears suddenly and grave symptoms appear, there are a few remedies which play a most important role. Stramonium is one of these. In a case calling for it you will find these symptoms: non-appearance of the rash; the child is hot, restless, and on falling asleep cries out as if frightened ; there are convulsive movements and the face is red. Cuprum is indicated in convulsion due to recession of the eruption. It has the same terror on awakening, but its symptoms are more violent than those of Stramonium and the face instead of being red is more apt to be bluish. Zincum has the same awakening from sleep as if terrified, but with Zincum there is much weakness, the child seems too weak to develop the eruption. Too slow development of the eruption with chest symptoms calls for it. Ant Tart is another remedy for retarded or repelled eruption. There will be great difficulty in breathing, rattling of mucus, bluish or purplish face, drowsiness and twitching.

Bryonia 6C to 30C - This remedy comes in well when the rash appears late, or runs an irregular course, and when inflammatory diseases of the chest accompany. The cough is dry and painful, there is soreness of the limbs and body, stitches in the chest, etc. Spasms from suppressed measles when the child is seized with great lassitude and debility, twitching of muscles or of single limbs or if the spasms are preceded by deep and violent coughing and oppressed respiration. For the chest complications a number of remedies may come into use. Sticta, if there be present an incessant dry and spasmodic cough, worse when lying down and a night ; it is a teasing, titillating cough. Phosphorus with its dry, exhausting cough with oppressed breathing. Rumex with its short tickling bronchial cough worse from cold air. Drosera with its whooping-like cough. All these may be indicated in measles. Sabadilla is the remedy when among the catarrhal symptoms there is violent sneezing attended with a frontal headache. It will corresponds to some epidemics and should not be overlooked.

Chickenpox

Cause - Chickenpox is an acute, systemic, usually childhood infection caused by the varicella-zoster virus. It usually begins with mild constitutional symptoms that are followed shortly by skin lesions appearing in crops and characterized by macules, papules, vesicles, and crusting. Chickenpox, which is extremely contagious and spread by infected droplets and is most infectious during the onset and early stages of the eruption. It is communicable from 48 hours before the first skin lesions appear until the final lesions have crusted. ☐Epidemics occur in winter and early spring in 3 to 4 year cycles. Some infants may have partial immunity, probably acquired from the womb, until aged 6 months. Infection provides lifelong protection.

Diagnosis - Chickenpox is suspected in patients with the characteristic rash, which is usually the basis for diagnosis. The eruption is characterized by appearing in successive crops. The temperature does not fall with the appearance of the rash. The rash may be confused with that of other viral skin infections.

Prevention - Vaccination provides effective prevention.

Symptoms - ☐Mild headache, moderate fever, and malaise may occur 11 to 15 days after exposure, about 24 to 36 hours before lesions appear. This onset is more likely in patients less than 10 years and is usually more severe in adults. The initial rash, a macular eruption which may be accompanied by an evanescent flush. Within a few hours lesions progress to papules and then vesicles, often intensely itchy, on red bases. Lesions initially develop on the face and trunk and erupt in successive crops; some macules appear just as earlier crops begin to crust. The eruption may be generalized (in severe cases) or more limited but almost always involves the upper trunk. Ulcerated lesions may develop on the mucous membranes in different parts of the body. In the mouth, vesicles rupture immediately and often cause pain on swallowing. Scalp lesions may produce tender, enlarged cervical lymph nodes. New lesions usually cease to appear by the 5th day and the majority are crusted by the 6th day, most crusts disappear in less than 20 days after onset. Pneumonia may complicate severe chickenpox in adults, newborns, and immune compromised patients of all ages but usually not in healthy young children. Myocarditis, transient arthritis or hepatitis, and hemorrhagic complications may also occur.

Prognosis - Chickenpox in childhood is rarely severe. Severe or fatal disease is more likely in adults, patients with depressed T-cell immunity and those receiving corticosteroids or chemotherapy. Those at risk of severe complications should receive postexposure prophylaxis with immune globulins, and, if disease develops, treatment with antiviral drugs.

Treatment - Mild cases require only symptomatic treatment. Relief of itching and prevention of scratching which may cause secondary bacterial infection may be difficult. Wet compresses, or, for severe itching, systemic antihistamines and colloidal oatmeal baths may help. To prevent secondary bacterial infection, patients should bathe regularly and keep their underclothing and hands clean and their nails clipped. Antiseptics should not be applied unless lesions become infected; infection is treated with antibiotics.

Herbal Treatment

Follow the directions given in The Acute Treatment Of Disease. If this has been done hopefully there will be no complications. The treatment is very similar to Measles but here we will make our main herb St Johns Wort for that is the specific herb for the Shingles virus which is a direct relation to the Chickenpox virus and its Action as a Nervine Antiviral is the best way to go. Some different herbs from measles to use are Burdock which is used for the fever and the eruption and can even be put on the eruption as a lotion. A very effective treatment for itching, that may avoid the complications of a secondary infections caused by scratching is Rosemary and Calendula Lotion mixed half and half in 1 to 10 parts water maybe soaked into a cloth to cover a large area and don't forget about Chickweed which is our main herb for itching use as a cream or lotion.

Homoeopathic Treatment

Antimonium Tartaricum 6C to 30C - Rattling of mucus with little expectoration, There is much drowsiness, debility and sweat, Thirst for cold water, little and often, and desire for apples, fruits, and acids generally. Pustular eruption, leaving a bluish-red mark. Great drowsiness. Worse, in evening; from lying down at night; from warmth; in damp cold weather; from all sour things and milk. Better, from sitting erect; from eructation and expectoration.

Belladonna 6c to 30C - has a marked action on the vascular system, skin and glands. Belladonna always is associated with hot, red skin, flushed face, glaring eyes, throbbing carotids, excited mental state, Heat, redness, throbbing and burning. Great children's remedy. No thirst with fever. Skin dry and hot; swollen, sensitive; burns scarlet, pustules on face. Worse, touch, jar, noise, draught, after noon, lying down. Better, semi-erect.

Ferrum Phos 6C to 12C - The remedy for first stage of all febrile disturbances and inflammations before exudation sets in; especially for catarrhal affections of the respiratory tract.

Kali Mur 6C to 12C - Should be taken as soon as the eruptions appear to help diminish scaring. May help to prevent the infection.

Mercurius Sol 6c to 30C - Where there is thick yellow discharges, offensive perspiration, odorous breath, and the patient is overly sensitive to heat and cold temperatures. In general the patient appears quite sick. Vesicular and pustular eruptions with itching worse from warmth of bed. All Mercury symptoms are worse at night.

Pulsatillia 6c to 30C - . It is pre-eminently a female remedy, especially for mild, gentle, yielding disposition. Sad, crying readily; weeps when talking; changeable, contradictory. The patient seeks the open air; always feels better there, even though he is chilly. Discharges thick, bland, and yellowish-green. Symptoms ever changing. Thirstless, peevish, and chilly. The fever has Chilliness, even in warm room and is without thirst. Worse, from heat, rich fat food, after eating, towards evening, warm room, lying on left or on painless side when allowing feet to hang down. Better, open air, motion, cold applications, cold food and drinks, though not thirsty.

Rhus Tox 6C to 30C - This is the most frequently indicated remedy. Great restlessness of mind and body. Warm bathing relieves itching. Worse, during sleep, cold, wet rainy weather and after rain; at night, during rest, drenching, when lying on back or right side. Better, warm, dry weather, motion; walking, change of position, rubbing, warm applications, from stretching out limbs.

Smallpox

Cause - Smallpox is a highly contagious disease caused by the smallpox virus, an orthopoxvirus. It causes death in up to 30%. The main concern for outbreaks is from bioterrorism. No cases of smallpox have occurred in the world since 1977, due to worldwide vaccination. In 1980, the World Health Organization (WHO) recommended discontinuation of routine smallpox vaccination. Because humans are the only natural host of the smallpox virus and because the virus cannot survive more than 2 days in the environment, WHO has declared natural infection eradicated.

Because immunity declines over time, nearly all people even those previously vaccinated are now susceptible to smallpox. Smallpox is transmitted person to person by direct contact or inhalation and contaminated clothing or bed linens can also transmit infection. The infection is most contagious for the first 7 to 10 days after the rash appears. Once crusts form on the skin lesions infectivity declines.

The attack rate is as high as 85% in unvaccinated people, and infection may lead to as many as 10 to 20 secondary cases from each primary case.

Disease Process - The virus invades the respiratory mucosa and multiplies in regional lymph nodes. It eventually localizes in small blood vessels of the dermis and the oropharyngeal mucosa. Other organs are seldom clinically involved, except for occasionally the CNS, with encephalitis. Skin lesions may develop secondary bacterial infection. It prevails more extensively in the winter months, declining in the spring and as the summer approaches. It prevails in the crowded regions of large cities. The severity of the attack in an individual patient does not depend so much upon the virulence of the infection, as upon the susceptibility of the individual. A typical case, however mild, may convey the disease at its worst.

Diagnosis - Diagnosis is confirmed by electron microscopy or viral culture of material scraped from skin lesions. It is only in the early stages of this disease that the diagnosis presents any difficulties. The presence of an epidemic, and the fact that the patient has been exposed, will suggest the possibility of the occurrence of this disease. The sudden onset, with severe illness from the first, the extreme backache and headache are characteristic. The absence of any soreness of the throat will exclude the probability of scarlet fever or diphtheria, as will also the absence of the peculiar abrupt vomiting, which is present at the onset of scarlet fever. In chicken pox the constitutional symptoms are very mild, and in impetigo the development of the disease begins with the appearance of single blebs or blisters which have none of the peculiarities of the developing smallpox pustule.

Prevention - Prevention involves vaccination, which, because of its risks, is performed selectively. Isolation of people with smallpox is essential. In limited outbreaks, patients may be isolated in a hospital in negative-pressure rooms equipped with high-efficiency particulate filters. In mass outbreaks home isolation may be required. Contacts should be placed under surveillance, typically with daily temperature measurement, and isolated at home for temperature less than 38° C or other sign of illness. The vitality of the virus remains for a long time after the death of the patient, and the bedding and furniture of a room will convey the disease for many days, unless thoroughly disinfected.

Symptoms - Variola major has a 10 to 12 day incubation period (range 7 to 17 days), followed by a 2 to 3 day prodrome of fever, headache, backache, and extreme malaise. Sometimes severe abdominal pain and vomiting occur. Following the prodrome, a maculopapular rash develops on the oropharyngeal mucosa, face, and arms, spreading shortly thereafter to the trunk and legs. The oropharyngeal lesions quickly ulcerate. After 1 or 2 days the cutaneous lesions become vesicular then pustular. Pustules are denser on the face and extremities than on the trunk and they may appear on the palms. The pustules are round tense and appear deeply embedded. The skin lesions of smallpox unlike those of chickenpox, are all at the same stage of development on a given body part. After 8 or 9 days the pustules become crusted. Severe residual scarring is typical. Mortality is about 30% due to a massive inflammatory response causing shock and multiple organ failure, and usually occurs in the second week of illness.

Variola minor results in symptoms that are similar but much less severe, with a less extensive rash. Mortality is less than 1%. About 10% of people with smallpox develop either a hemorrhagic or malignant variant. The hemorrhagic form is rarer and has a shorter, more intense prodrome followed by generalized erythema and cutaneous and mucosal hemorrhage. It is uniformly fatal within 5 or 6 days. The malignant form has a similar, severe prodrome, followed by development of confluent, flat, nonpustular skin lesions. In the rare survivors, the epidermis frequently peels.

Typical Symptoms From Herbalist Finley Ellingwood, M.D. 1910

Symptomatology:—From six to twelve days after exposure to the infection the first symptoms appear. The premonitory symptoms are a most severe **backache**, general **malaise**, extreme **muscular soreness** and an excruciating **headache**, usually frontal. Almost simultaneously with the occurrence of these symptoms is a severe **rigor** and the rapid development of a **high temperature**. The pulse becomes decidedly rapid, the respirations are increased and the patient has all the evidences of severe illness.

Other symptoms are **nausea, vomiting, loss of appetite** and usually obstinate **constipation**, although in a few cases an intractable **diarrhea** has appeared. The pulse at the onset is rapid, but it is usually full and strong until the eruption appears. The **temperature** at the onset may reach 105° F. within the first twenty-four hours, and perhaps 106° F. at the end of forty-eight hours. This high temperature is maintained with but little variation, until the **eruption** appears. At this point there is a rapid reduction of the temperature to perhaps 99° F. or perhaps 99.5° F., where it will remain until the pustular stage of the eruption occurs, when it will rise abruptly from 102.5° F. to 104° F. This is called the **secondary fever**. It has regular morning remissions, and if the disease progresses favorably it will ultimately end by lysis on the twelfth or fourteenth day. In some cases this secondary fever may be so mild as to be overlooked.

This disease is properly classified by the character of the eruption, into three distinct forms, the commonest of which, the discrete form, presents the symptoms which we have just given. The other forms are the confluent form, and the hemorrhagic form, known as black smallpox, or malignant smallpox.

In the **discrete form** of the disease, the eruption appears about the third day, in the form of coarse red spots, usually upon the forehead first, and at the edge of the scalp, and on the wrists. The macular appearance of the eruption soon develops into a distinct papule, somewhat elevated and hard upon pressure and conveying to the finger an indurated feeling, as if a single small shot was just beneath the skin. After perhaps twenty-four hours a tiny vesicle appears at the seat of the induration, which increases in size to the fifth day, when it is about the sixth or the fourth of an inch in diameter and contains a peculiar lactescent fluid. The vesicle does not collapse upon the escape of the fluid, and is surrounded by a distinct, narrow, bright red areola. The center of the vesicle becomes depressed, and by the sixth day it assumes the characteristic umbili-cated form. The fluid may become cloudy or purulent until, by the seventh or eighth day, it is distinctly pustular. The pus dries upon the surface of the eruption and forms a distinct scab, which is supposed to contain the characteristic infection of the disease.

There is a characteristic door from the pustule of smallpox which to those who are familiar with it, becomes diagnostic.

In the **confluent form** of this disease the symptoms at the onset are apt to be more severe and the eruption appears earlier, the papules are much more abundant, the bases approximate each other more immediately, and by the time the pustule has developed, the entire surface of the skin is covered with a suppurating eruption. So severe an involvement of the entire surface of the body produces most serious impressions. The nervous system becomes involved, the lymphatics are swollen with the inflamed condition of the skin, and symptoms of general pyemia, with extreme typhoid phenomena, will develop.

In the form known as **black smallpox** a change takes place in the character of the blood. Its coagulability is impaired and hemorrhages take place into the skin, the mucous membrane and the viscera. In the more benign form, hemorrhage occurs into the pustule only, especially in those of the lower extremities. In the more dangerous form, the hemorrhages occur from the eruption, and from various points on the mucous surface, and into the various organs of the body. When a distinct hemorrhagic diathesis develops, the blood becomes diffused beneath the skin also, and there are extensive ecchymoses. These may appear before the characteristic eruption shows itself; nose bleed, bleeding from the gums, bleeding from beneath the conjunctiva, from the palate or tongue, is common, as well as bloody vomit, bloody stools and hematuria. These cases are nearly all fatal.

A rash appears in some cases of smallpox, which may be general over the entire surface of the body, and mislead the physician in his diagnosis. In some cases it closely resembles the initial rash of scarlet fever, in others it is similar to that of measles. As these rashes disappear quickly on the development of the smallpox eruption they should not deceive the physician, if he is a close observer.

Prognosis - Causes death in up to 30%.

Treatment - Treatment is generally supportive, with antibiotics for the occasional secondary bacterial infection. Antivirals have never been used clinically. **The Following Is From Herbalist Finley Ellingwood, M.D. 1910** (I left the alcohol bit in, who am I to judge) The first and essential course to adopt with all patients, when known to have been exposed, or when the disease is anticipated, and it is not known that the patient has been exposed, is to have the patient immediately **vaccinated**, as this invariably modifies the course of the disease, if it does not prevent it. The patient must be **isolated**. This cannot be successfully done except in a well-equipped smallpox hospital, although in localities where the disease is not generally prevalent a small detached house can be secured and temporarily equipped to accommodate one or more patients. Good ventilation is important in the sick room, with the very best of nursing. Everything should be removed from the room, except the essential furniture, the patient should be allowed to drink **water** freely, and iced milk or **buttermilk**, with **lemonade** or **fruit jellies** dissolved in water, may be administered *ad libitum*. The administration of alcoholic beverages in regular small doses is essential during the period of the remission of the fever, and at any time when there seems to be a failure of the vital forces. (Alcohol in small doses is a stimulant)

Herbal Treatment

Follow the directions given in The Acute Treatment Of Disease. If this has been done hopefully there will be no complications and you really don't want complications with this one. Echinacea is the main specific for this disease throughout the whole disease and a lotion of it can be used with good results on the spots. Ellingwood says It stimulates the capillary circulation, promotes free elimination, antagonizes septic development of whatever character, inhibits to a marked degree the formation of pus, prevents gangrene and stimulates the skin in such a manner that the eruption is very mild, and in some cases the pustule heals with but little if any pock. Ellingwood also uses Bearberry with the Echinacea giving doses every 2 hours. Baptisia is our next main remedy not just for the fever but for its focus on the lymphatic system especially the glands. Along with this consider small doses of Poke Root to add to the work on the Lymphatic system. Think of Boneset for the fever and the aches and pains that come with the disease. Black Cohosh has been used in this disease for the extreme muscular and bone pains, and persistent aching in the muscles. The herb is a Alterative, Antispasmodic and Sedative and is good for nerve pains and should be considered along with Boneset. Ellingwood also says about this disease that the kidneys must not be over stimulated, and experience has proven that cathartics are worse than useless. Which is why he probably uses Poke Root instead of Cleavers. About using Echinacea as a lotion Ellingwood says. It may be used twice or three times daily with which to sponge the surface. A ten per cent solution is about the proper strength in mild cases. Where ecchymosis or gangrene are threatened it should be occasionally applied in full strength, over small areas, although there can be no objection to so applying it to the entire body. Regarding the spots we can use the treatment given in Measles and Chickenpox and to them we will add Lemon juice which helps to relieve the itching, dilute by half and treat just a small part of the body to determine the results and take it from there. Golden seal mixed with Vaseline and applied to the pitting is meant to prevent scaring as well as helping with the itching. Scaring is why I would use Calendula. Antivirals, Anti Inflammatories and Diaphoretic are three of the main Actions to keep under consideration in the treatment of this disease. I would keep in mind Lemongrass, Lemon Balm and Peppermint tea for its Antiviral and Fever Actions and would also consider St Johns Wort especially if the disease traveled to the nervous system or there were pains shooting along the nerve path ways which is one of the leading signs calling for this remedy but we mainly want it for its antiviral Action. We need Diaphoretics because we want the toxin to leave the body by the skin which is what the body is trying to do anyway so we will work with the body not against it. Use Licorice not only for pushing our formula into the body but also for its strong Anti-inflammatory Action I would also consider using high doses of vitamin C throughout the disease to try to tone down the inflammatory response.

Homoeopathic Treatment

Homoeopaths make what are called Disease Nosodes which are made from potentized disease products. Below is the Smallpox Nosode taken in a direct copy from Boerickes Materia Medica. As you can see this was made from the lymph fluid of a smallpox pustule. If one day you find yourself in an extremely bad position of having to cope with a disease outbreak a Nosode could save the day for you as well as your community and they are very easy to make.

VARIOLINUM
Lymph from Small-pox Pustule

Used for "internal vaccination." Seems to be efficacious in protecting against, modifying and aiding in the cure of smallpox.

Head - Morbid fear of small-pox. Deafness. Pain in occiput. Inflamed eyelids.

Respiratory - Oppressed breathing. Throat feels closed. Cough with thick viscid, bloody mucus. Feeling of a lump in right side of throat.

Relationship - *Excruciating backache. Aching in legs.* Tired all over with restlessness. Wrists pain. Pains shift from back to abdomen.

Fever - Hot fever, with intense radiating heat. Profuse, bad-smelling sweat.

Skin - Hot, dry. Eruption of pustules. *Shingles*.

Relationship - Compare: Vaccin (same action); *Malandrinum*--the morbid product of the grease of the horse (a prophylactic of small-pox and a remedy for the ill-effects of vaccination; chronic eczema following vaccination).

Dose - Sixth to thirtieth potency.

Aconite 6C to 30C - Sudden rise of temperature with high fever, thirst and restlessness are the chief indications for Aconite. Many confess to disappointment in the use of this remedy, and prefer Gelsemium in the initial stage, and indeed its pathogenesis more often corresponds to the trouble than that of Aconite. The aching in the back and limbs and the tight band headache of the disease are found under Gelsemium, and if dullness and apathy be present it is all the more indicated. Belladonna suits the congestive type, with the severe headache, backache and purplish face, a type often seen in young children. Hughes agrees with Baehr that Belladonna is more homoeopathic to the initial fever than Aconite. Veratrum viride may be called for in cases where the head is hot, and the extremities are cool and cyanotic; backache, fever and perspiration.

Bryonia 6C to 30C - Is also a first stage remedy; it has nausea, vomiting, severe headache, high temperature. The eruption is slow in coming to the surface and all the symptoms are worse by motion. It suits especially negroes. Cimicifuga, according to one observer, serves well in the intense backache and rheumatic pains. The body feels sore; the bed feels hard, the muscles feeling as though they had been pounded. Rhus has similar symptoms, restlessness, headache, and it is a useful remedy at the commencement of vesication, when the vesicles are small, and also when the pustules turn black from effusion therein, and diarrhea and dark bloody stools accompany. Much itching and swelling will call for Apis.

Antimonium Tartaricum 6C to 30C - Is a nearer simillimum to smallpox than any other remedy in the Materia Medica. Rokitansky proved the similarity of the smallpox pustule to those produced by Tartar emetic. Hughes recognizes it almost as a routine agent. With this remedy vesication and pustulation are marked. The mucous membranes are involved and bronchitis or broncho-pnuemonia is apt to be present, with the characteristic cough and expectoration symptoms. There are excruciating pains in the loins. It is especially adaptable to cases characterized by gastric irritation. It exercises a real abortive control over the variolous process and frequently covers the case from first to last.

Thuja 6C to 30C - Boenninghausen employed this remedy with success and believed it to be the best curative and preventive agent in smallpox. It suits especially the eruptive stage, with milky, flat, painful pustules upon a dark inflamed area. The pustulation is offensive. The remedy suits especially strumous and sycotic children. Hartmann recommended Sulphur as a preventive and curative. It belongs not only to the suppurative stage, but also to metastatic brain symptoms. Dr. Garth Wilkinson considered Hydrastis as much of a specific in variola as Belladonna is in scarlet fever. Variolinum 30th has been lauded by some observers as being especially useful at the stage where the vesicles change into pustules. Dr. Bishop, of Los Angeles, believes this remedy all sufficient in all cases. It quickly removes all dangerous symptoms, dries up the vesicles and prevents all scars. Dr. Zopfy mentions only Variolinum and Hepar in the disease. Arndt recommends it in the 6X and 12X triturations. Vaccinum 30 has been extensively used and with much benefit.

Arsenicum 6C to 30C - In unfavorable and hemorrhagic cases where there is much weakness, a burning heat, restlessness and irregularly developed eruption, the pustules become flat, livid, dusky and haemorrhagic, Arsenicum may be the remedy. Diarrhea is an attendant symptom. This, together with other Arsenicum symptoms, will make the choice easy. Lachesis, Crotalus and Baptisia will also be remedies to suggest themselves by typhoid and hemorrhagic symptoms. Dr. E. Williams reports of its favorable action in an epidemic occurring in England in 1872.

Hamamelis will also be found serviceable at times in the hemorrhagic variety. Anacardium. An eruption similar to variola is produced by Anacardium, and it often becomes useful in loss of memory as a sequel of smallpox. Sarracenia purpurea has also achieved considerable reputation in the treatment of smallpox.

Diphtheria

Cause - Diphtheria is an acute pharyngeal infection by Corynebacterium diphtheriae, some strains of which produce an exotoxin. Humans are the only known reservoir for C. diphtheriae. The organism is spread by respiratory droplets, direct contact with secretions or skin lesions. This is an acute infectious disorder, characterized by great prostration, a serious throat inflammation with an exudation and the formation of a false membrane.

Disease Process - Corynebacterium diphtheriae usually infects the nasopharynx (respiratory diphtheria) or skin. Diphtheria strains infected by a β-phage, which carries a toxin-encoding gene, produce a potent toxin. This toxin first causes inflammation and then necrosis of local tissues then damages the heart, nerves, and kidneys.

Diagnosis - Diagnosis is confirmed by culture. The appearance of the membrane confirms the diagnosis. Cutaneous diphtheria should be considered when a patient develops skin lesions during an outbreak of respiratory diphtheria. Swab or biopsy specimens should be cultured.

Prevention - Vaccination is the main preventative. During outbreaks poor personal and community hygiene contribute to the spread of cutaneous diphtheria.

Symptoms - Symptoms are either nonspecific skin infections or pharyngitis followed by myocardial and nerve tissue damage secondary to the toxin. Symptoms vary depending on infection site and whether toxin is produced. Most respiratory infections are caused by toxin-producing strains. Most cutaneous infections are caused by non–toxin-producing strains. Toxin is poorly absorbed from the skin; thus toxin complications are rare in cutaneous diphtheria.

Following an incubation period, which averages 2 to 4 days, and a prodromal period between 12 and 24 hours the patient develops mild sore throat, low-grade fever, and tachycardia. Nausea, emesis, chills, headache, and fever are more common in children. If a toxigenic strain is involved, the characteristic membrane appears in the tonsillar area. It may initially appear as a white, glossy exudate, but typically becomes dirty gray, tough, fibrinous, and adherent so that removal causes bleeding. Local edema may produce a visibly swollen neck (bull neck), hoarseness, stridor, and dyspnea. The membrane may extend to the larynx, trachea, and bronchi and may partially obstruct the airway or suddenly detach, causing complete obstruction. Skin lesions generally occur on the extremities and are varied in appearance, often indistinguishable from chronic skin conditions (eg, eczema, psoriasis, impetigo). In a few cases, it produces punched-out ulcers, occasionally with a grayish membrane. Pain, tenderness, erythema, and exudate are typical. If toxin is produced, lesions may be numb. Concomitant nasopharyngeal infection occurs in 20 to 40% of cases. Myocarditis is usually evident by the 10th to 14th day but can appear any time during the 1st to 6th week. Heart failure may develop.

Nervous system involvement usually begins in the 1st week of illness with bulbar palsy, causing dysphagia and nasal regurgitation. Peripheral neuropathy appears from the 3rd to 6th week It is both motor and sensory, although motor symptoms predominate. Resolution occurs over many weeks.

The Following Is From Herbalist Finley Ellingwood, M.D. 1910

The throat is at once complained of, with the chill. The fever rises quite rapidly, soon reaching 103° F. It has not the sudden high rise of some of the other infectious diseases, as the infection is progressive in its development. There is a wide difference in different cases, some are most violent at the onset, developing the entire train of classic symptoms within six hours, while in others mild symptoms may prevail for two or three days. A single small patch first appears, usually upon one tonsil. It is shaped like a grain of wheat and is grayish and sunken, with a narrow bright red areola of inflamed tissue. It sometimes forms on the back surface of an enlarged tonsil, or between the tonsil and the fauces. This patch rapidly increases in size, and the characteristic fetor of the breath appears. It assumes more of a dirty gray color and quickly spreads, involving both tonsils and the fauces. The edges are ragged and the approximate tissues are intensely red and angry in appearance.

With development of the membrane on the tonsils or upon the pharyngeal walls, the glands in the neck at the angle of the jaw become enlarged and often tender. This is not common in tonsilitis, nor in the non-specific forms of sore throat.

The symptoms of constitutional involvement increase as the toxins are absorbed. This occurs more or less rapidly, according to the severity of the infection. The temperature increases, the pulse becomes rapid, and perhaps irregular, and prostration occurs and increases rapidly. While the patient is usually dull, with perhaps a mild delirium, restlessness is almost invariably present, with signs of distress and general discomfort, the patient appearing severely ill. Convulsions seldom appear.

A rash is sometimes present in diphtheria, so closely resembling that of scarlet fever as to render a symptomatic diagnosis difficult. I have seen this rash exfoliate similarly to that of scarlet fever. Purpura and cyanosis appear in malignant cases. (I put Ellingwoods symptoms here because I wanted you to have a better description of the membrane and see the disease through his eyes)

Prognosis - Without specific treatment, the mortality of this disease is very high. The use of antitoxin has greatly reduced the mortality of this disease.

Treatment - Treatment is with antitoxin and penicillin or erythromycin. Childhood vaccination should be routine. Symptomatic patients should be hospitalized in ICUs to monitor for respiratory and cardiac complications. Isolation with respiratory and contact precautions is required and must continue until 2 cultures, taken 24 and 48 hours after antibiotics are stopped, are negative. Diphtheria antitoxin must be given without waiting for culture confirmation, because the antitoxin neutralizes only toxin not yet bound to cells. The use of antitoxin for cutaneous disease, without evidence of respiratory disease, is of questionable value because toxic squeal have rarely been reported, but some experts recommend it. Antibiotics are required to eradicate the organism and prevent spread; they are not substitutes for antitoxin.

Herbal Treatment

Follow the directions given in The Acute Treatment Of Disease. If this has been done hopefully there will be no complications and you really don't want complications with this one as it is not a very nice way to die at all. The Acute Treatment Of Disease mentioned gargling with Tea Tree oil, well for this condition we are going to add Poke Root to the gargle as it has a affinity to the tonsils while being a very strong Lymphatic herb with a Alterative Action. I would consider gargling every 2 hours and even increasing it to every 30 minutes if I started getting scared. Poke Root is also the specific for internal treatment along with Echinacea and Elecampane which has the Actions of Antibacterial, Alterative, Antitussive, Antiseptic and Astringent with its main use to inhibit the production of phlegm. Baptisia is another important herb that could be used along with Goldenrod which has a affinity for the throat and is Anti catarrhal, Anti Inflammatory and Antiseptic. Other throat herbs are Sage and Thyme. If there is breathing difficulties think of Eucalyptus as it is a strong Bronchodilator, put some oil and water in a humidifier or make your own steamer. Pine oil can also be added. If you start getting Heart Problems add Hawthorn to the formula. If bleeding problems happen use Witch Hazel which is a strong Astringent that is good for stopping bleeding. Golden Seal can be used on the start of recovery. Use lots of Vitamin C to try to detox the toxin and to reduce inflammation. For this condition you really need to lay on the Antibacterials as you really need to kill the infection before the toxin is produced. Other herbs to think of are Myrrh, Hyssop and Bayberry which can also be used as a gargle.

Homoeopathic Treatment

DIPHTHERINUM

Potentized Nosode

Adapted to patients prone to catarrhal affections of respiratory organs, scrofulous individuals. Diphtheria, laryngeal diphtheria, *post-diphtheritic paralysis*. Malignancy from the start. Glands swollen; tongue red, swollen; breath and discharge very offensive. Diphtheritic; membrane thick, dark. Epistaxis; profound prostration. Swallows without pain, but fluids are vomited or returned by the nose.

Relationship - Compare: *Diphtherotoxin* (Cahis) (Chronic bronchitis with rales. Cartier suggests it in the vago-paralytic forms of Bronchitis of the aged or in toxic bronchitis after grip).

Dose - Thirtieth, two hundredth or C. M potency. Must not be repeated too frequently.

(From Boerickes Materia Medica)

Mercurius Cyanatus 6C to 30C - Thus we have, as indications, great and sudden prostration and very high pulse. The weakness is extreme, collapse symptoms showing themselves even at the commencement of the disease. There is an exudation in the throat; at first it is white, but it may turn dark and threaten to become gangrenous. The tongue is brownish and blackish, with fetid breath, nose bleed, loss of appetite, profuse flow of saliva, etc. It is especially a remedy in the malignant type of diphtheria and when the disease invades the nostrils. The great prostration will serve to distinguish it from Kali bichromicum, which has the thick, tenacious exudation, also found under Mercurius cyanatus. Clinical experience with this remedy has proved that preparations below the 6th are less effective than the higher, and not as safe, since it produces a tendency to heart failure. The 30th potency seems to have been a favorite one. Dr. Villiers, of St. Petersburg, treated 200 cases of all sorts of severity without a single death, using the 6th to 30th potencies. Dr. Neushafer treated 85 cases with three deaths, using the 5th to 15th potencies hypodermically. Dr. Sellden, in 1879-82, reported in a district of Sweden 564 cases of diphtheria, of whom 523 died, a mortality of 92.7 percent. None treated with the cyanide of mercury. In 1883-86, 160 cases were reported, of whom 29 died. In 132 of these 160 cases the cyanide of mercury was used and only one case died. He and his colleagues have treated 1,400 cases with a mortality of 4.9 percent. A strength equal to the 2x was used.--London Lancet, April 24, 1888.

Kali Bich 6c to 30C - This remedy, which is perhaps more useful in the croupoid form of the disease, has marked symptoms. There is apt to be deep ulceration and a thick, tenacious exudation, often streaked with blood; the membrane is yellow looking and the cough is croupy and accompanied with pain in the chest. There is also swelling of the glands.

The indication for Kali bichromicum may be chiefly summarized as follows: 1. The yellow-coated or dry, red tongue. 2. The tough, tenacious exudation. 3. Pain, extending to neck and shoulders. These, and the fact that it is most useful in the later stage of the disease, when the line of demarcation has formed and the slough has commenced to separate, make the indication for the drug certain.

Kali Mur 6c to 30C - The indication for this remedy rest on a clinical basis, and it is one of the legacies of Schuessler to Homoeopathy. That it is a most excellent remedy and deserving of a high place in the treatment of diphtheria cannot be doubted by anyone who has ever tried it. The only indication we have are pain on swallowing, and white deposit in throat; but numerous well-marked cases of the disease have been treated with the remedy and symptoms like prostration, thick exudation over the tonsils, and entire soft palate, fetid breath, etc., have entirely disappeared. Perhaps like Kali bichromicum, it will be found to be better adapted to the croupoid form. Kali chloratum or the chlorate of potash is useful in diphtheria when gangrenous spots appear; ulcers with foul secretions and offensive discharges. It is one of the best remedies to prevent extension to the nasal mucous membrane.

Kali Permanganicum 6C to 30C - This is another of the potashes which has achieved some reputation in diphtheria, where there is ulceration, gangrenous suppuration and fetid odor. The indication for its use are, throat swollen both inside and outside. The throat is oedematous and the membrane is horribly offensive; there is a thin discharge from the nose and a Lachesis difficulty of swallowing and regurgitation. In many respects it resembles Apis, but the extreme fetor will distinguish. Dr. Van Lennep considers it almost a specific.

Apis 6C to 30C - Edema stands first among the indications for this remedy. Stinging pains, and sore, blistered tongue are also characteristic. The throat has a glossy-red appearance as if varnished. Membrane forms on either tonsil and is grayish, dirty-looking and tough. Swallowing is most difficult owing to the oedema. The throat is swollen externally and there is much prostration, dry, hot skin and restlessness. Suppression of the urine is a complication that will call for Apis.

Lachesis 6C to 30C - Lachesis is a wonderfully good remedy in diphtheria. Great sensitiveness of the throat will always bring it into mind. Further indications are the appearance of the disease first on the left side of the throat, spreading to the right. Extremely painful and difficult swallowing, violent prostration and great fetor, the patient sleeping into an aggravation of all symptoms. The dyspnoea is so marked that the patient must sit up to breathe. Gangrenous tendency and specific condition. There is a purplish throat and much swelling and infiltration externally, here resembling Apis. Very similar symptoms are obtained under two other of the snake poisons, namely, Crotalus and Naja. A characteristic symptom of Lachesis is that the throat feels worse from empty swallowing.

Phytolacca 6C to 30C - Pain in the back and limbs, a general aching all over with great prostration are general characteristics of this remedy, and if we get, in addition to these, highly-inflamed throat, which is much swollen, so sore and sensitive that deglutition is almost impossible, pain shooting to ears, thick-coated tongue, fetid breath, swollen glands, high, rapid and weak pulse and a grayish membrane, we have a picture of diphtheria that Phytolacca will cure. Great burning in the throat is also an indication, and chilliness as the disease commences. Drs. Burt and Bayes recommend the tincture and also the use of a gargle. Other observers also consider the remedy as specific, and it probably is with the foregoing indications.

Arsenicum 30C - Last, but not least, we have Arsenicum, and it may save when no remedy will. It is mainly a remedy indicated by its general symptoms alone, such as low fever, prostration, restlessness, thirst, foetid breath, etc., hence it is not a true diphtheria remedy. It is most useful in the later stage of the disease when indicated by these very symptoms, and when, when, perhaps, in spite of other remedies, the patient has been constantly going downhill, until the very adynamic condition, met so well by Arsenicum, has been reached. The throat will be much swollen inside and out, the membrane will be dark, and there will be much fetor, and there will be present considerable edema. It may correspond to the prodromal stage also, with the tired-out feeling, thirst and feverish flush. Arsenic iodide may prove curative for the septic conditions and hoarseness which sometimes remain after diphtheria.

Whooping Cough

Cause - Pertussis is a highly communicable disease occurring mostly in children and teenagers that is caused by the bacteria Bordetella pertussis. Symptoms are initially those of a respiratory infection followed by spasmodic coughing that usually ends in a prolonged, high-pitched, crowing inspiration (the whoop). Pertussis is endemic throughout the world. In a given unimmunised locality, it becomes epidemic. It occurs at all ages, but 71% occurs in children less than 5 years, and 38% of the cases including nearly all deaths, occur in infants less than 6 months old. It is also serious in the elderly. Transmission is airborne from infected patients, particularly in the catarrhal and early paroxysmal stages and causes disease in 90 to 100% of close contacts. Transmission by contact with contaminated articles is rare. Patients usually are not infectious after the 3rd week of the paroxysmal phase.

Disease Process - A specific infectious disease occurring epidemically, and characterized by a peculiar, spasmodic, paroxysmal cough, ending in a whoop. The whoop is caused by the air rushing through the contracted larynx during a prolonged inspiration which follows a paroxysm of coughing, the air in the lung being completely exhausted by the effort. The disease usually attacks children under ten years of age, though no age is exempt. It is also characterized by catarrh of the respiratory tract. The disease begins with a cold and a mild cough. After this, the typical coughing bouts set in. The coughing continues until no air is left in the lungs. The patient will eventually cough up some phlegm and these attacks may well be followed by vomiting. The child's temperature is likely to remain normal. A bout of whooping cough can be very distressing for both the child and the parents who feel unable to help. Coughing attacks may occur up to 40 times a day and the disease can last for up to eight weeks.

Diagnosis - Diagnosis is by nasopharyngeal culture. The diagnosis is readily made after the characteristic whoop develops; before this we may not be positive, although the catarrhal symptoms, hoarseness and spasmodic cough, are suggestive of the trouble.

Prevention - Active immunization is part of standard childhood vaccination. Immunity after natural infection lasts about 20 years.

Symptoms - The incubation period averages 7 to 14 days (maximum 3 weeks). B. pertussis invades respiratory mucosa increasing the secretion of mucus which is initially thin and later viscid and tenacious. Uncomplicated disease lasts about 6 to 10 weeks and consists of 3 stages, catarrhal, paroxysmal, and convalescent.

The catarrhal stage begins insidiously generally with sneezing, lacrimation, or other signs of coryza; anorexia; listlessness; and a troublesome, hacking nocturnal cough that gradually becomes worse. Fever is rare.

After 10 to 14 days, the paroxysmal stage begins with an increase in the severity and frequency of the cough. Repeated bouts of less than 5 rapidly consecutive forceful coughs occur during a single expiration and are followed by the whoop a hurried, deep inspiration. Copious viscid mucus may be expelled or bubble from the nostrils during or after the paroxysms. Vomiting is characteristic. In infants, choking spells (with or without cyanosis) may be more common than whoops.

Prognosis - Mortality is about 1 to 2% in children aged less than 1 year and is highest in the 1st month of life. Most deaths are caused by bronchopneumonia and cerebral complications. Respiratory complications are most common, including asphyxia in infants. Otitis media occurs frequently. Bronchopneumonia (also common in the elderly) may be fatal at any age. Seizures are common in infants but rare in older children. Hemorrhage into the brain, eyes, skin, and mucous membranes can result from severe paroxysms and consequent anoxia. Cerebral hemorrhage, cerebral edema, and toxic encephalitis may result in spastic paralysis, mental retardation, or other neurological disorders. Umbilical herniation and rectal prolapse occasionally occur. Symptoms diminish as the convalescent stage begins, usually within 4 weeks of onset. The average duration of illness is about 7 weeks (ranges from 3 weeks to 3 months). Paroxysmal coughing may recur for months.

Treatment - Treatment is with macrolide antibiotics. Hospitalization with respiratory isolation is recommended for seriously ill infants. Isolation is continued until antibiotics have been given for 5 days. In infants, suction to remove excess mucus from the throat may be lifesaving. O_2 and tracheostomy or nasotracheal intubation is occasionally needed. Expectorants, cough suppressants, and mild sedation are of little value. Because any disturbance can precipitate serious paroxysmal coughing with anoxia, seriously ill infants should be kept in a darkened, quiet room and disturbed as little as possible. Patients treated at home should be quarantined, particularly from susceptible infants, for at least 4 weeks from disease onset and until symptoms have subsided.

Antibiotics given in the catarrhal stage may ameliorate the disease. After paroxysms are established, antibiotics usually have no clinical

Herbal Treatment

Follow the directions given in The Acute Treatment Of Disease. If this has been done hopefully there will be no complications and you really don't want complications with this disease. This is a good example of why you must start treatment as soon as symptoms begin. This disease comes on like a cold then you have Whooping Cough. Herbalist David Hoffman gives the following formula for Whooping Cough 2 parts Mouse Ear, 1 part Sundew, 1 part Coltsfoot, 1 Part Thyme and 1 part White Horehound. This is a good formula, look up the individual herbs and see why, Horehound is and was the main remedy for coughs. For this condition I like Wild Cherry Bark which has a direct action on the cough reflex nerve. Most of the Expectorants we use for this condition are Antispasmodic and Anticatarrhal, concentrate on the ones that are also Antibacterial. Some of the specifics for this condition are Aniseed, Black Cohosh, Blood Root, Coltsfoot, Elecampane, Eucalyptus, Grindelia, Lobelia, Mullein, Passion Flower, Red Clover, Sundew, and Thyme. Be sure to concentrate on the Antibiotic herbs as a direct attack against the bacteria even consider gargles if the patient is old enough. Don't forget that Garlic is one of our best Respiratory herbs as it exits the body via the lungs putting its Actions just where we need them. For babies and the very young the Homoeopathic Remedies mat be your only option.

Homoeopathic Treatment

PERTUSSINUM
Coqueluchin
(PERTUSSIN)

Taken from the glairy and stringy mucus containing the virus of whooping-cough. Introduced by John H. Clarke for the treatment of whooping-cough and other spasmodic coughs.

Relationship - Compare: *Drosera; Corallium; Cuprum; Naphthal; Mephitis; Passiflor; Coccus Cacti; Magnes phos.*

Dose - The thirtieth potency.

(From Boerickes Materia Medica)

Drosera 6C to 30C - Drosera is one of the remedies praised by Hahnemann; indeed, he once said that Drosera 30th sufficed to cure nearly every case of whooping cough, a statement which clinical experience has not verified. Drosera, however, will benefit a large number of the cases, if the following indications be present: a barking cough in such frequent paroxysms as to prevent the catching of the breath; worse in the evening. All efforts to raise the phlegm end in retching and vomiting. The attacks are especially worse after midnight; the child holds its epigastrium while coughing. The drosera child cries a great deal. Arnica has crying before coughing because recollection or previous soreness and pain in present. Bayes says: "Drosera is more useful in whooping cough than any other remedy in our Materia Medica." Unlike Hahnemann, however, he claims that the higher dilutions are powerless, and he prescribes the first. Drosera acts better in pure, uncomplicated whooping cough, and while it will correspond to some epidemics it will fail in others.

Cuprum 6C to 30C - In whooping cough accompanied with convulsions, or when the paroxysms are long and interrupted, Cuprum will be the remedy. Spasms of the flexor muscles predominate. The cough is very violent and threatens suffocation. This remedy will come in sometimes very nicely after Drosera and do good work. The patient coughs up a tough, gelatinous mucus, there is much rattling in the chest, and the face and lips are bluish. A great characteristic of the remedy is the relief from a swallow of cold water. Hale mentions the usefulness of Cuprum in cases accompanied with spasms, clenched hands, etc.

Corallium Rubrum 6C to 30C - This is a very useful remedy in severe cases of whooping cough. Before the cough there is a smothering sensation. The child gapes and becomes black in the face. It is a remedy for that shot, quick, ringing cough known as the "minute gun" cough. The smothering shows itself in the form of gasping, crowing inspirations. After each attack of cough the child sinks back perfectly exhausted. No other drug produces such a violent paroxysm. It is perhaps oftener indicated in the later stages of the affection, but the neurotic element must be present, and also the constriction of the chest before the attacks.

Coccus Cacti 6C to 30C - This remedy has paroxysms of cough with vomiting of clear, ropy mucus, extending in thick, long strings even to the floor. This is sometimes seen in children who cough and cough with this tenacious mucus stringing from mouth and nose, waving to and fro until it finally gives way. The paroxysms come on in the morning, and accompanying them there is often vomiting of a clear, ropy mucus. Eructations of wind following cough are an indication for Ambra grisea. Coccus is a useful remedy for the protracted bronchial catarrhs remaining after whooping cough. The excessive secretion of mucus under Coccus is marked and causes the child to strangle. The choking is most characteristic, even more so than the strangling.

Mephitis 3C - Mephitis is useful in a cough with a well-marked laryngeal spasm, a whoop. Cough is worse at night on lying down, there is a suffocated feeling, and the child cannot exhale. Farrington observes that this remedy will often apparently make the patient worse, while it really tends to shorten the course of the disease. The catarrhal symptoms calling Mephitis are slight, but the whoop is prominent. The smothering comes on with cough, while with Corallium rubrum it comes on before the cough, and is followed by great exhaustion. There is not much expectoration with Mephitis. There are many spasmodic symptoms with this remedy, such as cramping of the legs at night.

Belladonna 6C to 30C - In sudden violent paroxysms of whooping cough, without any expectoration, and the symptoms of cerebral congestion, Belladonna will be found useful. Epistaxis may accompany, and the patient is worse at night. Boenninghausen says that it is suitable mostly in the beginning of the disease, or, later, when there is fever. Often in the beginning of the disease it use will shorten and modify the disease. Another indication for belladonna is present when the attacks terminate by sneezing. The cough is excited by a tickling in the throat, as if from down. Retching and vomiting and pain in the stomach are prominent symptoms, but when Belladonna is the remedy the congestive symptoms will be present and active, the onset sudden; the child grasps at the throat and clings to its mother, as if frightened.

Ipecac 6C to 30C - Convulsive cough, where the child becomes blue or pale and loses its breath, great nausea and relief from vomiting are prominent symptoms for Ipecac. A "gagging cough" is a good indication for the remedy. The discharge of mucus is copious and tenacious, and the patient is very weak after the attacks. Violent shattering coughs following each other in quick succession, not permitting recovery of breath, indicate Ipecac. The child is limp and weak, and there is free perspiration. Sulphur is also an excellent remedy for vomiting after the paroxysmal cough.

Antimonium Tart 6C to 30C - With this remedy the child is worse when excited or angry, or when eating; the cough culminates in vomiting of mucus and food. There is much rattling of mucus in the chest, but the expectoration is slight. The child demanding Antimonium tartaricum will be irritable and cross, and will cry, when approached; the tongue will be white and weakness will be present. If diarrhea be present with great debility and depression of vital forces, or if the child vomits its supper shortly after midnight, Antimonium tartaricum will be the remedy. It also has marked aggravation form warm drinks.

Cina 6C to 30C - This is not always a worm remedy. It is a most excellent remedy in whooping cough. It has the same rigidity as Ipecac, the child stiffness out and there is a clucking sound in the oesophagus when the little one comes out of the paroxysm. Grinding of the teeth during sleep will further indicate Cina. It, is of course, specially indicated by symptoms of worms and in children who are predisposed there to.

Mag Phos 6C to 30C - This is the prominent Schuesslerian remedy for whooping cough, which begins as does common cold. The attacks are convulsive and nervous, ending in a whoop. Clinically, I have found this remedy, used in the 30th potency, to act marvelously in certain epidemics. While associated with Dr. William Boericke, of San Francisco, it was not an uncommon thing for a patient to come to us for "some of our whooping cough remedy," which was nothing else than Magnesia phosphorica 30th. It seemed especially adapted to the then prevailing epidemic. The indications may be stated as cough in severe paroxysms, with blue or swollen and livid face, with a severe whoop. Kali sulphuricum will also at times be found useful.

Kali Bich 6C to 30C - This remedy suits cases where there is a hoarse cough; child breathes superficially and rapidly to prevent attacks of coughing. It is a coarser cough than that of Hepar, worse from eating and on inspiring deeply; there is a general catarrhal involvement of the nose, throat and frontal sinus, and the expectoration is yellow, tough and stringy, differing from that of Coccus cacti which is being yellow.

Scarlet Fever

Cause - Scarlet fever is caused by group A streptococcal Pyogene (and occasionally other) strain that produce a toxin, leading to a diffuse pink-red cutaneous flush that blanches on pressure. The rash is seen best on the abdomen or the lateral chest, as dark red lines in skin folds. A strawberry tongue (inflamed papillae protruding through a bright red coating) is another common symptom. The upper layer of the previously reddened skin often desquamates after the fever subsides. Other symptoms are similar to those in streptococcal pharyngitis. Scarlet fever is uncommon today.

Children from two to six years of age are more susceptible. Infection is caused by direct contact with patient or contact with clothes or any other infected articles of the patient.

Disease Process - An acute highly infectious self-limiting disease of childhood, epidemic and endemic in occurrence, with symptoms of initial vomiting, a typical fever, sore throat and a highly characteristic eruption.

The disease varies in severity in different cases and in different epidemics. It may exhibit only a mild rash, with a slight fever and an absence of throat symptoms, the patient not being confined to the bed, or it may exhibit violent and serious symptoms at its onset, which increase in severity rapidly, with a malignant sore throat, extreme toxaemia, enlarged glands, especially of the throat and neck, swollen tissues, delirium and sordes. This disease has a tendency to complications. The disease is uncommon in the tropics.

Diagnosis - Can be made when the Rash along with the strawberry tongue is seen. The rash starts on the neck and upper chest and spreads over the body sometimes in a few hours affecting most the flexor surfaces of the elbows and knees and the inner thighs. The rash is bright scarlet with scattered red spots. The skin is smooth at first then rough.

The symptoms of scarlet fever are clearly marked in a typical case that a diagnosis is not difficult. These are the abrupt vomiting, with sudden high temperature, rapid, hard pulse, sore throat and the characteristic redness of the skin after about thirty-six hours, which can be pressed out entirely by the finger, leaving a very white skin, to which the redness slowly returns. There is a characteristic appearance of the tongue in scarlet fever patients which is known as the strawberry tongue. There is a white, thin coat at first on the tongue surface which is in sharp contrast to the bright red appearance of the mucous membrane and mouth. Soon the papillae of the upper surface of the tongue becomes elongated and clubbed, as it were, on their tips and stand up above or through the white coating like the surface of a ripe strawberry.

Prevention - Infection is highest in the beginning and rash forming stages of the disease then falls rapidly, few are infective after the 4th week. Quarantine period for contacts is 10 days.

Symptoms - Simple Scarlet fever has three stages the Invasion, Eruption and Desquamation. The onset can be sudden with sore throat with tenderness on swallowing. Vomiting is early and constant. The sore throat is commoner in adults while the vomiting is common in children. Temperature rises rapidly often at 103 to 104 when first taken. Face is flushed, tongue furred and pulse rapid especially in children. In the **Eruption stage** the rash appears 24 to 36 hours after disease onset and the symptoms worsen with the throat more painful and swollen along with the strawberry tongue and the temperature can go higher. Symptoms increase for 2 or 3 days then the rash disappears and the symptoms improve. The **Desquamation stage** starts as the rash starts to go and the skin is stained and rough. Desquamation or peeling starts at the neck or follows the order of the rash and occurs last on palms and soles. On the face it begins in numerous places and separates as powder, on the abdomen as scales and on the soles of the feet as large flakes. This is most marked in the second week and usually complete in the 4th week.

Complications can be nephritis which can occur at the end of the 3rd week, Otitis Media especially in children up to 15 years, Arthritis which is very common in adults but rare in children.

Prognosis - Scarlet fever was very virulent in the 18th and first half of the 19th century with a death rate of about 20% with 15% alone caused from kidney complications. Modern treatment with antibiotics and hospitalization for complications has reduced this to nearly nil except in third world countries.

Treatment - The following treatment is from **Finley Ellingwood, M.D. Treatment of Disease, 1910.** The patient should be effectually quarantined in a large, well ventilated room, with an experienced nurse, who will carefully change her clothes before mingling with others outside. Every means must be taken to prevent the patient becoming chilled or the hands and feet or surface of the body from becoming cold, as this prevents a free development of the rash. This same care must be continued throughout the entire course of the disease to the end of convalescence in order to prevent renal congestion, which is always imminent. This threatening danger may be averted in most cases if it is never forgotten. A mild infusion of **Couchgrass** will often supply an additional quantity of water to keep the kidneys flushed and to retain the mass of debris excreted, in perfect solution. This can be iced and drunk *ad libitum* during the fever, and fruit juices, or fruit jellies may be dissolved in the infusion to impart a pleasant taste and nutritious properties. The **food** should be liberal, but nutritious and readily digestible, or in part predigested. Milk in various forms may be given with eggs, which may be beaten together and to which, in prostrate cases, brandy may be added to advantage. Broths, gruels and jellies are of much service with toast during the fever. Upon its abatement the diet may be increased with care, including the usual articles of plain food.

Herbal Treatment

As always follow the directions given in The Acute Treatment Of Disease. If this has been done hopefully there will be no complications and you really don't want complications with this disease. Diaphoretics are very important in this disease so as to get the toxins to leave the body via the skin as much as we can so as to avoid potential kidney problems later on. The kidneys filter the blood and when you have Scarlet Fever it is a very toxin laden blood so we must try to take the weight off the kidneys first with Couchgrass as mentioned in the treatment above and with Echinacea which we always use for toxins cruising the system along with Baptisia which will add its Anti-microbial Action to that of Echinacea and also help with the fever. A good Diaphoretic to use which would help with the vomiting would be Peppermint but don't be in too much of a hurry to stop the vomiting as we want all toxins out of the body so concentrate more on the nausea. Other diaphoretics to think of are Chamomile, Elder, Garlic, Ginger which are all good for use on the young and maybe Yarrow which has a Urinary Antiseptic Action as well. For the sore throat at the beginning gargles should be considered, think of Thyme, Sage or Pokeroot which are specifics for the throat or Tea Tree Oil. Generally for skin diseases more so in the Chronic diseases Herbalists always tend to use the Alteratives which are the blood cleansers. Let the disease run its course and try to prevent complications. Specifics used in the past for Scarlet Fever have been Valerian for restless children, Hyssop, Pleurisy Root, Cayenne, Baptisia, Poke Root, Bayberry, Black Cohosh and Eucalyptus.

Homoeopathic Treatment

Belladonna 6C to 30C - This remedy corresponds to the asthenic type, with a bright red rosy hue to the skin, a bright red throat, pain in the epigastrium, the strawberry tongue and the glandular swellings. Thus it is seem that it corresponds to the smooth bright red, Sydenham variety of scarlet fever. It has no correspondence with a miliary rash or with malignant symptoms. There are usually present in a well-marked Belladonna case symptoms of cerebral irritation, such as delirium, twitching of muscles, uneasy sleep. Mercurius will be indicated in certain epidemics by its characteristic throat symptoms, but Belladonna is more often called for. Aconite may be needed at the onset if its symptoms be present, though this remedy usually finds no place in the treatment of conditions due to a poisoned state of the blood. Hahnemann's discovery that **Belladonna is a prophylactic** in scarlet fever has been abundantly verified in practice. Sulphur is also a most useful remedy to use in scarlet fever, but its especial field is for the sequelae bursting forth upon a scrofulous diathesis.

Gelsemium 6C to 30C - Here the patients are quiet and listless; they are prostrated and stupid; the pulse is throbbing but compressible, and at the onset of the disease it suits cases where neither Aconite nor Belladonna are indicated. The asthenic form, with great prostration is more often met with in poorly nourished children, and here Gelsemium is often the remedy. If the case develops any special malignancy of symptoms other remedies will be needed.

Bryonia 6C to 30C - Bryonia is a remedy often of great value. When we recall its headache, white then brownish tongue, the characteristic thirst, the sharp pains in the tardy development of the rashes, occurring perhaps in blotches and resembling that of measles, or a disappearing rash with possibly delirium on waking, Bryonia will do good service.

Ailanthus 6C to 30C - This is a most potent antidote to malignant scarlet fever and suits especially severe cases. The patient lies in a stupor, the rash is imperfect, dark and purplish; swollen, livid throat and infiltration of the cellular tissue about the neck; excoriating nasal discharge, drowsiness and prostration, violent vomiting, severe headache and dizziness, small quick pulse, the stools thin, bloody and offensives and there is much foetor to all the discharges. It will save life oftentimes in the most desperate cases. Arum triphyllum has excoriating discharges from the nose, swollen tongue, sore throat; the child is restless and irritable, he tosses about. The extreme soreness of the throat is characteristic of Arum; the lips and nose are irritated and the child picks at them until they bleed.

Rhus Tox 6C to 30C - A most useful remedy in adynamic forms of scarlet fever. Here the child is restless, drowsy, has a red and smooth tongue, oedematous fauces, the parotids are especially apt to swell or suppurate, the eruption does not come out well, and when it does come out is miliary. The great depression, weakness and bodily restlessness and the supervening of rheumatic symptoms late in the disease will serve to indicate Rhus. Apis mellifica must be carefully distinguished from Rhus. This remedy has high fever, restlessness and nervous agitation; the mouth and throat are red and the tongue blistered; there is early prostration and scanty urine, drowsiness, miliary rash. It is a remedy; only occasionally useful in scarlet fever; it stands midway between Belladonna and Rhus toxicodendron; there will generally be present an oedematous condition of the skin and throat, and the skin will prick and sting. It comes in well, however, in albuminuria following scarlet fever.

Lachesis 8C to 30C - This remedy suits forms of the disease having a malignant tendency; the child is drowsy and the rash comes out imperfectly and slowly, is dark interspersed with a miliary rash; the throat is inflamed, the cervical glands are swollen, the tongue is dirty yellow. It suits cases core adynamic than those calling for Rhus. Hydrocyanic acid is also sometimes indicated in scarlet fever of a malignant type, and Muriatic acid suits malignant cases oftentimes better than either Rhus or Lachesis. With this acid the rash comes out sparingly and is interspersed with petechiae or bluish spots; the child is restless, throws off the bedclothes; the skin takes on a purple hue and there is great weakness and prostration, delirium, a rapid intermitting pulse, foul breath, acrid nasal discharge and sore, bleeding ulcerations in the mouth. Under Arsenicum the rash comes out imperfectly; the child is thrown into convulsions and then relapses into a stupor.

Ammonium Carb 6C to 30C - This is also a useful remedy in scarlet fever. The throat is swollen internally and externally, the glands are enlarged, the tonsils are swollen and bluish and the child is drowsy. The drowsiness, miliary eruption and dark throat will distinguish from Belladonna.

Zincum 6C to 30C - Zincum will be needed in certain enervated children who become restless and delirious, or else are quit and unconscious and very weak, too weak in fact to develop an eruption, and as a result of this non-development of the eruption brain symptoms, such as meningitis with sharp pains through the head, supervene. In these cases it will often bring out the eruption and save the child. Cuprum may be needed in troubles from a suppressed rash and Calcarea carbonica must be thought of for scrofulous children with an undeveloped or receding rash. Kali sulphuricum is a remedy for the stage of desquamation.

Mumps

Cause - Mumps is an acute, contagious, systemic viral disease, usually causing painful enlargement of the salivary glands, most commonly the parotids. The causative agent is a paramyxovirus which is spread by droplets or saliva. The virus probably enters through the nose or mouth. It is in saliva for up to 6 days before salivary gland swelling appears. It is also in blood and urine and in the CSF (spinal fluid) if there is CNS (central nervous system) involvement. One attack usually confers permanent immunity. The disease occurs at any age, but most usually between 5 and 10 years of age and is unusual in children under 2 years of age.

Disease Process - An acute contagious disease of childhood and early adult life, characterized by inflammation of the parotid glands, which may also involve all of the salivary glands, and be conveyed to the mammae in the female, and to the testicles in the male.

Diagnosis - Mumps is suspected in patients with salivary gland inflammation and typical systemic symptoms, particularly if there is parotitis or a known mumps outbreak. Mumps is also suspected in unexplained aseptic meningitis or encephalitis during mumps outbreaks.

Prevention - Vaccination is highly effective. It is endemic in certain heavily populated areas but may occur in epidemics when people are crowded. It occurs mainly in unimmunized populations, with peak incidence during late winter and early spring.

Symptoms - After a 14 to 24 day incubation period, most people develop headache, anorexia, malaise, and a low to moderate grade fever. Involvement of salivary glands occurs 12 to 24 hours later, accompanied by fever up to 39.5 or 40° C. Fever persists for 24 to 72 hours. Glandular swelling peaks about the 2nd day and lasts for 5 to 7 days. Involved glands are extremely tender during the febrile period.

Parotitis is usually bilateral. Pain on chewing or swallowing, especially on swallowing acidic liquids such as vinegar or citrus juice, is its earliest symptom. It later produces swelling beyond the parotid in front of and below the ear. Occasionally, the submandibular and sublingual glands also swell, more rarely, these are the only glands affected. Submandibular gland involvement produces neck swelling beneath the jaw, and suprasternal edema may develop, perhaps due to lymphatic obstruction by enlarged salivary glands. With sublingual gland involvement, the tongue may swell. The oral duct openings of the affected glands are edematous and slightly inflamed. The skin over the glands may become tense and shiny. Mumps may involve organs other than the salivary glands, particularly in post pubertal patients. About 20% of post pubertal male patients develop testicular inflammation (orchitis), usually unilateral, pain, tenderness, edema, erythema, and warmth of the scrotum. In females, gonadal involvement (oophoritis) is less commonly recognized, far less painful, and does not impair fertility. Meningitis, typically with headache, vomiting, stiff neck, and, occurs in 1 to 10%. Encephalitis, with drowsiness, seizures, or coma, occurs very rarely. About 50% of CNS mumps infections occur without parotitis.

Pancreatitis, typically with sudden severe nausea, vomiting, and epigastric pain, may occur toward the end of the first week. These symptoms disappear in about 1 week, leading to complete recovery.

Prognosis - Uncomplicated mumps generally resolves itself although a relapse can occur rarely after about 2 weeks. Complications may include orchitis, meningoencephalitis, and pancreatitis.

Treatment - Treatment of mumps and its complications is supportive. The patient is isolated until glandular swelling subsides. A soft diet reduces pain caused by chewing. Acidic substances (eg, citrus fruit juices) that cause discomfort should be avoided.

Herbal Treatment

Follow the directions given in The Acute Treatment Of Disease. If this has been done hopefully there will be no complications and you really don't want complications with this disease. The main specific for this disease is Poke Root which is used internally (only 1ml doses at a time) and as a gargle which can be mixed with the other throat specific herbs like Thyme and Sage. To Poke Root think of adding another strong Lymphatic System herb such as Baptisia or Cleavers. For the fever use the Diaphoretics with Peppermint being a good choice because of its flavor and also its Action on nausea and sickness, Chamomile could be added for a calming effect. These two herbs are very good for children. For the pain on swallowing think of Antiinflammatory and Demulcent herbs with Mullein and Licorice covering both of these Actions and again giving a nice flavor. The specifics for this disease are Poke Root, Mullein, Burdock, Calendula (Glandular Swellings), Cramp bark, Echinacea, Lemon Balm and Pennyroyal.

Homoeopathic Treatment

Belladonna 6C to 30C - This is unquestionably the most important remedy, corresponding to vascular engorgement, fever and nervous irritability so common in this disease. The glands are swollen, hot and sensitive to pressure, worse on the right side. The pains are flying and lancing and extend to the ear. It is useful when the swelling suddenly subsides, and is followed by throbbing headache and delirium.

Rhus Tox 6C to 30C - Rhus corresponds to dark red swellings, with tendency to erysipelatous inflammation. There is much aching in the limbs, the patient is restless and the symptoms are worse at night. It is our best remedy in secondary parotitis. The left side is more apt to be affected. Lachesis corresponds to left-sided mumps, with purplish swellings and aggravation after sleep.

Mercurius 6C to 30C - This is one of our best remedies in mumps, as if has a specific action on the salivary glands. There is slight fever and it is useful in the later stages. The special symptoms are tenderness, salivation, offensive breath and threatening suppuration. Pilocarpine muriate 3x is what Burnett terms his "big shot in mumps." It seems to affect especially the parotid gland.

Pulsatillia 6C to 30C - Especially useful in orchitic and mammary complications. The tongue is thickly coated, the mouth is dry and the pain is worse evenings and after lying down. For metastasis to the ovaries Pulsatilla may be the remedy. Conium is indicated by excessive hardness of the swelling. Clematis and Aurum may be useful in orchitic complications.

Meningitis

Cause - Meningitis is an inflammation of the meninges, the membranes that cover the brain and spinal cord. Meningococcus causes meningitis and septicemia. Meningitis and septicemia account for more than 90% of meningococcal infections. Local outbreaks occur mostly in in sub-Saharan Africa between Senegal and Ethiopia, an area known as the meningitis belt. Transmission generally occurs via direct contact with respiratory secretions from a carrier. Carrier rates rise dramatically during epidemics. After invading the body Meningococcus causes meningitis and severe bacteremia in both children and adults. Children between 6 months and 3 years are the most frequently infected. Other high-risk groups include adolescents, military recruits and college freshmen living in dormitories. Infection or vaccination confers type-specific immunity. The disease is most common among children and those of early youth, but it attacks adults up to perhaps twenty years of age quite commonly. No age however is free from liability to attacks during an epidemic.

Disease Process - Meningitis is usually caused by bacteria or viruses (viral meningitis is called aseptic meningitis). Less common causes include fungi, protozoa, and other parasites. Meningitis is a severe acute inflammatory disorder involving the meninges of the brain and spinal cord;

epidemic endemic and sporadic in occurrence; characterized by an abrupt onset, with chill, fever, headache, pain in the spinal column, stiffness and contraction of the muscles of the neck and back, and, in violent cases with impairment of the brain and mental function, mild coma or delirium, dullness of the eyes and irregularly contracting pupils, or pupils irresponsive to light

Diagnosis - Diagnosis is clinical, confirmed by culture. Guiding symptoms can be the rash, photophobia and stiff neck.

Prevention - Isolate patient. Vaccination is recommended for military recruits and travelers to endemic areas. Close contacts of people with meningococcal disease are at increased risk for acquiring the disease and should receive a prophylactic antibiotic.

Symptoms - Symptoms are usually severe and include headache, nausea, vomiting, photophobia, lethargy, rash, multiple organ failure and shock. Patients with meningitis frequently report fever, headache, and stiff neck. Other symptoms include nausea, vomiting, photophobia, and lethargy. A maculopapular or hemorrhagic petechial rash often appears soon after disease onset.

The Following Is From Herbalist Finley Ellingwood, M.D. 1910

The following is a far better description of the symptoms so I have added it here.

In the epidemic form, as a rule, there are no prodromes, the patient being suddenly stricken down, from previous good health. Usually there is a chill, which is almost immediately accompanied with headache and dizziness, with an abrupt development of fever. The temperature usually is not high, but severe cases will reach 104° F. and hold that point steadily, with but slight variations for from twenty-four to thirty-six hours. A temperature of 102.5° F. is more common, and is usual with the milder cases, or with those of slow development. In many cases there is no marked variation in the temperature, often there is no change for a long period, but a reduction or increase of one degree perhaps within twelve or eighteen hours is not uncommon. There are no intermissions and but slight remissions, with no regularity in their appearance.

The headache, which is one of the first symptoms, rapidly increases until it becomes almost unbearable. This is accompanied with severe pain in the spinal cord, involving the muscles of the back. These muscles soon become rigid and the tenseness involves the muscles also of the thighs, arms and neck. Brain symptoms appear quickly, and consciousness is soon lost, the patient becoming dull and stupid and developing a mild delirium. In other cases the patient lies with the eyes open, but takes no notice of things around him and is soon found to be partially unconscious. In other cases there is great restlessness, with a high degree of nervous excitability.

A profound convulsion may occur early, usually in the form of opisthotonos, although this is rare. Commonly the stiffness occurs in the muscles of the back of the neck, the head is drawn backward and forced into the pillow, the head can be moved from side to side, but flexion and extension will result in excruciating pain, the posterior cervical muscles are hard and in a state of tonic contraction from irritation of the anterior roots of the cervical nerves. In infants the constant movement of the head from side to side, with the crowding of the occiput into the pillow, is almost a classic symptom.

The **eruption** of meningitis occurs in perhaps one-half of the sporadic or endemic cases. In epidemics it is present in the larger number of cases. The eruption by far the most common is the petechial eruption, from which the disease has the name of spotted fever. This occurs in the form of irregular purpuric spots, which may be diffused or limited to a small area. At first the eruption is quite red, later it occasionally becomes dark and appears as ecchymoses.

To those who are experienced, the appearance of the eye assists greatly in diagnosis. Most commonly the eye is dull, with a dilated pupil. The eye may be very bright, with contracted pupil, or the pupils may be unequal in size, and in all cases not readily responsive to light. The conjunctivae usually assumes an injected or chemosed appearance, and photophobia is common

In the isolated cases, dullness of the mind, with somnolence, or stupor may occur early. In fatal cases this increases to coma, with no recurrence of consciousness. With the dullness there may be mild delirium, or nocturnal delirium only may occur, independent of any tendency to stupor. Active delirium with violent manifestations is not uncommon in the early stage. This may be accompanied with hallucinations, and in the female with hysterical manifestations.

Vomiting is not an uncommon symptom. It is often of cerebral origin, but may be induced by faults of the stomach. The tongue is usually thick and pale, but slightly coated, and the appetite is early lost, but later the tongue becomes dark and dry, the secretions are all suppressed and sides appears. Constipation is apt to be present, with tympanitic distension of the bowels.

At first the patient passes a large quantity of pale urine of low specific gravity. Later it is reduced in quantity, until but little is passed, which has a high specific gravity. Retention, suppression and incontinence are not uncommon during the later stages of the disease, and albumen and sugar are found in rare isolated cases.

Prognosis - Infection is associated with a mortality rate of 10 to 15%. Of patients who recover, 10 to 15% have serious sequel, such as permanent hearing loss, mental retardation, or loss of phalanges or limbs. In **Finley Ellingwoods** time the death rate in severe epidemics was from fifty to seventy-five per cent. In mild epidemics from twenty to thirty per cent were fatal. In sporadic cases the mortality was very high, especially in young children.

Treatment - Treatment is penicillin or a 3rd-generation cephalosporin. Corticosteroids decrease the incidence of neurologic complications in children. When corticosteroids are used, they should be administered with or before the 1st dose of antibiotics. Dexamethasone is given for 4 days. **Ellingwood says** the patient must be confined in an isolated room, away from confusion and noise of every kind, with a most careful and conscientious nurse, and the room should be darkened. The patient should receive a concentrated and highly nutritious diet. The disease is rapidly exhausting in its character and all measures must be adopted that will sustain the strength. Milk, eggs, beef juice, rice, and fruit juices must be given freely. When the active symptoms have abated, the physician should in no wise relax his assiduous attention, as the period of convalescence is apt to be long and recovery very slow.

Herbal Treatment

This is another good example of beginning treatment before you know what the disease is because by the time you have figured this one out it is really too late to do that much. The herbs that Ellingwood was using in his time are far too dangerous for us to use now especially with our lack of experience with them for he was using them close to the toxic doses in serious diseases such as this. Safe specifics we can use that were used in the past are Baptisia, Boneset, Lobelia and Passion Flower for the pain. Basically concentrate on the strong Antibacterials especially those that work in and on the blood stream. As we should never really give up there is something else we can try. Essential Oils can cross what is known as the Blood Brain Barrier and get into the spinal fluid, now that we have that handy bit of information lets act upon it. First of all we will give heaps of Garlic oil internally in a serious case I would do it in 5 to 10 capsules of oil at a time. Next we will use a selection of Antibacterial and Antiseptic Essential Oils, choose from Tea Tree Oil, Garlic (puncture some Garlic Oil capsules), Eucalyptus, Rosemary, Lavender, Juniper, Bergamot and Sandalwood. Mix your formula with a carrier oil and apply to the neck and down the spine area till about the top of the hips. Essential Oils work by medicating the blood stream via the skin so care must be taken not to overdo it as it throws a load on the liver whose job it is to detox the blood, this is why caution should always be used using Aromatherapy. In our case we are concentrating on the spine and neck trying to get the oil into the cerebrospinal fluid so it can travel to the meninges and have a direct Antibacterial Action.

Homoeopathic Treatment

Belladonna 6C to 30C - Corresponds to the initial stages, where there is intense heat of the body, strong pulse, bright red face and delirium, where the cerebral irritation is marked by intense pain in the head, starting out of sleep crying out, grinding teeth. For simple meningitis, not the tubercular form, when everything is acute and intense; when effusion commences, however, it ceases to be the remedy. Aconite. Meningitis from heat of the sun's rays after long exposure thereto, or cerebral congestions from anger. It is only useful at the onset. Fear is a marked symptom. Veratrum viride. Intense cerebral congestion, rapid pulse, tendency to convulsion, followed by prostration. Elliot considers Veratrum viride in the lower potencies our best remedy in acute meningitis. Coldness of the surface loss of consciousness, dilated pupils, labored, slow, irregular pulse. Gelsemium. Is hardly homoeopahtic to pain as its action is wholly motor, but it may be indicated in meningitis by its general symptoms. It is less often indicated and hence less valuable than Belladonna. Yet Spalding has used the remedy as a basic one in the cerebro-spinal variety with uniform success, losing but one case.

Bryonia 6C to 30C - Suits well cerebral effusions with a benumbed sensorium. The following will be useful indications upon which to prescribe Bryonia. Constant chewing motion with the mouth; when moved screams with pain; child stupid, abdomen distended; tongue white, pains are most sharp and stitching, and the patient drinks greedily; there is a livid flushed face, high temperature, copious sweats. Thus it is seen that Bryonia produces a characteristic image of meningitis and suits especially cases caused by suppressed eruption.

Apis 6C to 30C - Here nervous agitation predominates; there are shrill cries, stabbing pains; the child puts its hand to its head and screams. There is an oedematous face, scanty urine, and the patient is thirstless, it suits especially infantile cases and especially the tubercular form due to an developed eruption. Cicuta is useful in the irrigative stage when there are general convulsions, twitching in fingers and unconsciousness. It also markedly controls the effusion. The head is spasmodically drawn back with stiff neck. Violent jerks in any part of the body. Strangles on drinking, dilated pupils and staring look, trismus; one of our best remedies, having a fine clinical record.

Helleborus 6C to30C - Mental torpor marks this drug; a sensorial apathy, there is want of reaction. It corresponds to a later stage of the disease, when effusion has taken place; then symptoms such as wrinkling of one arm and one leg are indicative of Helleborus. There are shooting pains in the head, sudden crying out, screaming, boring head into the pillow. The cries have a most pitiful sound. Camphora. In the fulminant variety where the poison falls on the patient like a thunderbolt and collapse approaches speedily. The patient is cold, pale and pulseless, eyes sunken, face livid. Patient cold, but does not want to be covered.

Zincum Met 6X - This remedy corresponds to the subacute form, especially if tubercular and due to suppressed eruptions. Febrile disturbance is absent or slight, there are marked twitching jerkings and hyperaesthesia of all the senses and skin, and tremulousness of the feet. At the beginning there are sharp lancinating pains and great exhaustion of nerve force. The 6X trituration is recommended. Sulphur is useful in tubercular meningitis; the child lies in a stupor with cold sweat on forehead , jerking of limbs, spasms and suppressed urine. Clarke advises Bacillinum 100th, which he claims is very prompt in its action. Cuprum suits cases marked with violent convulsions, thumbs clenched, loud screaming, face pale with blue lips. No remedy equals it in these conditions, but it is of more use in the later stages.

Tuberculosis

Cause - TB is caused by Mycobacterium tuberculosis. TB occurs almost exclusively from inhalation of a droplet containing M. tuberculosis. They are dispersed primarily through coughing, singing, and other forced respiratory maneuvers by a person with active pulmonary TB. Tuberculosis is a chronic progressive infection with a period of latency following initial infection. It occurs most commonly in the lungs. Pulmonary symptoms include productive cough, chest pain, and dyspnea. Tuberculosis is the leading infectious cause of morbidity and mortality in adult's worldwide, killing about 2 million people every year. People with pulmonary cavitary lesions are especially infectious. Droplet nuclei containing tubercle bacilli may float on room-air currents for several hours, increasing the chance of spread. About a quarter of household contacts acquire the infection. Transmission is enhanced by overcrowding thus people living in poverty or in institutions are at particular risk. Once effective treatment begins the cough rapidly decreases, and within weeks, TB is no longer contagious.

Disease Process - TB of the tonsils, lymph nodes, abdominal organs, bones, and joints was once commonly caused by ingestion of milk infected with M. bovis, but such infection has been largely eradicated in developed countries by slaughtering cows that test positive on a tuberculin skin test. Tubercle bacilli initially produce a primary infection, followed by a latent (dormant) phase and, in some cases, by active disease. Infection is not transmissible in the primary and latent phases. Primary infection: Airborne droplet nuclei lodge predominantly in the lower lung, usually in only one site. Tubercle bacilli replicate inside macrophages ultimately killing them, inflammatory cells are attracted to the area, causing a tubercle and sometimes pneumonitis. In the early weeks of infection, some infected macrophages are borne to regional lymph nodes. Blood can spread it to any part of the body, particularly the lower portions of the lungs, epiphyses of the long bones, kidneys, vertebral bodies, and meninges. In 95% of cases, after about 3 weeks of uninhibited growth, the immune system suppresses bacillary replication before symptoms or signs develop. Foci of infection in the lung or other sites resolve into epithelioid cell granulomas, which may have caseous and necrotic centers; tubercle bacilli can survive in this material for years, the host's resistance determining whether the infection ultimately resolves without treatment, remains dormant, or becomes active.

Foci may leave nodular scars in the apices of one or both lungs (Simon foci), calcified scars from the primary infection (Ghon foci), or calcified hilar lymph nodes.

In about 10% of patients overall, latent infection develops into active disease, although the percentage varies significantly by age and other risk factors. In 50 to 80% of those who develop active disease, TB reactivates within the first or second year, but it can occur decades later. Any organ initially seeded may be a site of reactivation, but reactivation occurs most often in the lungs. Tuberculosis development within the structure of the lungs is characterized by hectic fever, cough, progressive emaciation, night sweats, diarrhea and great prostration.

Diagnosis - Diagnosis is by sputum culture along with a chest x-ray. The tuberculin skin test is a common method used to determine if people have come in contact with TB and is fast to do in large groups of people.

Prevention - Vaccination and isolation of the infected. When a patient is suffering from the disease and remains in contact with other individuals, he must sleep alone, in a thoroughly ventilated room, and all of the sputum must be expectorated directly into a proper spit cloth, or into soft cloths that have been treated with some antiseptic solution, and these must be hygienically disposed of. The floor of the patient's room must be devoid of carpets, and the walls of hangings, and everything that can possibly be dispensed with must be removed. Most important of all is the complete isolation of the patient.

Symptoms - In active pulmonary TB, even moderate or severe disease, the patient may have no symptoms except "not feeling well" or may have more specific symptoms. Cough is most common. At first, it may be minimally productive of yellow or green sputum, usually on rising, but the cough may become more productive as the disease progresses. Drenching night sweats are a classic symptom but are neither common in nor specific for TB. Painful breathing may develop. Hemoptysis occurs only with cavitary TB.

The Following Is From Herbalist Finley Ellingwood, M.D. 1910

In a large proportion of cases the development of this disease extends over quite a period of time. There is a history of impaired health, from causes that seem to be well understood, but the treatment of which has been unsatisfactory.

In other cases there is a history of exposure, with an acute inflammation, most commonly some one of the forms of acute lung involvement, which during a protracted and unsatisfactory convalescence develops a hectic fever, night sweats, greatly increased prostration, emaciation and a return of cough, though perhaps it differs in character from that which previously existed. The cough of severe bronchitis may continue in spite of all treatment, until hectic fever, chills and night sweats appear, and lead to a diagnosis of developing phthisis.

It is observed in the cases of slower development that there is increasing debility, an incapacity for continued labor, or for any persistent active exercise, and an inclination to be chilly on slight exposure or from a draft. There may at first be no cough, but in the larger proportion of cases a persistent cough is present, which varies in character at different times, but is always unyielding to any of the usual methods of treatment. Occasionally there is much improvement at the first, but the condition suddenly increases without known cause and becomes very severe, and the sputum may be streaked with blood, or there may be a slight hemorrhage. This always causes alarm and usually results in a thorough investigation, disclosing the real character of the disease.

With the occurrence of the chilliness, if the temperature be taken, it will be found that there is a slight elevation above the normal all the time, perhaps less than a degree, or even a fraction of a degree, at the lowest point, increasing, with an increase of chilliness, at a given time each day, usually in the evening, to perhaps 101 1/2° F.

The fever is seldom persistently high; in fact, 103.5° F. is probably the point of its highest development. It varies from 99.5° F. to 101.5° F. in the milder cases, or in the incipient stage, to from 101.5° F. to 103° F. in the severe cases, or in the stage of complete development. In the later stages of this disease there may be septic or pyemic infection, which will increase the temperature and alter somewhat its previous character. At other times, in the erratic temperature changes, it may become sub-normal for a short time, as low as 96° F. in some cases, for brief periods. The chilliness is more apparent in the developing stage. When the disease has reached its full development and a higher temperature persists, the chilliness disappears, or only occurs on actual exposure. The fever is always more or less irregular in character and may be temporarily influenced by antipyretic remedies, but ultimately increases and persists in spite of the treatment.

The cough varies greatly in the time of its appearing, and in its character. It is, of course, the result of the progressive changes. At first, if nervous irritation, or bronchial irritation, with deficient secretion, are present, it will be dry and irritating, perhaps hoarse and barking and almost constant. It is apt to be worse on lying down at night, or on the least exposure to cold. If bronchitis coexists, distinct thick mucus, or muco-purulent bronchial secretion, will appear shortly, which will materially change the character of the cough. It will occur in paroxysms and will be loose, with a "rattling" respiration. When, in the progress of the disease, softening and disintegration occur in the process of the formation of cavities, the cough is protracted and very "hard" on attempting to rise in the morning, and continues until large quantities of sputum of varying character is expectorated from the tubes and from the cavities, in which it has accumulated during the night. This may induce nausea and vomiting, and result in temporary faintness or exhaustion. The taking of food may induce a paroxysm of cough, which may also result in vomiting. When the cough induces hemorrhage, active efforts for its restraint must be adopted, and it must be controlled also when it induces irritation, sleeplessness and exhaustion. As has been stated, there may be no expectoration at the onset. This may account for the absence of cough in a few cases, as the cough may be only necessary to clear the air passages. The first sputum is usually composed of mucus alone, and, unless there is a coexisting bronchitis, it will be colorless, in which case it will assume the greenish or yellowish green, thick and tenacious character of the bronchial exudate. Very soon, however, it becomes grayish yellow in character, somewhat watery in appearance, and is distinctly muco-purulent. As the cavities develop and disintegration of tissue progresses, the sputum is thin and filled with very small greenish gray or yellowish gray masses. Later, pus will be found in the expectoration, and in some cases, from decomposition within the cavities, the sputum is of a sweetish and offensive taste, and fetid and offensive odor. If, in the development of a cavity, hemorrhage occurs, the blood will not be uniformly intermingled in the sputum, as is the case in pneumonia, but it is thrown out independently. The quantity of the sputum expectorated, during the earlier stages of the disease, increases slowly until the formation of cavities begins, when it increases greatly for a short time, and from that time on will be irregular in quantity, depending upon the course of the breaking down of tissue within the cavity. In some cases only a few drams will be expectorated in twenty-four hours. In the later stages it may amount to from eight to twelve ounces. In childhood and in the aged there may be but little expectoration throughout the entire course of the disease.

Pain:—It is not common for a tubercular patient to suffer pain unless there are rheumatic or neuralgic complications, or unless the pleura is involved. When this appears, the pain occurs on inspiration and is increased by deep breathing and by coughing. In an occasional case there may be a steady pain through the diseased area. Usually it is lateral, or at the base of the lung, or beneath or between the scapulae. These patients are quite subject to muscular rheumatism of the chest walls, or to intercostal neuralgia.

Respiration:—There is increased frequency of Respiration with the onset of this disease, and as the disease progresses, the respirations vary from twenty-four to thirty-six, and the latter point usually continues during the latter stages of the disease. When the tubercular deposits are miliary in character and thus are more general in their involvement of the lung tissues, the respirations become still more frequent, and in the later stages of the disease cyanosis may develop. Dyspnoea is by no means as common as in acute pulmonary troubles. It occurs in the later stages when the respiratory area has been seriously reduced in quantity.

Hemorrhage occurs in a majority of the cases of phthisis, especially in those that are ulcerative in type. It is much more frequent in males than in females. In the majority of cases it occurs at first as a single streak of blood in the sputum, or a tiny red clot, later a small mass of frothy blood will be brought up, bright red in color, to be followed soon by other streaks or small clots. While in a few cases the increase in quantity may be very gradual, there is apt to be soon after the first appearance, quite a free hemorrhage. These continue irregular in quantity and at very irregular intervals throughout the entire course of the disease. As has been stated, in an exceptional case quite a free hemorrhage may occur before the disease has been recognized, and sometimes this may be very severe and prostrating. With all hemorrhages, especially those occurring early, there is a flush of heat over the body, some vertigo or faintness, a sweet or sweetish salty taste in the mouth, and increased rapid breathing, with sudden weakness, which in the severe cases amounts to extreme prostration or even collapse.

Sweating:—A symptom that occurs early in the disease is sweating. This occurs with the development of the fever, and is commonly nocturnal or occurs only during sleep. From the first it is apt to be very profuse in quantity, and later is the immediate cause of weakness, which is very apparent to the patient. The sweats are caused by the conditions that induce the fever—an effort on the part of the system to rid itself of the toxic elements—and occur when the system is in a state of relaxation. When they produce exhaustion they must be controlled, in order that the strength may be preserved, although the treatment is known to be only temporary in its influence.

Emaciation:—Loss of flesh and consequently of weight occurs from the onset of this disease, in part from the same causes which I have just named, as those which induce anemia. The patient loses strength because the irritating causes which are present in the disease, such as fever, sleeplessness, loss of appetite and persistent cough, with occasional hemorrhage, all interfere with nutrition and restoration. These contribute equally in the reduction of the weight of the patient. When the disease is established the loss of weight may early be quite rapid, amounting to an average of from eight to twelve ounces per day. The rapidity of the loss depends somewhat upon the severity of the disease, and if the pathologic processes are arrested there is a stay in the emaciation, and if a gain in flesh can be secured, this is indeed encouraging.

Prognosis - In healthy patients with drug-susceptible pulmonary TB, even severe disease and large cavities usually heal if appropriate therapy is used and completed. Still TB causes or contributes to death in about 10% of cases often in those who are debilitated for other reasons. Disseminated TB and TB meningitis may be fatal in up to 25% of cases despite optimal treatment. TB is much more aggressive in immune compromised patients and if not properly and aggressively treated may be fatal in as little as 2 months from its initial symptoms. This is especially true of Multiple Disease Resistant TB, in which mortality can approach 90%.

Treatment - Treatment is with multiple antimicrobial agents mentioned previously at the front of the book under Disease Resistant Antibiotics.

The Following Is From Herbalist Finley Ellingwood, M.D. 1910

Treatment of Pulmonary Tuberculosis:—In the treatment of pulmonary tuberculosis a strictly systematic course must be adopted with reference to the following facts, the necessity for which course is now being established by incontrovertible proofs from the united observations of the entire profession:

- 1. An immediate recognition of the real character of the disease and

the prompt adoption of a systematic course and plan of life, for its cure, are of the first and of vital importance.
- 2. The bacillus tuberculosis must be destroyed.
- 3. The vital forces of the patient must be sustained and improved by—
  - (a) A care-free, out-of-door life, with a correct climatic adjustment and physical exercise, fitted to each individual patient.
  - (b) The utmost care of the stomach and intestinal apparatus, to secure the ingestion, the digestion, the appropriation and assimilation of the largest possible quantity of highly nutritious foods. A careful watchfulness through the entire course of the disease for this purpose, until health is unquestionably established.
  - (c) Attention to the nervous system to retain its vigor and prevent the continuance of any irritation of any character.
- 4. Drugs alone will not cure the disease and must not be depended upon for that purpose, but conditions are constantly arising which materially decrease the resisting power of the patient, reduce his vital force and permit and encourage the development and progress of the disease, which can be overcome entirely, or greatly modified, by medicines, which must then be carefully prescribed.

A proper restraint upon all the developing processes of the disease will exercise a controlling, an inhibiting power upon the influence of the bacillus and will retard its destructive operations. This can be accomplished with medicine. With prompt attention to these conditions tuberculosis in its early stages is certainly curable. Statistics now prove that at least 75 per cent of the incipient cases should recover.

Pure Air and Sunlight:—The first essential in the destruction of the bacillus tuberculosis is an abundance of pure air. The attainment of this alone has resulted in the improvement of the case otherwise unfavorably situated. The patient should spend as much as possible of the twenty-four hours in the open air. Those who have discovered the onset of the disease before their physical strength was materially abated and have wandered off into the woods and have roughed it, sleeping in the open air at all reasonable temperatures, and especially in pine woods, have observed a rapid improvement. Others have adopted a cowboy's life, doing at first only such work as the strength would permit, but sleeping always in the open air, riding on horseback and increasing the amount of enjoyable labor as strength improved.

Amelioration of the symptoms is effected at home, by the patient spending the days in the sunlight, and the nights in a large open room, freely ventilated, or upon a veranda, or on the house top, as is done in large cities in an occasional case.

At all resorts for such patients provision is now made for exposed sleeping rooms and for sunbaths in the open air. Much has been said of the benefit of cool air, to properly* protected patients, but the consensus of opinion now is that temperature is of less importance than pure air and sunshine. A temperature which is steady and uniform, devoid of sudden changes or of contrasts between the night and day temperatures is most desirable. Provision is now made for the construction of small portable houses where a patient can have all essential conveniences, with light and constant, perfect, thorough ventilation by day and night, provision also being made for heating and the preservation of a pleasant and equable temperature when desired.

Nutrition:— In adapting the food to the patient, while the highest nutrition must be preserved, the individual articles must be selected with reference to existing conditions and idiosyncrasies. Because of the rapid progress of the emaciation and because of the demand for nutrition in the reconstructive and restorative processes, the feeding must be generous in the extreme. Exercise and out-of-door air increase nerve force and promote an appetite. These can also be further increased with medicines properly adjusted. The appetite must be satisfied with fresh raw eggs, given in a fixed quantity at stated intervals; milk similarly given, meat juices and rare meat, as raw beef properly prepared and seasoned. These may be made very palatable, and should be given about five times a day at stated intervals. It is well for the patient upon awakening in the morning, before being disturbed, to drink slowly a pint of hot milk, to which has been added a pinch of salt. He should compose himself upon his right side, to sleep again if possible, or to remain perfectly quiet and undisturbed for perhaps half an hour, when this will, in most part, have passed through the pylorus and have been absorbed without actual digestion. He may take a raw egg with this.

In the course of about two hours he should have a cereal breakfast with cream, and perhaps a small juicy steak, and toast, with oranges or other fruit. At midday the patient should have a full strong meal, with roast meat, vegetables or macaroni, a dessert of rice, tapioca, corn starch or Indian pudding. It is often of much advantage to give a simple digestive after each meal, however small, for a time until the exact digestive power of the stomach can be determined. This may be the essence of pepsin, papaw, some diastatic ferment or pancreatin, as shall be indicated. Soups, oysters and fish are all of value and acceptable under proper circumstances.

It is necessary to give the patient a light meal again late in the afternoon, and at suppertime strong food, but that easy of digestion, must be selected. Oysters, raw or stewed, raw eggs, or eggs soft boiled, should be taken at this meal, with creamed toast and perhaps baked potatoes or baked apples.

In the selection of a beverage the patient may be permitted to drink sparingly of either tea, coffee or cocoa, properly prepared. It is well to heat cream or milk, a half teacup full, and then fill the cup with the other beverage and season as is desired. If possible, milk should be adjusted as the most reliable restorative beverage. Buttermilk or matzoon and kumyss all are palatable and nutritious beverages and will be accepted when the acids in the system are deficient and when the stomach is feeble.

The use of fruit juices, or jellies dissolved in water, or cider, are all in place under proper circumstances. The author is not in favor of alcoholic beverages in this disease, believing that but little, if any, good has come from them. He has permitted, occasionally, an egg nog made with port or sherry wine, in the advanced stages of the disease.

As has been suggested, the amount of food at each meal and the character of the food must be adjusted with reference to conditions that then exist and no rule of general and continued application should be laid down, as in no disease do conditions change more readily, or are more easily influenced than in this. In the morning, after having spent a quiet, undisturbed, restful night, a much stronger breakfast can be taken than after broken, disturbed sleep and an unrefreshed awakening. Food in quantity must be avoided immediately after exercise, when the patient is exhausted, or after a fit of anger or worry. A nutritious beverage or a stimulant may be first given and followed by a period of rest, after which food properly selected may be given.

Herbal Treatment

As usual we should have begun treating this as soon as we saw the first symptoms. As this is the last of our contagious diseases we shall do this differently. Ellingwood believes there is a deficiency of acids in the fluids and treatment should begin with a tonic for the Nervous and Digestive system. So to start consider giving Swedish Bitters to stimulate the digestive system. Swedish Bitters was made up by a monk in the late 16th century and is a formula made up of the most bitter herbs all but together, I will leave you to find more information about this yourself, use the net or go to a health shop and get a brochure. Bitters are very good for people losing weight or those with digestive problems, do not forget to always check and correct the diet. What I am going to do now is give you the herbs and why I am using them I will leave it to you to see why I picked them and as usual I will be using more than just a single Action in each herb, try to figure out how much each herb covers the whole disease. All the Herbs Given will be specifics for TB. Remember the main Action we need for this disease is Antibacterials with the best being Garlic as it exits the body via the lungs and could probably just by itself cause the TB bacteria to wall itself up in the bottom corner of the lung just to escape it until it goes away, this is the main problem with TB.

For The Cough we can use Elecampane (I can think of 7 useful Actions from this herb), Blood root, Coltsfoot, Eucalyptus, Grindelia, Horehound, Hyssop, Irish Moss, Lobelia, Marsh Mallow, Mullein, Pine, Plantain, Pleurisy Root, Red Clover, Sundew, and Thyme. In cases of bleeding from the lungs think of Black Cohosh, Elecampane, Coltsfoot, Eucalyptus, Hyssop, Mullein, Plantain plus add to these some of the strongest Astringents if it gets severe such as Shepherds Purse, Cranesbill or Witch Hazel. For the digestive system think of Golden Seal, Hops and Vervain. For the Wasting Away and the Fatigue think of Aloe Vera, Asparagus, Fenugreek, Ginkgo Biloba, Ginseng, Golden Rod, Gotu Kola, Nettles, Pau D' arco, Schizandra, Shitake and Slippery elm, to add to these think of the Adaptogens, Tonics and Rejuvinatives. As mentioned these are just the specifics so add what else you feel is needed using these as the back bone of your formulas.

Homoeopathic Treatment

Phosphorus 6C to 30C - Phosphorus corresponds especially to TB in the rapidly growing young who are brilliant in mind but have a heredity tendency to weak lungs and take cold easily. The chief symptoms are great hoarseness with evening aggravation, weak chest, cough, copious sputum with hectic fever and especially its blood streaked expectoration and tightness across the chest. Cavities form rapidly and there is increasing hectic fever and flushing of the face especially towards evening and another useful symptom is a burning between the shoulder blades. This is considered the nearest specific for Pulmonary TB. The cough of Phosphorus arises from irritation in the trachea. It is tickling which is lower down than the irritation calling for Belladonna It is made worse by talking or using the voice; in fact, any change in breathing causes the cough. It is at first dry and tight and then with expectoration of tenacious purulent mucus. It is worse from a change to cold air, the chest feels dry, and there is a constriction across the upper part of the chest. Continued hoarseness with a distressing, dry cough. Coughing blood. It is also a remedy for stomach or hepatic coughs, anemic coughs, and in reflex coughs, being here similar to Ambra grisea. Phosphorus follows Belladonna well. Belladonna relieves the soreness, tenderness and fever, but the hoarse, rough voice yields to phosphorus. A dry cough is an important indication for Belladonna.

Calc Carb 6C to 30C - TB is a constitutional disease and therefore needs a constitutional remedy so be sure to math more so than the symptoms. The Calc Carb picture is fair fat and flabby and produces the following TB like symptoms. Nosebleed, throat symptoms of irritation and rawness, eruptive skin conditions, sweat from least exertion profuse and exhausting, mental state of hope, eye and ear symptoms, falling of hair, fullness across the chest with spitting of blood.

Nitric Acid 6C to 30C - A TB remedy for before lung cavities are formed. Hectic fever, soreness of chest, frequent hemorrhages, profuse and of bright red blood, dyspnea, hoarseness which is much worse in the morning, diarrhea which is also worse in the morning, a sharp stitching through the right chest to the scapula. There is a weak heart and much palpitation. The sweat is worse at night and towards the morning and exhausts the patient. The skin is cold towards the morning, there is a tickling cough which annoys the patient all night, sometimes the cough is dry, other times loose and rattling, the rales are loud, the expectoration is offensive, dirty green, bloody and purulent. Worse for warmth.

Silica 6C to 30C - Is used in the suppurative stage of TB. Patient finds it impossible to keep warm, the cough at first is dry, racking, but afterwards loosens; there is copious rattling in the chest and expectoration of offensive muco-pus. the purulent character of the expectoration indicating abscess formation in the lungs is characteristic and is more profuse after exertion.

There are large cavities in the lungs, profuse night sweats and hectic or suppurative fever. There is no better remedy in the treatment of exhausting night sweats.

Bryonia 6C to 30C - This remedy becomes of use when the pleura of the lungs become inflamed or involved. Inability to take a deep breath on account of sharp pains. The cough of Bryonia is generally dry and concussive. It seems to come from the region of the stomach, and is preceded by a tickling in the epigastrium. During the cough the patient holds the sides of the chest with his hands, as the cough not only shakes the chest, but also hurts distant parts of the body. It is induced also by coming from the open air into a warm room and is accompanied by bursting headache. The expectoration is scanty, tough and sometimes bloody.

Water Bourne Diseases

Water borne diseases are caused by water that has been contaminated by human or animal wastes and includes diseases such as cholera, typhoid, shigella, polio, meningitis, and hepatitis A and E. Humans and animals can act as hosts to the bacteria, viral or protozoa organisms that cause these diseases. In countries with inadequate sewer systems human wastes are disposed of in open latrines (which can overflow in rains), ditches and canals or are used as fertilizer on croplands resulting in extensive diarrheal diseases. Worldwide the lack of sanitary waste disposal and clean cooking, drinking and washing water leads to over 12 million deaths per year.

The risk of diarrheal disease outbreaks following natural disasters is higher in developing than in developed countries though this can change if there is massive damage to infrastructure such as damage to main sewerage treatment plants or pipes or the loss of power stopping the pumps that send the waste to the treatment plants.

Rehydration Formulas

Dehydration, and severe diarrheal diseases particularly in epidemics are massive killers in the third world especially among children. The death rate is dramatically reduced now due to the use of Oral Rehydration Solutions (ORS) packed into millions of sachet and sent around the world by WHO.

Many diseases can dehydrate you not only from diarrhea but also from the fever and vomiting alone so great care must always be paid to dehydration in any disease. In the western world hospitals they don't use ORS but use the IV drips instead but if there is a massive pandemic then we all have to look after ourselves so let's get used to the idea of making and using Oral Rehydration Solutions now and of always keeping an eye open for the possibility of Dehydration in any condition. Remember when you make your own ORS that ingesting plain water does not help restore the salt content of the body. But ingesting water with too much salt will draw fluids from the body, and make the dehydration worse.

Sugar is also added to the ORS solutions for two reasons. First because sugar helps with the transport of fluids across the cellular membranes in the bowel and second because sugar also provides needed calories to keep the strength up but as with salt too much sugar can be detrimental, it can promote diarrhea and make the loss of fluids worse.

Symptoms of dehydration can be weakness, headache, and fainting, dryness of the mouth, decreased saliva, lack or very decreased urine that is dark in color and highly concentrated, sunken eyes, loss of the elasticity of the skin, low blood pressure especially upon sitting up or rising from the sitting to the standing position and a fast pulse when laying or sitting up.

Formulas

1. The simplest formula is 3 Tablespoons of sugar and 1 teaspoon of salt dissolved in 1 quart (946 mls) of potable water.
2. An alternative simple formula is 8 teaspoons of sugar and 1 teaspoon of salt dissolved in 1 quart of potable water. This basic formula has been used effectively for more than 30 years by WHO.
3. A slightly more complicated formula may be used to replace lost potassium, and to help control diarrhea. This formula is from Dr. Steven J. Greenwald and is designed specifically to help people who were being threatened with extreme diarrhea.

ORAL REHYDRATION FLUID FORMULA
1/4 teaspoon Salt (common table salt - sodium chloride)
1/4 teaspoon Salt Substitute or "Lite Salt" (potassium chloride)
1/4 teaspoon Baking Soda
2 ½ tablespoons Sugar
Combine these ingredients and dissolve them in 1000 ml (1 liter) of sterile water.

Chemists will be able to help with any problem here.

Gastroenteritis Bacterial Infections

The bacteria most commonly implicated are: Salmonella, Campylobacter ,Shigella and E. coli

Gastroenteritis is inflammation of the lining of the stomach and small and large intestines. Most cases are infectious, although gastroenteritis may follow ingestion of drugs and chemical toxins. Gastroenteritis is usually uncomfortable but self-limited. Electrolyte and fluid loss is usually little more than an inconvenience to an otherwise healthy adult but can be grave for people who are very young, elderly, or debilitated or who have serious concomitant illnesses. Worldwide, an estimated 3 to 6 million children die each year from infectious gastroenteritis.

Bacterial gastroenteritis is less common than viral. Bacteria cause gastroenteritis by several mechanisms. Certain species eg, Vibrio cholerae, enterotoxigenic strains of Escherichia coli adhere to intestinal mucosa without invading and produce enterotoxins. These toxins impair intestinal absorption and cause secretion of electrolytes and water by stimulating adenylate cyclase, resulting in watery diarrhoea.

Some bacteria (eg, Staphylococcus aureus, Bacillus cereus, Clostridium perfringens) produce an exotoxin that is ingested in contaminated food. The exotoxin can cause gastroenteritis without bacterial infection. These toxins generally cause acute nausea, vomiting, and diarrhea within 12 hours of ingestion of contaminated food. Symptoms abate within 36 hours.

Other bacteria (eg, Shigella, Salmonella, Campylobacter, some E. coli subtypes) invade the mucosa of the small bowel or colon and produce microscopic ulceration, bleeding, exudation of protein-rich fluid, and secretion of electrolytes and water. The invasive process and its results can occur whether or not the organism produces an enterotoxin.

Campylobacter is occasionally transmitted from dogs or cats with diarrhea. Salmonella can be transmitted by undercooked eggs and by contact with reptiles. Species of Shigella are the 3rd most common bacterial cause of diarrhea in the US and are usually transmitted person to person, although food-borne epidemics occur.

Several Vibrio species (eg, V. parahaemolyticus) cause diarrhea after ingestion of undercooked seafood. V. cholerae sometimes causes severe dehydrating diarrhea in the developing world. Listeria causes food-borne gastroenteritis

Parasites: The parasites most commonly implicated are Giardia and Cryptosporidium

Certain intestinal parasites, notably Giardia lamblia adhere to or invade the intestinal mucosa, causing nausea, vomiting, diarrhea, and general malaise. Giardiasis occurs throughout the world. The infection can become chronic and cause a malabsorption syndrome. It is usually acquired via person-to-person transmission (often in day care centers) or from contaminated water. Cryptosporidium parvum causes watery diarrhea sometimes accompanied by abdominal cramps, nausea, and vomiting. In healthy people, the illness is self-limited, lasting about 2 weeks. In immunocompromised patients the illness may be severe, causing substantial electrolyte and fluid loss. Cryptosporidium is usually acquired through contaminated water.

Gastroenteritis Viral Infections

Gastroenteritis is inflammation of the lining of the stomach and small and large intestines. The viruses most commonly implicated are Rotavirus and Norovirus

Rotavirus is the most common cause of sporadic, severe, dehydrating diarrhea in young children. Rotavirus is highly contagious; most infections occur by the fecal-oral route. Adults may be infected after close contact with an infected infant. The illness in adults is generally mild. Incubation is 1 to 3 days. Norovirus most commonly infects older children and adults. Infections occur year-round. Norovirus is the principal cause of sporadic viral gastroenteritis in adults and of epidemic viral gastroenteritis in all age groups; large waterborne and food-borne outbreaks occur. Person-to-person transmission also occurs because the virus is highly contagious. Incubation is 24 to 48 h.

Astrovirus can infect people of all ages but usually infects infants and young children. Infection is most common in winter. Transmission is by the fecal-oral route. Incubation is 3 to 4 days.

Adenoviruses are the 4th most common cause of childhood viral gastroenteritis. Infections occur year-round, with a slight increase in summer. Children less than 2 years are primarily affected. Transmission is by the fecal-oral route. Incubation is 3 to 10 days.

In viral infections, watery diarrhea is the most common symptom; stools rarely contain mucus or blood. Rotavirus gastroenteritis in infants and young children may last 5 to 7 days. Vomiting occurs in 90% of patients, and fever more than 39° C (102.2° F) occurs in about 30%. Norovirus typically causes acute onset of vomiting, abdominal cramps, and diarrhea, with symptoms lasting only 1 to 2 days. In children, vomiting is more prominent than diarrhea, whereas in adults, diarrhea usually predominates. Patients may also experience fever, headache, and myalgias. The hallmark of adenovirus gastroenteritis is diarrhea lasting 1 to 2 weeks. Affected infants and children may have mild vomiting that typically starts 1 to 2 days after the onset of diarrhea. Low-grade fever occurs in about 50% of patients. Astrovirus causes a syndrome similar to mild rotavirus infection.

Disease Causing Organisms In Food

Disease	Where You Find It
Campylobacter jejuni	Raw meat and poultry, non-pasteurized milk
E. coli	Raw Beef
Clostridium botulinum	Poorly processed canned low acid foods or vacuum packed smoked fish.
Clostridium perfringens	Food made from poultry or meat
Listeria monocytogenes	Raw meat and sea food, raw milk, some fresh cheeses
Salmonella bacteria	Poultry, meat, eggs, dried foods, dairy products.
Staphylococcus aureus	Custards, salads such as egg, chicken and tuna.

Antibiotics Used For These Bacterial Infections

Organism	Antibiotic	Dose
Vibrio cholerae	Ciprofloxacin Doxycycline	1 g once 300 mg single dose
Clostridium difficile	Metronidazole Vancomycin	500 mg tid for 10 days 125–250 mg qid for 10 days
Shigella	Ciprofloxacin	500 mg po bid for 5 days
Giardia lamblia	Metronidazole Nitazoxanide	250 mg tid for 5 days 500 mg bid for 3 days
Entamoeba histolytica	Metronidazole	750 mg tid for 5–10 days
Campylobacter *jejuni*	Ciprofloxacin Azithromycin	500 mg bid for 5 days 500 mg once/day for 3 days500

Shigellosis

Cause - Shigellosis is an acute infection of the intestine caused by Shigella sp. Shigella is a bacteria that is distributed worldwide and is the cause of inflammatory dysentery for 5 to 10% of diarrheal illness in many areas and kills about 700.000 people per year with 60% of that figure being children. Shigella is divided into 4 major subgroups: A, B, C, and D.

The source of infection is the faeces of infected people or convalescent carriers. Direct spread is by the fecal-oral route. Indirect spread is by contaminated food. Flies serve as vectors. Epidemics occur most frequently in overcrowded populations with inadequate sanitation. Shigellosis is particularly common in younger children living in endemic areas. Adults usually have a less severe disease. Infection imparts little or no immunity.

Disease Process - All species of Shigella cause a acute bloody diarrhea by invading and causing patchy destruction of the colon which leads to the formation of small ulcers and inflammation.

Diagnosis - Diagnosis is confirmed by stool culture. The mucosal surface, as seen through a proctoscope, is red with numerous small ulcers.

Prevention - Hands should be washed thoroughly before handling food, and soiled garments and bedclothes should be immersed in covered buckets of soap and water until they can be boiled. Proper isolation techniques (especially stool isolation) should be used with patients and carriers. Ensure there is safe water to drink and control flies.

Symptoms - Symptoms depend on the strain of bacteria, A, B and C cause a milder illness while D produces the Shiga toxin which causes a more severe and prolonged illness. Symptoms can include fever, nausea, vomiting and diarrhea that is usually bloody. The incubation period is 1 to 4 days. The most common presentation is watery diarrhea; it is indistinguishable from other bacterial, viral, and protozoan infections except maybe by the blood and ulceration. In adults, initial symptoms may be episodes of gripping abdominal pain, urgency to defecate, and passage of formed faces that temporarily relieves the pain. These episodes recur with increasing severity and frequency. Diarrhea becomes marked, with soft or liquid stools containing mucus, pus, and often blood. Rectal prolapse and consequent fecal incontinence may result from severe tenesmus (unproductive painful straining). Sometimes some adults may present without fever, with non blood and no mucoid diarrhea, and with little or no tenesmus. In young children, onset is sudden, with fever, irritability or drowsiness, anorexia, nausea or vomiting, diarrhea, abdominal pain, distension, and tenesmus. Within 3 days, blood, pus, and mucus appear in the stools. The number of stools may increase to more than 20 per day, and weight loss and dehydration become severe. If untreated, a child may die in the first 12 days. If the child survives, acute symptoms subside by the second week.

Prognosis - The disease usually resolves spontaneously in adults, with mild cases in 4 to 8 days, severe cases can take 3 to 6 weeks. Significant dehydration and electrolyte loss with circulatory collapse and death occur mainly in debilitated adults and infants less than 2 years old. Secondary bacterial infections can occur especially in debilitated and dehydrated patients. Other complications are uncommon but can be toxic neuritis, arthritis, myocarditis, and rarely intestinal perforation.

Treatment - Treatment is supportive, mostly with rehydration and antibiotics (Eampicillin or Trimethoprim-sulfamethoxazole). Fluid loss is treated symptomatically with oral or IV fluids Antibiotics can reduce the symptoms and shedding of Shigella but are not necessary for mild illness in healthy adults. However children and the elderly, debilitated and those with severe disease generally should be treated.

Herbal Treatment

Treatment should have begun at the first sign of the symptoms and would of hopefully made the condition a more milder form of the disease. Some of the main herbs for this condition are Goldenseal, Barberry, Baptisia and Yarrow. Let's take a look now at the main herbs used for Dysentery as Dysentery is worse than diarrhea because it is clinically characterized by the presence of mucous and blood in the stool along with abdominal pain and tenesmus. Some of the main herbs for Dysentery are Avens, Bayberry (different from Barberry), Bistort, Black Catechu, Cranesbill, Turmeric and Witch Hazel. With these look at the Anti inflammatorys and Demulcents. Also look at the Carminatives and Antispasmodics so as to try and reduce the tenesmuses. Always monitor the blood loss from the dysentery and if worried crush up a natural type of iron pill and mix it in well with the rehydration formula to allow for maximum absorption. Wild Yam is a good herb for anyone nearly bent double clutching their tummy in pain. A example **Formula Might Be**

Goldenseal - Is a gut antibiotic that focuses on mucous membranes.

Astringent.

Baptisia - For its antimicrobial and lymphatic action.

Licorice - Pushes the formula into body. Demulcent, Antispasmodic anti-inflammatory.

Cranesbill - Our main Astringent, Anti inflammatory

Peppermint - Carminative, Antispasmodic, Analgesic

You could even change the last remedy to something else and you could also give the patient Peppermint and Chamomile tea to help with the abdominal spasms, pains and as part of the rehydration. As this disease might be releasing toxins into the system we can use Vitamin C to act on the toxins so as to hopefully reduce their effect and damage and also consider Echinacea for the same reason.

Homoeopathic Treatment

Dysentery is a more serious form of diarrhea, where the stools are tinged with blood and mucus. Dysentery is inflammation of the bowel resulting from infection. There are two kinds – dysentery caused by a bacterial germ (bacillary dysentery or shigellosis), and amoebic dysentery, caused by an amoeba called Entamoeba histolytica.

Mercurius Corrosvus 6C to 30C - All the preparations of mercury act on the intestines, producing bloody stools with tenesmus, and, of course, all may be indicated in dysentery. Mercurius Corrosivus is the one usually thought of in this affection, as its symptoms corresponds to many severe cases especially the severe and extreme tenesmus; this is the great characteristic of the remedy.

Arsenicum Album 30C - Arsenicum is a valuable remedy in dysentery. There are scanty stools, burning in the rectum, thirst, and after the stool there is great prostration, but there is not the tympanitic distention of the abdomen found under Lycopodium and Carbo vegetabilis; though the patient is restless and thirsty, water is borne badly. Stools which are undigested, slimy and bloody, indicate Arsenicum. Blackish brown, horribly offensive stools also indicate well the remedy. The tenesmus and burning of the anus and rectum continue after stool. If Arsenicum be well indicated its characteristic thirst and restlessness must be present.

Aconite 6C to 30C - In the first stages of dysentery Aconite has proved a useful remedy, and it comes in especially well when the days are warm and the nights are cold. , The stools are frequent and scanty with tenesmus, the skin is hot and dry and general Aconite symptoms are present. Ferrum phosphoricum comes in cases less acute than Aconite; there is more blood with the stool, but tenesmus contra-indicates the remedy. Mercurius follows both well. Belladonna is especially suitable to the dysentery of children and plethoric young persons. Cowperthwaite recommends the 3X.

Cantharis 6C to 30C - This remedy, which produces such an intense vesical tenesmus, also produces a like condition in the rectum. Its characteristics are bloody and slimy discharges which look like the scrapings of the intestines, which are nothing but the fibrous exudations from the disease. Tenesmus is marked, and always with Cantharis there is a painful urination, and there is present a colic-like pain doubling the patient up, being here similar to Colocynth, which has a number of the same symptoms. Thus both have the above symptom of being doubled up by pain, both have slimy and bloody stools, worse from eating or drinking; but under Colocynth the pains cease after stool and the patient is relieved by bending double. Cantharis has more inflammation, Colocynth more nervous symptoms. Colchicum is also similar, the tenesmus and constriction of anus following stool is more tormenting than the urging during stool; tympany also strongly indicates Colchicum. Kali bichromicum follows Cantharis when the scrapings become jelly-like. The thirst with Cantharis is unquenchable.

Sulphur 6C to 30C - For persistent or chronic cases of dysentery Sulphur is the remedy; the tenesmus continues, in fact there is a sort of tenesums all the time, the stools are slimy and there is frequent sudden urging to stool. Sometimes this condition is present without the tenesums. In Nux the tenesums ceases after stool and the pains are relieved for a short time; it is similar to Sulphur in its frequent urging, the stools are bloody, slimy, scanty and watery, and the patient is worse in the morning. Tearing pains down the thighs as an accompaniment of dysentery would indicate Rhus toxicodendron. Great offensiveness of stools and constriction of the anus would suggest Lachesis. Baptisia is useful where there is tenesums but no pain which indicates vital depression, offensive discharges are also present. It is especially useful in dysentery of old people with fevers. Aloes is also a useful remedy in dysentery. The stools are of a jelly-like mucus, and covered with blood and accompanied by griping in the epigastric region, the amount of mucus expelled is large, and, like Sulphur, it is useful in chronic cases. It is also a splendid remedy in purely inflammatory dysentery and follows Aconite well. Ipecac may be useful in cases where large quantities of mucus are expelled. In haemorrhoidal dysentery, which is really a phlebitis of the haemorrhoidal veins, Aloes and Hamamelis are the remedies.

Rotavirus

Cause -Rotavirus is a common and contagious virus that causes vomiting and diarrhea. Rotaviruses are a group of viruses that can cause severe viral gastroenteritis in infants and young children. The incubation period is approximately 2 days. A rotavirus has a characteristic wheel-like appearance when viewed by electron microscopy. Rotaviruses are nonenveloped, double-shelled viruses. The primary mode of transmission is fecal-oral. Because the virus is stable in the environment, transmission can occur through ingestion of contaminated water or food and contact with contaminated surfaces.

Rotavirus is one of the most common causes of diarrhea in children. Worldwide the virus causes over 600,000 deaths a year, mostly in developing countries. By five years of age, almost every child will have been infected with rotavirus.

In temperate climates rotavirus diarrhea occurs in seasonal peaks during cooler months. In tropical climates cases occur throughout the year. Adults can become infected but serious illness is rare.

Disease Process - The primary site of infection is the duodenum and jejunum of the intestinal tract. The mucosal cells that line these areas become infected with the virus and the resultant damage reduces their absorption abilities.

Diagnosis - Samples of stool are sent for a rapid antigen test.

Prevention - Practicing good hygiene is the best preventive measure. A sick child and the people in the household should wash their hands frequently. In addition, a new oral vaccine to prevent rotavirus infection is now recommended to be given at ages 2, 4, and 6 months.

Rotavirus infections are spread when infected people do not wash and dry their hands adequately after going to the toilet. Contaminated hands then spread the virus to other people and surfaces that may be touched by others. Hands can become contaminated while changing the nappy of an infected infant.

Symptoms - Onset is often sudden and the illness mainly affects infants and young children under 3 years of age. The disease is characterized by vomiting and watery diarrhea for 3 to 8 days, and fever and abdominal pain occur frequently. If fluid losses are not replaced, dehydration develops. Dehydration makes the child weak and listless, with a dry mouth and rapid pulse. Immunity after infection is incomplete, but repeated infections tend to be less severe. Adults can also be infected, though disease tends to be mild.

Prognosis - Most children will recover on their own if provided with adequate fluid replacement. However some children will become very ill and require hospitalization for rehydration treatment. Severe diarrhea and dehydration occurs mainly among children 3 to 35 months of age.

Treatment - There is no specific treatment for rotavirus. Most children get better with fluid replacement by mouth. Seriously ill children require intravenous fluids. About one in 40 children with rotavirus gastroenteritis will require hospitalization for intravenous fluids. As the diarrhea subsides the child can be moved to a BRATY diet which consists of, Bananas, Rice, cereal, Apple sauce, Toast and Yoghurt. These foods are easy to digest and gives the tummy a bit of a rest.

Herbal Treatment

Follow the directions given in The Acute Treatment Of Disease. It was reported recently in a medical journal that Tormentil *(Potentilla tormentilla a good Astringent)* was of benefit to take in Rotavirus. Those taking tormentil root extract had a shorter duration of diarrhea and did not require as much intravenous or oral rehydration fluids. In another study published in 2001, Stevia was found to have antiviral effects against the rotavirus. Secondly, Stevia shows a strong ability to kill a wide range of food-borne bacteria. With this being mainly a child's disease we will try to use the herbs more suitable for children with the best 3 for this condition being Agrimony, Chamomile and Peppermint. Agrimony is a specific for childhood diarrhea It is Astringent, Cholagogue and a good tonic herb. Chamomile with its Anti-inflammatory and Carminative actions is a specific for childhood gastritis. Peppermint will help on the side of vomiting and fever being Antiemetic, Diaphoretic and also a Carminative. These two herbs are both pain killers. The strong Astringents for this condition are Cranesbill and Witch Hazel which should control the condition, add your other herbs to one of these. You could consider giving a tea of any mixture of these herbs sweetened with Stevia and maybe honey as part of the rehydration treatment as well.

Homoeopathic Treatment

Aethusa Cynapium 6C to 30C - Describes a situation of violence, violent vomiting, violent diarrhoea, violent abdominal colic. This remedy is frequently used in children especially those who collapse easily and will probably need medical attention, Intolerance to milk, face shows anxiety and pain.

Argentum Nitricum 6c to 30C - Is quite similar to Arsenic in many ways. The stools are green, slimy and bloody, like chopped spinach in flakes, with the stool there is a discharge of flatus and much spluttering, the stools are worse from any candy, sugar, or from drinking. The children are thin, dried up looking, and it seems as if the child had but one bowel and that extended from the mouth to the anus. Another characteristic is its use in diarrhea brought on by great mental excitement, emotional disturbance, etc.

Arsenicum Album 30C - Sufferers can have vomiting and diarrhea at the same time, restless, anxious, feels very cold, great prostration after diarrhea, burning pains, symptoms worse between midnight and 2am. Thirst for small quantities and often.

China 6C to 30C - The characteristic Cinchona diarrhea is a painless one, of a cadaverous odor. It is slimy, bilious, blackish and mixed with undigested food; it is worse at night and after eating, with a rapid exhaustion and emaciation, diarrhea is worse after eating

Croton Tiglium 6C to 30C - Is one of the great homoeopathic remedies for diarrhea. Its characteristics are a yellowish, watery stool pouring out like water from a hydrant, and especially associated with nausea and vomiting and aggravated by eating and drinking and to this we may add the quite common accompaniment of nausea, preceded by a little pain in the abdomen, diarrhea associated with a lot of anal urging. worse by the slightest touch.

Ipecacuanha 6C to 30C - Constant nausea with vomiting, the diarrhea smells offensive and contains a lot of undigested food

Phosphorous 6C to 30C - It has green mucous stools worse in the morning, often undigested and painless. The stools pass as soon as they enter the rectum, and contain white particles like rice or tallow. Diarrhea that causes a burning sensation when being passed. One of the characteristics of Phosphorous is the vomiting of what has been drunk as soon as it becomes warm in the stomach.

Sulphur 6C to 30C - The diarrhea of sulphur is very characteristic. It has changeable stools, yellow, watery, slimy, and in scrofulous (lack of resistance) children may contain undigested food. It is worse in the morning about four or five O'clock, when it wakens the patient and drives him out of bed in great haste. The whole remedy picture is full of burning sensations, the anus becomes red and itches a lot. Patients easily become hot and stick feet out of bed clothes to cool down.

Aloes 6C to 30C - Aloes is a remedy whose chief action is on the rectum. It produces a constant desire to stool, and the passages are accompanied with a great deal of flatus. The great characteristic of the drug feeling of uneasiness, weakness, and certainly about the rectum; there is a constant feeling as if stool would escape, the patient dares not pass flatus for fear of the escape of faeces. This condition is met with in children sometimes; they pass faeces when passing flatus. The stool themselves are yellow and pasty or lumpy and watery, and before the stool there are griping pains across the lower part of the abdomen and around the navel. These pains also continue during stool and passage usually relieves them. The essentials are, the lumpy, watery stool, the intense griping across the lower parts of the abdomen before and during stool, leaving after stool, and the extreme prostration and perspiration following.

Norovirus

Causes - Noroviruses are a group of viruses that can cause gastroenteritis with diarrhea, stomach pain and vomiting. They are found in the faces or vomit of infected people. People can become infected with the virus in several ways, including eating food or liquids that are contaminated, touching surfaces or objects contaminated and then placing their hand in their mouth, small airborne particles from projectile vomiting; having direct contact with another person who is infected and showing symptoms or sharing foods or eating utensils with someone who is ill. There are many different strains of norovirus, which makes it difficult for a person's body to develop long-lasting immunity. Therefore, norovirus illness can recur throughout a person's lifetime. These viruses thrive on cruise ships because they are very hardy and highly contagious. They can survive temperature extremes in water and on surfaces.

Disease Process - Once someone is infected from contaminated food, the virus can quickly pass from person to person through shared food or utensils, by shaking hands or through other close contact. A day or two after being exposed to the virus typical symptoms may be nausea, vomiting (more often in children), watery diarrhea (more often in adults), and stomach cramps.

Diagnosis - Specific diagnosis of norovirus is routinely made by polymerase chain reaction (PCR) assays or real-time PCR assays, which give results within a few hours

Prevention - People working in day-care centers or nursing homes should pay special attention to children or residents who have norovirus illness. This virus is very contagious and can spread rapidly throughout such environments. Both faeces and vomit are infectious. Particular care should be taken with young children in nappies who may have diarrhea. People infected with norovirus are contagious from the moment they begin feeling ill. It is important for people to continue to use good hand washing and other hygienic practices. People infected with norovirus should not prepare food while they have symptoms and for 48 hours after they recover from their illness. Infections occur year-round.

Treatment - Currently, there is no antiviral medication that works against norovirus and there is no vaccine to prevent infection.

Symptoms - Symptoms of illness usually begin about 24 to 48 hours after ingestion of the virus, but they can appear as early as 12 hours after exposure. Illness usually includes nausea, vomiting, diarrhea, and some stomach cramping. Sometimes people also have a low-grade fever, chills, headache, muscle aches, and a general sense of tiredness. The illness often begins suddenly, and the infected person may feel very sick. The illness is usually brief, with symptoms lasting only about 1 or 2 days, but can last longer. In general, children experience more vomiting than adults. Dehydration is the most serious health effect that can result from norovirus infection, and it is a particular concern in young children, the elderly, and people with weakened immune systems.

Prognosis - Norovirus is usually not serious, although people may feel very sick and vomit many times a day most people get better within 1 or 2 days, and they have no long-term health effects related to their illness. The main complication to watch out for and treat is dehydration.

Herbal Treatment

With this condition we have to treat it as we see the symptoms and as it affects the young and old the most we have to choose the more gentle herbs. Consider Ginger and Peppermint for the nausea and vomiting. Licorice can be considered for its anti-viral, anti-inflammatory and demulcent actions as well as its flavoring. Think of Chamomile for tummy pains and cramps and also for calming children. Agrimony is the main specific for childhood diarrhea though also consider Meadowsweet especially if the condition feels acidy.

Homoeopathic Treatment

Arsenicum Album 30C - Arsenicum is a valuable remedy in dysentery. Vomiting and diarrhea with great mental restlessness and anxiety with profound fear of death. Thirst for small sips of water thirst, after the stool Burning pain after stool. Aggravated by sight, smell or even the thought of food. Exhaustion which can be sudden and extreme. There can be a faint feeling, with a fever alternating chills. Cold sweat on forehead during and prostration after. Worse after midnight. Good remedy for food poisoning. If Arsenicum be well indicated its characteristic thirst and restlessness must be present.

Chamomilla 30C - Along with the vomiting will be diarrhea that looks greenish. You may feel very irritable and contrary.

Ipecac 30C - Nausea and vomiting predominate when Ipecac is needed. Constant nausea and frequent vomiting, however vomiting gives no relief from the nausea, worse at night. Sleepy after vomiting. Worse for any movement, after eating and for smell of food. Hot or cold sweat. Stomach feels relaxed, as if hanging down; clutching, squeezing, griping, as from a hand, each finger sharply pressing into intestines; worse from motion. Flatulent, cutting colic about umbilicus. The tongue will be clean, not coated.

Phosphorus 30C - Frequent vomiting. Great thirst for water and ice cold drinks but vomits up shortly afterwards. Vomits even the smallest amount of food and drink. Vomiting will often occur 15 minutes after drinking. Diarrhea gushes out painlessly. Has green mucous stools worse in the morning, often undigested and painless. The stools pass as soon as they enter the rectum, and contain white particles like rice or tallow. Diarrhea that causes a burning sensation when being passed. One of the characteristics of Phosphorous is the vomiting of what has been drunk as soon as it becomes warm in the stomach.

Podophyllum 6C to 30C - Painless diarrhea. Diarrhea worse early in morning continues through forenoon, and accompanied by sensation of weakness. Fear he is going to be very ill. Diarrhea like gushing out. Thirst for large quantities of cold water. The tongue is coated white or yellow.

Veratrum Album 30C - Copious vomiting and nausea; worse least motion. Great weakness after vomiting. Nausea, with profuse salivation and violent thirst. Vomiting with suffocating sensation, redness and heat in face. Cold feeling in stomach and abdomen. Stomach as if weak, with internal sensation of coldness. Diarrhea is frequent, watery, gushing; cutting pain in stomach; prostrating, cold sweat on forehead during and prostration after. Excessive vomiting with nausea and great prostration; worse after drinking and by motion; great weakness after.

Cholera

It is a highly contagious disease that is transmitted by contaminated food, water and flies. Cholera can be very aggressive and kill within 24 hours if not treated. The disease is very common in tropical countries in Asia, South America and Africa but can occur as epidemics in the colder countries generally starting when it heats up.. In the river deltas of India and Bangladesh cholera remains endemic and may cause up to 500,000 deaths a year. Cholera often affects large numbers of people especially after natural disasters when the water becomes contaminated. Cholera is characterized by purging, muscular cramps and rapid collapse.

Causes - Caused by ingesting food or water contaminated with the bacteria Vibrio Cholerae. Cholera epidemics spread easily in areas where human faces pollute the water supply. Shellfish and plankton may serve as a natural reservoir.

Disease Process - Cholera bacteria that survive the stomach acid bath invade the small intestines and then start producing a toxin that inflames the intestinal walls and causes the body to release tremendous amounts of water. Untreated Cholera has a 50 percent death rate.

Diagnosis - Is by a sample of stool checked for the bacteria. Diagnosis is easier in epidemics while in sporadic cases confusion can arise.

Prevention - The main method of stopping the spread of cholera is to stop the drinking water becoming contaminated with sewage. People who have Cholera must be quarantined or isolated and all of their waste products must be burned or disinfected. Patient's utensils and clothing must also be sterilized after each use so as to prevent disease transmission to others. Travelers into the area must be Vaccinated (only lasts a few months) and bring their own water and food.

Symptoms - We will divide the symptoms into stages. The first stage is **The Stage Of Evacuation**. Cholera begins with a few loose stools usually within hours turning into severe diarrhea or purging, vomiting which often becomes incessant, muscular cramps especially in the legs which may become agonizing, progressive exhaustion, thirst becomes extreme, stools at first yellow become like rice water when frequent they become odorless, temperature drops below normal, exhaustion and collapse increase. With the purging the body can lose as much as a liter of fluid an hour. With adequate fluid replacement severe cases can lose up to 20 liters per day.

Stage Of Collapse - The face looks pinched with the eyes sunken and the skin wrinkled, there is restlessness and maybe cyanosis, clammy perspiration, semi consciousness or coma, involuntary passing of watery motions. Pulse rapid or hard to find. If the body loses to much fluid shock and death result from loss of blood pressure and the thickening of the blood, then the temperature starts to falls and the organs start to fail. Death can occur in 24 hours without treatment.

Stage Of Conclusion - In favorable cases there is rapid improvement, consciousness returns, skin becomes warm, bile appears in the motions and the motions become less frequent. There is usually some fever and erythema is common. Some people can be infected and show no symptoms these are known as carriers. The illness subsides spontaneously in 3 to 6 days. Infection with V. cholerae gives long term immunity to the disease.

Prognosis - Unfavorable with very rapid onset and low temperature.

Treatment - Bed rest and warmth. The main treatment is to replace the fluids as quickly as possible using a rehydration formula so as to replace the sugars and salts. A simple oral rehydration formula is a table spoon of sugar and a tea spoon of salt to a pint of water (600mls), Give water by mouth frequently and in small amounts. If this cannot be done fast enough orally then it can be done intravenously. Antibiotics can help shorten the duration of the disease.

Herbal Treatment
Follow directions as given in The Acute Treatment Of Disease. Below is a well-documented formula used in the treatment of Cholera, it is made by combining the following herbal tinctures in equal quantities.

Prickly Ash
Ginger
Bayberry
Oregon Mountain Grape or Coptis Chinensis
Cranesbill
Cayenne
Dosage of this formula is 2 tsp to 1 tbsp in water every 4 hours

These herbs contain the Actions of Stimulants, Astringents, Antibacterials, Antispasmodics, Carminatives, Diaphoretics and many more but the first are the main actions we need for this disease. Other Cholera Specific herbs are Barberry, Garlic, Galangal, Geranium, Goldenseal, Grapefruit Seed, Juniper, Prickly Ash, Saffron, Sandalwood,

Homoeopaths have traditionally used tincture of Camphor for the prevention of Cholera the dose is 2 drops of tincture in a teaspoon of sugar without water.

Another preventative is the juice of lemon or lime which can kill **cholera** bacilli within a very short time so consider adding this to the rehydration formula. Onions have also been used in the past for the treatment of cholera. For this grind about 30 gm of onions to pulp with 5 to 7 black peppers dose as an infusion twice a day.

Homoeopathic Treatment

Arsenicum Album 30C - Debility, exhaustion, restlessness, fear and worry, burning pains, cannot bear the sight or smell of food, nausea, retching, vomiting after eating or drinking, Cholera with intense agony, prostration and burning thirst, body cold as ice, cramps in calves, worse after midnight and cold foods and drinks, better from heat and warm drinks.

Camphora 30C - One of the specifics for Cholera in the first stages. Sudden sinking of strength, pulse small and weak, sudden attacks of vomiting and diarrhea, cold, low blood pressure, appears anxious, face bluish, cholera with cramps in the calves, great weakness, collapse, insomnia, extreme restlessness, worse at night and with motion, does not like cold air, better for warmth.

Carbo Veg 30C - The typical carbo patient is fat, sluggish and lazy and has a tendency of chronic complaints. Body becomes blue and icy cold, for states of collapse in Cholera, must have fresh air, bluish appearance, abdomen greatly distended, desire to be constantly fanned. This remedy has been known from it use in plagues as the corpse restorer.

Cuprum Met 30C - Use for the spasmodic stage, the specific for cholera with cramps in the calves and abdomen, painful cramps in the calves, bluish appearance, frequent vomiting, nausea, has a strong metallic taste in the mouth, neuralgia of abdominal viscera, worse from vomiting, better from cold water.

Ipecac 30C - For the first symptoms of cholera where vomiting and nausea predominate. Persistent nausea and vomiting, cutting pains across the abdomen.

Veratrum Album 30C - This is the third specific for Cholera. A perfect picture of collapse with coldness, blueness and weakness, vomiting, purging, cramps in the extremities. Face very pale, blue, collapsed and cold. thirst for cold water but is vomited as soon as swallowed, cold feeling in abdomen, diarrhea forcefully evacuated followed by great prostration sometimes coming out of both ends at the same time, worse at night, better for warmth.

Typhoid Fever

Typhoid fever and Paratyphoid are similar diseases but the second is milder then the first and caused by a slightly different bacteria though they both can be called Enteric Fever. The disease can be characterized by inflammation, fever and generally by sloughing of Peyer's glands, swelling of the mesentery and engorgement of the spleen.

Historically the disease seems to prefer autumn and prefers it victims between 10 to 30 years of age.

Causes - Typhoid is spread mainly through the ingestion of food and water contaminated with S.typhi especially dairy products and shellfish. The bacteria can survive in water for up to 2 weeks and can survive in ice. It lives and multiplies in milk without changing the appearance. There are human carriers of this disease mainly older women who have had gallbladder damage in the past as this is the area that S. typhi colonizes in carriers. Infected food handlers can spread the disease as well. Throughout history Armies and refugees have been susceptible to Typhoid but in modern countries with sewage control and control of milk production the disease has now become rare.

Disease Process - Once the bacteria make it to the small intestines they attack what is known as the Peyers Patches which are small lymphatic opening running along the small intestines, through these they gain access to the bodies lymphatic system and travel to the liver and from there to the blood stream infecting macrophages in the lymph nodes, bone marrow and spleen.

Diagnosis - The beginning stage gives us our main clues, one, two, or three weeks of listlessness, tiredness, headache, loss of appetite, general depression and maybe blood nose, with these progressively increasing until the patient takes to bed, are the most characteristic symptoms of this fever, and the regular step-ladder rise in temperature with daily remissions, the peculiar dullness of intellect, the marked prostration. If to this we add tenderness and gurgling in the right iliac region, enlargement of the spleen, diarrhea, the presence of the rash the diagnosis is complete. Typhoid should be suspected in temperate climates if a fever lasts a week without falling.

Prevention - The Homoeopathic remedies Baptisia and Pyrogen may abort this disease

Symptoms - Be aware that the Typhoid toxins are slowly poisoning the system and may sometimes attack one system more then another such as the lungs, kidneys or the nervous system, this can be confusing when trying to diagnose. In describing the symptoms we will use the old method and go through the stages. The first stage is **The Stage Of Incubation** - commonly 10 to 15 days usually with no symptoms but the patient can start getting tired, depressed, not refreshed from sleep and maybe headaches come on. The next stage is the **Period Of Onset** - Initial symptoms can be varied and include headache which can become severe and persistent, malaise, blood nose, abdominal pain, loss of appetite, diarrhea or constipation, chilly sensations, pains in the joints, bronchitis and a daily stepwise elevation in the temperature up to 105 degrees or more in the coming weeks. Pulse rate can be slow compared with the temperature. The day the patient puts themselves to bed is regarded as the first day of the first week. Between the 7th and 10th day two important events can occur, the spleen becomes enlarged and a rash appears on the abdomen or chest. **Second Week** - Headache goes, pale face with a dull expression and an occasional flush with dilated pupils and dry lips. Can be deafness, temperature remains constantly high, dry tongue, abdominal pains increase, can have obstinate constipation or if dysentery it looks like pea soup. Delirium in severe cases especially at night. Death may occur with pronounced nervous symptoms. Hemorrhage and perforation may occur towards the end of the week. **Third Week** - In ordinary cases symptoms remains the same as the previous week, loss of flesh and weakness is now marked, in the mild cases the symptoms begin to subside. In severe cases other problems like pneumonia or perforation of the small intestine can set in. **Fourth Week** - In ordinary cases convalescence begins, appetite returns and temperature becomes normal, general condition is extremely weak. Patient can recover over the next 2 to 8 weeks.

Prognosis - Is good for those without complications, a severe onset is not a good sign. Mortality is higher in hot weather especially in the obese or those with preexisting conditions or diseases such as diabetes or alcoholism.

Treatment - Confine to bed until covalence which is about three weeks after the temperature becomes normal. Good nursing is essential, keep turning over to prevent bed sores. Only give very easily digestible foods which are nourishing and are low in fat as it is the lymphatic system that transports the fat from the intestines, diarrhea needs stricter dieting. Give plenty of fluids. After the temperature has been normal for 3 days start to very slowly get the diet back to normal over a week or more. Try to keep temperature to safe levels during fever. If untreated 10 to 20 % of patients die usually of complications such as pneumonia.

Herbal Treatment

Follow the directions given in The Acute Treatment Of Disease. If this has been done hopefully this will now be a milder form of the disease. The specifics for this disease are Echinacea and Baptisia. As this is such a long and drawn out disease you will have to think in the actions needed as different symptoms come and pass especially if the disease moves into other body systems such as The Respiratory System (Pleurisy Root), but always keep in mind that it is the toxins (Vitamin C) of the bacteria traveling through the blood that is our main problem so for whatever action you choose try to find a herb that also has the Actions of a Alterative or a Antimicrobial along with the Action or Actions you require at the time. One of the main groups of herbs we should look at is the Lymphatic herbs as this disease is using the Lymphatic system to get into the body. The best herb to choose from here is Calendula for the following reasons, this herb is used for wounds and to stop bleeding along with being a major germicide so all these actions will be having a direct effect on the wounds on the Peyers Patches in the small intestines, this herb also has an action on the liver and is a lymphatic so as you can see a lot of this herbs actions focus on the areas we need. Passion Flower is a good herb that can be used to help induce sleep if needed. Herbs in the past that have been used for Typhoid are Baptisia, Bayberry, Eucalyptus, Fringe Tree, Garlic, Ginkgo, Horehound, Juniper, Magnolia, Pleurisy Root, Prickly Ash.

Homoeopathic Treatment

Arnica 3 to 30C - Arnica frequently fits this disease. It has many symptoms common to Baptisia and Rhus, yet its individual symptoms are marked. It is a remedy that is not so likely to be indicated early as Baptisia. There is a stupor, and indifference to everything, patients do not know that they are sick, and care less; they go to sleep while answering questions; the head is hot the body cool, and all over there is a bruised feeling; the patient tosses about the bed to find a soft spot; the stools and urine are in involuntary; there are bed sores, petechiae appear all over the body; finally a condition of stupor arrives characterized by dropping of lower jaw. Worse from touch and motion.

Arsenicum Album 30C - This is one of the remedies for typhoid fever when the case begins to looks "bad"; but it is hardly ever indicated in the beginning of the disease. The terrible prostration so characteristic is accompanied by irritability and anxiety. The patient is faint and weak, exhausted, perhaps with cold sweat and delirium; the mouth and teeth are covered with sordes; the mouth is sore; there is a diarrhea of dark, offensive stools, intense fever and the characteristic Arsenicum thirst. Like Rhus, there is restlessness, but it is rather a "prostrated restlessness" than a "rheumatic restlessness." All the symptoms of Arsenicum are worse after midnight. An extremely red tongue has always been a guiding and characteristic symptoms of this remedy. Worse from cold drinks, Better Heat.

Baptisia 6C - Use from 6C and upward in potency. Perhaps no remedy presents a clearer picture of a typical case of typhoid fever than Baptisia which is also the main herbal remedy for this condition as well. Baptisia suits poisoned blood conditions, and is applicable to any stage of the disease, a dull, dark besotted countenance. Has a drowsy, stupid state, has a black or brownish coated tongue, patient falls asleep while answering questions, bed feels too hard, seems as if intoxicated this is very characteristic. The patient feels tired and bruised all over; is restless, and tosses about the bed to find a soft spot, but his restlessness is rather due to the mental rather than to the physical condition. Delirium is often present, profound prostration; the breath is fetid, and all exhalations and discharges from the patient are exceedingly offensive. The temperature is high, and so is the pulse, and there is tenderness in the ileo-caecal region. If the characteristic expression of countenance, the characteristic mental condition and the characteristic offensiveness of all discharges are taken into consideration.

Bryonia 12 to 30C - This is one of the great typhoid fever remedies, and is sooner or later, indicated in a majority of cases of the disease. The characteristic symptoms are great soreness over the body, tired feeling, irritable, every exertion fatigues, dread of all motion. A splitting ,agonizing frontal headache, worse from motion. The face gets red towards evening. There is a fullness of the head in the morning, which is followed by nose bleed. The patient drinks large quantities at long intervals. This thirst of Bryonia, when present is characteristic. The bowels are generally constipated; indeed some writers claim that Bryonia ceases to be of value when diarrhea sets in. Most pains feel like stitching and tearing and are better from motion. Worse from warmth, morning and motion, Better from pressure, lying on painful side

Gelsemium 30C - A remedy often indicated in the first stage especially in mild cases. The patient feels sore and bruised all over, as if pounded, there is also a dread of motion, headache, drowsiness, red face; the nervous symptoms are predominant., lack of muscular coordination. Patient is characteristically dull and apathetic, looks and feels as if going to have a fit of sickness; but does not care much, never worries over condition. Drooping eyelids is characteristic, it shows general languor and malaise. There is chilliness, full and flowing pulse. Gelsemium usually precedes Baptisia, its symptoms being similar but milder. Baptisia leads when soreness is most prominent, and Gelsemium when prostration is most marked. The mind is clouded with Baptisia, not so much so with Gelsemium.

Rhus Tox 6 to 30C - Restlessness and muscular soreness, all of which are found under Baptisia, but the restlessness of Rhus is to relieve the muscular soreness. The mental symptoms of Rhus in this disease are a muttering delirium, and, perhaps, refusal to take the medicine for fear of being poisoned. The imagination is active. There is often headache and nosebleed, which relieves the headache. There is diarrhea of yellowish-brown stools of offensive odor which may be involuntary. The abdomen is tympanitic and sensitive over the ileo-caecal region. There are pains in the back and limbs. It is especially indicated for backache that is severe. The spleen is also sensitive. There is apt to be, when Rhus is indicated, some pulmonary congestion. The characteristics are the restlessness, the red-tipped tongue, the offensive discharges the trembling of the chin and involuntary stools. Worse from cold and rest, Better from warmth and motion.

Giardia

Causes - Giardiasis is a infection with the flagellated protozoa Giardia lamblia. Waterborne infection is the major source of giardiasis. Transmission can also occur by direct person-to-person contact, especially in institutions and day care centers or between sex partners. Symptoms appear on average 7 days after infection. Giardia cysts remain viable in surface water and are resistant to routine levels of chlorination. Wild animals may also serve as reservoirs. Thus, mountain streams as well as chlorinated but poorly filtered municipal water supply systems have been found to be the cause of outbreaks. Many cases are asymptomatic. However, asymptomatic people can pass infective cysts.

Disease Process - Giardia protozoa firmly attach themselves to the small intestines and begin to multiply usually every 5 hours. In prolonged infections it destroys the villi of the small intestines which are responsible for absorbing food and malnutrition can be a result. Some organisms transform into environmentally resistant cysts that are spread by the fecal-oral route.

Diagnosis - Diagnosis is by identifying the organism in fresh stool. Characteristic trophozoites or cysts in stool are diagnostic, but parasite excretion is infrequent and at low levels in chronic infections. Thus, diagnosis may require repeated stool examinations.

Prevention - For asymptomatic infections, metronidazole is the drug used. Water can be decontaminated by boiling. Giardia cysts resist routine levels of chlorination. Disinfection with iodine-containing compounds is variably effective and depends on the turbidity and temperature of the water and duration of treatment. Good sanitary practices can help avoid the onset of giardiasis, simple steps such as cleaning the hands and fingers well with soap and water before touching foodstuffs or before meals are a very effective way to counteract the possibility of giardiasis. Other sanitary steps can also be taken. While washing and drying oneself, a simple option is to use a single dedicated towel as a personal toilet item without sharing it with anyone else.

Symptoms - Infection can be asymptomatic or cause symptoms ranging from intermittent flatulence to chronic malabsorption. Symptoms of acute giardiasis generally appear 1 to 2 weeks after infection. They are usually mild and include watery malodorous diarrhea, abdominal bloating, greasy stools that tend to float, abdominal cramps and distension, flatulence and eructation, intermittent nausea, epigastric discomfort, and sometimes low-grade malaise and anorexia. Acute giardiasis usually lasts 1 to 3 weeks. Malabsorption of fat and sugars can lead to significant weight loss especially for children in severe cases. A small group of infected patients develop a more chronic form of the disease with diarrhea of foul stools from failure to absorb digested food, abdominal distension, and malodorous flatus. Substantial weight loss may occur. Chronic giardiasis occasionally causes failure to thrive in children.

Treatment - Take care of dehydration and ensure the patient doesn't become malnourished. For symptomatic infections the drugs used are Metronidazole or Tinidazole which is as effective as, and less toxic than, metronidazole. Nitazoxanide is available in liquid form for children.

Herbal Treatment

Goldenseal and Barberry are the main herbs for this condition as they contain the chemical berberine which is active against Giardia. Barberry is listed as Anthelmintic and Amoebicidal while Goldenseal is not. Other herbs used for this condition are Grape Fruit Seed and Papaya. Protozoa are single-celled organisms that can multiply within the body, while worms can't multiply in the human body, which means that they usually clear up with treatment without reinfecting you. So with Giardia you have got to be sure that you have killed them all so we shall continue the attack via the diet.

These are some dietary recommendations often suggested to support the intestinal parasite cleansing process: Temporarily avoid coffee, refined sugar, alcohol, and refined foods. Eat anti-parasitic foods. Try eating more raw garlic. Pineapple contains the digestive enzyme bromelain. A diet rich in pineapple can help to clear certain parasites such as tapeworms. Papaya seeds contain enzymes that help to digest protein. They can be chewed, but watch out, they are as hot as mustard seeds. Carrots, sweet potatoes, and squash are some foods that are rich in beta carotene, a precursor for vitamin A. Vitamin A is thought to increase resistance to penetration by larvae. Vitamin C and zinc also support the immune system. Probiotics such as Lactobacillus acidophilus, Bifidobacteria, and L. bulgaricus can help to rebuild beneficial intestinal bacteria. Now go look at the Action of Anthelmintics and start adding some of the herbs listed there to the diet especially Garlic and Wormwood.

Homoeopathic Treatment

I have only given 2 remedies as Giardia is a living parasite so here it's better to concentrate on destroying the cause rather than on the end results.

China 6C to 30C - The diarrhea of this remedy has a lot of wind associated with it. The abdomen is often bloated with gas, this may be trapped or passed easily up or down but the person feels no relief for letting it go. Stools are passed with a lot of gas, spluttering and spraying. They are often yellow, frothy and watery. They smell foul and may also contain undigested food; the stools may also be bloody. Good for the intestinal protozoan parasite called Giardia. As the diarrhea progresses the person may become greatly weakened due to the loss of fluids, they become cold, sweaty and drowsy. The person is worse for touch or examination, noise and pressure on the abdomen. They feel better for bending double and warmth. The symptoms may also show periodicity e.g. the diarrhea seems to get better then worse on alternate days.

Colocynthis 6C to 30C - This is another common diarrhea remedy. It has a lot of abdominal pains associated with it; they can be violent, cutting, gripping, grasping, clutching or radiating and colicky. All of the pains come in waves over the person. The patient is often very thirsty. The stools are frothy, watery, yellowish and often passed with a lot of flatulence. The person feels worse for the least food, but better for doubling over clutching the abdomen or rubbing it quite firmly. Gentle motion, perhaps rocking, makes them feel better too.

Cryptosporidiosis

Cause - Cryptosporidiosis is infection with Cryptosporidium. Cryptosporidia are protozoa that replicate in the small-bowel epithelial cells. C. parvum and C. hominis are responsible for most human cases. Infections results from fecally contaminated food, water or surfaces, direct person-to-person contact, or zoonotic spread especially from farm animals into rivers and lakes especially after strong rains. The disease occurs worldwide.

Disease Process - After replication in the small intestines infective oocysts are shed into the lumen and passed in stool. After ingestion by another vertebrate, the oocyst releases sporozoites that transform into trophozoites in epithelial cells, replicate, and then produce oocysts that are released into the lumen of the intestine to complete the cycle. Thin-walled oocysts are involved in autoinfection.

Diagnosis - Identifying the oocysts in stool confirms the diagnosis, but conventional methods of stool examination are unreliable. Oocyst excretion is intermittent, and multiple stool samples may be needed.

Prevention - Stools of patients with cryptosporidiosis are highly infectious; strict stool precautions should be observed along with good personal hygiene. Boiling water is the most reliable decontamination method. Wash and peel foods and always wash hands before preparing food.

Symptoms - The primary symptom is watery diarrhea often with other signs of GI distress such as stomach cramps. Illness is typically self-limited in healthy patients. The incubation period is about 1 week, with clinical illness occurring in 80% of infected people. Onset is acute, with profuse watery diarrhea, abdominal cramping, and less commonly, nausea, anorexia, vomiting, fever, and malaise.

Prognosis - Symptoms generally persist 1 to 2 weeks and then abate. Fecal excretion of oocysts may continue for several weeks after symptoms have subsided. Asymptomatic shedding of oocysts is common among older children in developing countries.

Treatment - Treatment, when necessary, is with Nitazoxanid but it is usually only used for immune impaired people. Look out for and treat dehydration.

Herbal Treatment

Herbal treatment is the same as Giardia as this is also a protozoa parasite infection to. Here are some more Antiprotozoal Herbs - Albizia lebbeck, Barberry, Calendula, Chinchona and Garlic.

Homoeopathic Treatment

This is the same as Giardia.

Leptospirosis

Cause - Leptospirosis includes all infections caused by Leptospira. Leptospirosis is a bacterial animal disease occurring in many domestic and wild animals that people can get, it may cause unapparent illness or a serious, even fatal, disease. Warm moist environments favor the survival of the bacterial spirochetes so the incidence of this disease is greater in the tropics. A carrier state exists in which animals shed leptospires in their urine for months. Dogs and rats and farm animals are common probable sources. Human infections are acquired by direct contact with infected urine or tissue, or indirectly by contact with contaminated water or soil. Abraded skin and exposed mucous membranes (conjunctival, nasal, oral) are the usual entry portals into the body. The incubation period ranges from 2 to 20 (usually 7 to 13) days.

Diagnosis - Diagnosis is by darkfield microscopy, culture, and serology. Similar symptoms can result from viral meningoencephalitis and other spirochetal infections. Leptospirosis should be considered in any patient with fevers of a unknown origin who might have been exposed to leptospires and with a reddish coloration of the conjunctiva

Prevention - Cover wounds and always wear shoes in suspect areas. Remove food wastes to keep rodents away, always drink boiled water.

Symptoms - You can get a mild or severe form of this disease with only about 10% getting the severe form. There are 2 phases with the septicemic phase starting abruptly, with headache, severe muscular aches, chills, and fever sometimes with kidney or lung problems. There is a reddish coloration of the conjunctiva which can be used to confirm diagnosis that usually appears on the 3rd or 4th day. This phase lasts 4 to 9 days, with recurrent chills and fever that often spikes to more than 39° C. and then the fever drops. Then all of a sudden the symptoms can get better or disappear for a few days and then the second phase of the disease begins. The second or immune, phase occurs between the 6th and 12th day of illness and means it is a more severe infection. Fever and earlier symptoms recur, and sometimes includes hepatic, renal, and meningeal involvement.

The severest form of the disease is called Weil's Syndrome which has the same as the first but is more severe and is likely to have complications with the liver and kidneys. With liver problems jaundice will come on and the whites of the eyes may go yellow while with the kidney problems urine output will decrease and may even stop and there would be edema seen in the face and feet, with lung involvement there could be in mild cases coughing which on getting worse leads to coughing of blood an then breathing problems. There can be bleeding problems with this disease such as petechial (flat small spots on the skin), nose bleeds and bleeding from the lungs.

Prognosis - Mortality is nil in patients with the mild form. With jaundice, the mortality rate is 5 to 10%; it is higher in patients over 60 years.

Treatment - Treatment is with Doxycycline or Penicillin.

Herbal Treatment

This is one disease where you should start treatment as mentioned in Disease Fighting Herbs right away for you definitely do not want to deal with the complications of this disease, you want it to run the mildest course possible and end soon. This is a hard disease to treat as it involves lots of different body systems and Actions along with having a bleeding problem (Astringents) in most body systems as well. Good herbs to start with are Boneset and Guaiacum as they are both Diaphoretics (fever) and good for muscle aches and pains. The bacteria in this disease must be cruising the blood stream to have such an effect on so many different body systems so we will attack it with Antibiotic Alteratives with our main one being Garlic because it's all these as well as being a Diaphoretic. Other to consider are Baptisia and Echinacea. Guaiacum is also an Alterative. Think of Milk Thistle for protecting the liver especially if the disease heads in that direction. For the Kidneys think of Cleavers as this will help with the skin as well. For problems with the eye think of Eye Bright. Another worry about this disease is what it must do to the inside of blood vessels especially capillaries when you consider its bruising like effects on the skin so we shall also think about the herb Yarrow which helps with fevers, circulation and wound healing as well as having a strong Action on the urinary system.

Homoeopathic Treatment

Leptospirosis Nosode - Nosodes are disease products that are turned into potencies and used to treat a disease or prevent it. In Cuba recently they had a big outbreak and used this disease nosode with great success.

Aconite 6C to 30C - Used for diseases with a sudden and sometime violent onset especially of fever. This remedy can sometimes abort a disease so it is one of the best to start with. There is physical and mental restlessness, fright, complaints from very hot weather, red inflamed eyes, in the fever it feels as if cold waves pass through them.

Crotalus Horridus 6C to 30C - A very good remedy for controlling liver complications and reducing hemorrhages and jaundice.

Berberis 30C - Suitable for the milder case, will control liver dysfunction and has a action on the kidneys, blood in urine, frontal headache,

Phosphorus 30C - Another valuable liver remedy, will control the tendency to hemorrhages, faces are generally clay colored.

Ipecacuanha 30C - A good anti hemorrhagic, eyes inflamed, for those with nausea and vomiting.

Lycopodium 30C - Useful remedy for the convalescent stage when emaciation or loss of condition is apparent, will restore liver function and aid digestion.

Lachesis 30C - Delirium tremens with much trembling and confusion. Very important for patients of a melancholic disposition. Ill effects of suppressed discharges. Cannot bear anything tight anywhere. In fever they are chilly in back; feet icy cold; hot flushes and hot perspiration. Upper part of windpipe very susceptible to touch. Sensation of suffocation and strangulation on lying down, particularly *when anything is around throat*; compels patient to spring from bed and rush for open window. Cough; dry, suffocative fits, tickling. Little secretion and much sensitiveness, Boils, carbuncles, ulcers, with bluish, purple surroundings. Purpura, with intense prostration. There is a bleeding tendency running all through this remedy.

Hepatitis A

Cause - Hepatitis A virus is a single-stranded RNA picornavirus. It is the most common cause of acute viral hepatitis and is particularly common among children and young adults. In some countries more than 75% of adults have been exposed.

The disease spreads primarily by fecal-oral contact and may occur in areas of poor hygiene. Waterborne and food-borne epidemics occur, especially in underdeveloped countries and refugee camps. Eating contaminated raw shellfish is sometimes responsible. Sporadic cases are also common, usually as a result of person-to-person contact. Fecal shedding of the virus occurs before symptoms develop and usually ceases a few days after symptoms begin; thus, the disease has no known chronic carrier state and does not produce chronic hepatitis or cirrhosis.

Disease Process - Unlike hepatitis B and Hepatitis C, Hepatitis A does not cause chronic (ongoing, long-term) disease. Although the liver does become inflamed and swollen, it heals completely in most people without any long-term damage. Once you have had Hepatitis A, you develop lifelong immunity and cannot get the disease again. Because of the way the disease is spread, the hepatitis A virus tends to occur in epidemics and outbreaks.

Diagnosis - A blood test will be done for antibodies to hepatitis A. The test will show whether you have been exposed recently to Hepatitis A.

Prevention - Good hygiene in handling food and avoiding contamination of water supplies is important. Vaccination against hepatitis A is recommended for all children. It is also recommended for adults at high risk of exposure to the infection:

Symptoms - Many people with Hepatitis A have no symptoms at all. Sometimes symptoms are so mild that they go unnoticed. Older people are more likely to have symptoms than children. Symptoms of hepatitis A usually develop between 2 and 6 weeks after infection. The symptoms are usually not too severe and go away on their own, over time. The most common symptoms are vomiting especially in children, loss of appetite, a yellow discoloration of the skin and whites of the eye, urine is very dark in color like tea, pain in area of liver. Symptoms usually last less than two months, although they may last as long as nine months. About 15% of people infected with hepatitis A have symptoms that come and go for 6-9 months.

Prognosis - Recovery from the acute infection is usually complete except when the infection is very severe.

Treatment - There are no specific medicines to cure infection with hepatitis A. Most people require no treatment except to relieve symptoms.

Take the weight off the liver by having low fat food as bile is needed for digestion of fat food. Eat easily digested foods and limit as much as possible the chemicals and toxins going into the body especially alcohol for the livers normal job is to neutralize toxins. In other words give the poor thing a rest.

Herbal Treatment

As usual you should of started off with our main Disease Fighting Herbs which have hopefully made this a much milder version of the disease. The main herb for the treatment of Hepatitis is Milk Thistle. Its strong Antioxidant Action helps to protect the liver from further damage and its regenerative properties help to speed up the healing process. Dandelion is a herb that works well with Milk Thistle. If this turns out to be a long term disease where you can feel tired and exhausted all the time we will add a Adaptogen to the formula called Astragalus, this should help in the return of strength and it also has a good Antiviral action. Schizandra is a Adaptogen which is close to being a specific for hepatitis and also is a immune stimulant. Eliminative support must be given especially if there is jaundice to help the body as a whole deal with the systemic problems caused by the liver dysfunction. Laxatives, Diuretics and Diaphoretics are the most important ones to consider. Read the Treatment part about the diet as the less rubbish put in the less the liver has to deal with for when one organs starts to fail all the others have to work harder to do its job. Treat symptoms as they come and go trying to use herbs that support the liver as well so, try to choose most of your herbs from the Cholagogues

Homoeopathic Treatment

Bryonia 6C to 30C - When there are stitching pains in the right liver region, Bryonia is the first remedy to be thought of, though for these pains we have other remedies, such as Chelidonium and Kali carbonicum. Under Bryonia the liver is swollen, congested and inflamed; the pains in the hypochondriac region are worse from any motion, and better from lying on the right side, which lessens the motion of the parts when breathing. It is one of the chief remedies for jaundice brought on by a fit of anger. Chamomilla has this symptom, but the Chamomilla patient gets hot and sweats, while the Bryonia patient is apt to be chilly, though he appears hot. There is a bitter in the mouth and the stools are hard and dry, or , if loose, papescent and profuse and associated with a colic. Berberis has stitching pains from the liver to the umbilicus. Chelidonium is distinguished by the character of the stools. Bryonia is pre-eminently a gastro-hepatic remedy, and has pain in right shoulder, giddiness, skin and eyes slightly yellow

Mercurius 6C to 30C - This remedy has much sensitiveness and dull pain in the region of the liver; the patient cannot lie on the right side. The liver is enlarged. The skin and conjunctiva are jaundiced. The stools are either clay-colored from absence of bile, or yellowish-green bilious stools passed with a great deal of tenesmus. There is a yellowish white coated tongue which takes the imprint of the teeth and there is a foetid breath, loss of appetite and depression of spirits. Leptandra has aching and soreness in the region of the liver and is especially indicated in the lazy livers of city men; but is distinguished from Mercurius in the stools, which are pitchlike and black, accompanied with no tenesmus, but rather a griping and the pains of Leptandra are dull, aching and burning in the posterior part of the liver. The character of the diarrhea will also distinguish Mercurius from Magnesia muriatica, which is useful in the enlarged livers of puny and rachitic children. It is a splendid remedy for "torpid liver." It suits well simple jaundice in children.

Podophyllum 6C to 30C - The principal use of Podophyllum is in liver affections. Primarily, it induces a large flow of bile, and, secondarily, great torpidity, followed by jaundice. It is indicated in torpid (sluggish or inactive) or chronically congested liver, when diarrhea is present. The liver is swollen and sensitive, the face and eyes are yellow and there is a bad taste in the mouth. The tongue is coated white or yellow and the bile may form gall stones. There is a loose watery diarrhea, or if constipation be present the stools are clay-called. It somewhat resembles Mercurius; it is sometimes called "vegetable mercury." There are a number of drugs having the symptom that the tongue takes the imprint of the teeth, namely; Mercurius, Podophyllum, Yucca, Stramonium, Rhus and Arsenic. Another symptom of Podophyllum is that the patient constantly rubs the region of the liver with the hand. Functional torpor of the portal system and the organs connected there with indicates Podophyllum. There is constipation, clay-coloured stool, jaundice and langour.

Chelidonium 6C to 30C - The liver symptoms of Chelidonium are very prominent. There is soreness and stitching pains in the region of the liver, but the keynote for this drug in hepatic diseases is a pain under the angle of the right shoulder blade, which may extend to the chest, stomach, or hypochondrium; there is swelling of the liver, chilliness, fever, jaundice, yellow coated tongue, bitter taste and a craving for acids and sour things, such as pickles and vinegar. The stools are profuse, bright yellow and diarrhea; they may be clayey in color. It is remedy to be used in simple biliousness and jaundice, and in hepatic congestion or inflammation the character of the stools will distinguish Bryonia. Taken altogether, Chelidonium is perhaps our greatest liver remedy; it causes the liver to secrete thinner and more profuse bile than any remedy; it is a useful remedy to promote the expulsion of gall stones, and to prevent their formation. In simple catarrhal jaundice it is often all sufficient. It affects the left lobe of the liver much less than does Carduus marianus.

Nux Vomica 6C to 30C - In liver affections occurring in those who have indulged to excess in alcoholic liquors, highly seasoned food, quinine, or in those who have abused themselves with purgatives, Nux is the first remedy to be thought of. The liver is swollen hard and sensitive to the touch and pressure of clothing is uncomfortable. The first remedy in cirrhosis of the liver. Colic may be present. Jaundice induced by anger also calls for Nux, also jaundice from abuse of quinine, in the former cases reminding of Chamomilla , which is an excellent remedy for biliousness of nervous, irritable women. In the enlarged liver of drunkards, Sulphur, Lachesis, Fluoric acid, Arsenic and Ammonium muriaticum must also be borne in mind, together with Nux. Juglans cinerea causes a jaundice like Nux vomica, with stitching pains about the liver and under the right scapula, bilious stools and occipital headache. Nux must be compared with China, Pulsatilla in liver affections from over-eating. Iris seems to have a solvent action upon the bile, it is especially useful in torpid liver and when gastric disorders result from perversion of hepatic and intestinal functions. Jaundice and constipation. Aloes has biliousness from torpor of the portal system, distension of the liver, bitter taste and jaundice.

Lycopodium 6C to 30C - Lycopodium acts powerfully on the liver. The region of the liver is sensitive to the touch, and there is a feeling of tension in it, a feeling as if a cord were tied about the waist. Cirrhosis. The pains are dull and aching instead of sharp and lancinating, as under Chelidonium. Fullness in the stomach after eating a small quantity. There are no real icteric symptoms, but there is a peculiar sallow complexion. Natrum sulphuricum is useful when the patient has a bad, slimy taste in the mouth and "thinks he is bilious." There is apt to be weight and aching in the liver; he can lie on that side, but on turning to the left side the liver seems to pull and draw. Natrum sulphuricum is the greatest Schuessler specific for liver affections, and clinically it has often worked well. Dr. Alfred Pope claims that Lycopodium is more useful than any other remedy in old hepatic congestions. Pain in back and right side from congestion will often yield to the remedy.

Sulphur 6C to 30C - Sulphur is suitable to chronic affections of the liver; it increases the flow of bile and there is much pain and soreness in the liver. Sulphur often completes the cure commenced by Nux. Liver complaints from abuse of mercury will oftentimes call for Sulphur. If the stools are colorless and if much jaundice or ascites be present Sulphur is contra-indicated. Lachesis, however, has jaundice, as do all snake poisons, and is useful in the enlarged livers of drunkards, with tenderness on pressure and throbbing in the right side.

Animal And Insect Bourne Diseases
Vector-borne Diseases

Vector borne diseases basically mean that the carrier or host of the disease is a animal or insect good examples being dogs (rabies), rats (plague), rodents in general, mosquitos (dengue), flies, lice (typhus) etc. Natural disasters, particularly meteorological events such as cyclones, hurricanes and flooding, can affect vector breeding sites and vector-borne disease transmission. While initial flooding may wash away existing mosquito breeding sites, standing-water caused by heavy rainfall or overflow of rivers can create new breeding sites. This can result (with some weeks delay) in an increase of the vector population and potential for disease transmission, depending on the local mosquito vector species and its preferred habitat. To make matters worse especially in floods both people and animals especially flooded out rats will all head to high ground where they live closely together for a while creating a situation for disease transmission. With Climate Change a lot of the vector borne diseases could move to new areas and higher altitudes as the temperature heats up and they find life more comfortable in new areas.

Populations of humans are getting larger and suburban sprawl is concentrating what's left of the wildlife together especially in countries like South America where there are lots of species that we don't even know exist, just imagine what unknown diseases they could be host to and how many of them are going to be able to cross over to humans whose immune systems have never dealt with such a disease, then a newly infected person goes for a sales trip around the world.

Below is a list of just a few of the mosquito vector diseases from all over the world.

Mosquito Diseases - Dengue Fever, Yellow Fever, Murray Valley Encephalitis, Ross River Fever, Japanese Encephalitis, West Nile Virus, ST Louis Encephalitis, Venezulan Equine Encephalitis Virus, Eastern Equine Encephalitis Virus, Western Equine Encephalitis Virus, Chikungunya Virus, Rift Valley Fever and of course you can't leave out the obvious one Malaria. For Our Natural Treatment Of Diseases we shall start with the first four on the list as this will give us a fairly good idea how to treat the others.

Dengue Fever

Cause - Dengue is a mosquito-borne disease caused by a flavivirus. Dengue is endemic to the tropical regions of the world in latitudes from about 35° north to 35° south. Outbreaks are most prevalent in Southeast Asia but also occur in the Caribbean, including Puerto Rico and the US Virgin Islands, Oceania, and the Indian subcontinent, more recently, Dengue incidence has increased in Central and South America and Australia as the climate changes. The causative agent is a flavivirus with 4 serogroups and is transmitted by the bite of *Aedes* mosquitoes.

Disease Process - An acute, specific, fever, occurring epidemically in tropical and subtropical climates, and characterized by two severe paroxysms of fever, separated by an intermission at half time, great muscular and arthritic pains, and attended usually by a skin eruption.

Diagnosis - Dengue fever is suspected in patients in endemic areas who develop sudden fever, headache, myalgias, and adenopathy, particularly with pain behind the eyes which worsens with movement and the characteristic rash or recurrent fever. Evaluation should rule out alternative diagnoses, especially Malaria and Leptospirosis. Diagnosis involves PCR and serologic testing.

Prevention - People in endemic areas should try to prevent mosquito bites and mosquito breeding. To prevent further transmission by mosquitoes, patients with dengue should be kept under mosquito netting until the second bout of fever has resolved. Vaccines are being evaluated.

Symptoms - Dengue fever usually results in the abrupt onset of high fever, headache, myalgias, arthralgia's, lymphadenopathy, and a rash that appears with a 2nd temperature rise after a period of no fever. Respiratory symptoms, such as cough, sore throat, and rhinorrhea, can occur. Dengue can also cause potentially fatal hemorrhagic fever with bleeding tendency and shock.

After an incubation period of 3 to 15 days symptoms of chills, headache, retro-orbital pain with eye movement, lumbar backache, joints are red, slightly swollen, and stiff; there is also general muscular soreness and severe prostration begin abruptly. Extreme aching in the legs and joints occurs during the first hours, which accounts for the traditional name of breakbone fever. The temperature rises rapidly to up to 40° C, with hypotension and relative bradycardia. Cervical and inguinal lymph nodes are usually enlarged. Although the temperature is extremely high, there is rarely delirium or unconsciousness to relieve the excruciating pain. The lymphatics become painful and swollen. Fever and other symptoms persist 48 to 96 hours followed by a rapid break in the fever with profuse sweating.

Patients then feel well for about 24 hours, after which fever usually occurs again, typically with a lower peak temperature than the first. Simultaneously, a maculopapular rash spreads from the extremities to cover the body except the face or to cover the trunk and extremities in a patchy distribution. The palms and soles may be bright red, swollen, and itchy.

Mild cases of dengue, usually lacking lymphadenopathy, get better in less than 72 hours. In a more severe disease, debility may last several weeks. Death is rare. Immunity to the infecting strain is long-lasting, whereas broader immunity to other strains lasts only 2 to 12 months.

Dengue Hemorrhagic Fever

Dengue Hemorrhagic Fever in children less than 10 years of age living where dengue is endemic requires prior exposure to the dengue virus. It is suspected in children with a sudden fever that stays high for 2 to 7 days with hemorrhagic manifestations, petechiae, purpura , bleeding gums, vomiting of blood, and hepatomegaly.

Dengue Hemorrhagic Fever in adults begins with abrupt fever and headache and is initially indistinguishable from classic dengue. Shock and increasing illness may develop rapidly 2 to 6 days after onset. Bleeding tendencies occur, usually as purpura, bruising, petechiae, or sometimes as vomiting of blood, blackening of the faeces from blood, or blood nose and occasionally as bleeding of the brain lining. Enlargement of the liver is common, as is bronchopneumonia. Myocarditis can occur.

Prognosis - Death is rare in Dengue but in Hemorrhagic Dengue mortality ranges from 6 to 30% with most deaths in infants.

Treatment - Treatment is symptomatic. **Aspirin and Brufen should be avoided in Dengue as this increases the bleeding tendency and stomach pains.**

Herbal Treatment

Keep the initial fever within safe limits (see Fevers) especially in children for lots of them have convulsions from the high temperature. With the disease being self-limited, the objective of our treatment will is to reduce the febrile state, ease the intense pain, and make the patient as comfortable as possible. To do this think of Peruvian Bark as our main Febrifuge and Boneset which is historically the specific for this diseases as it name derives from break bone fever. Boneset is a febrifuge but we are using it for the pains and aches of the disease. Lemon balm and Lemongrass could be mixed together and used in a Diaphoretic tea to constantly sip during the fever, and another reason for their use is that both of these herbs are Antiviral, Peppermint could be added to improve the flavor. Rest in bed should be emphasized, and the diet should be fluid in character; milk and rich broths being best suited to sustain the patient's strength. If the disease heads for the lymphatic system the herbs to think of are Baptisia and Poke Root (never use more than 1ml doses of Poke Root). For the pains in the eyes think of Eye Bright which is also a strong Astringent which is the next action we shall need especially if bleeding occurs. Agrimony is a good astringent which would help with any bleeding in the Digestive and Urinary Systems use the list of Astringents to find a herb that matches the systems bleeding along with some of the other symptoms. If there seems to be blood coming from everywhere add one of the strong Astringents Cranesbill, Witch Hazel or Shepherds Purse.

Homoeopathic Treatment

Eupatorium Perfolatum 30C to 200C - This will probably be the major remedy of choice and is used as a preventative for the disease. It comes from the herb, Thoroughwort and is known as "Bone-Set." It was used in the 1800 and 1900's by homeopaths when Dengue became epidemic during those time periods.

MENTAL/EMOTIONAL: Person feels as if they are losing their minds. Anxious feeling, along with moaning. Restless and cannot sit or lie still, although they wish they could (every movement hurts them).

HEAD: Throbbing pain, as if a cap of metal were pressed over the entire skull ,pushing downward. Vertigo with falling to the left. Top and rear of head painful. Headache may be periodical--every 3rd and 7th day. Upon lying down, the rear of the skull (occipital region) feels very heavy and there's a weighted feeling to it.

EYES: soreness of the eyeballs. Worse: light of any kind. Even the lids feel sore.

MOUTH: tongue has a thick yellow coat. Cracks or soreness at corners of mouth. Very thirsty for cold liquids. Bitter taste in mouth.

STOMACH: Liver region sore to touch. Vomit may contain bile, green color. Vomiting preceded by being very thirsty. Hiccups. Doesn't want any tight clothing around the waist or stomach region.

STOOL: diarrhea, green, watery with cramps.

RESPIRATORY: Sneezing. Hoarseness with cough, worse: morning, and a sore chest. Great soreness of muscles and bones of chest. Cough is relieved by getting down on hands and knees. Cough worse from 2am to 4am. Worse breathing in. Unable to lie on left side. Worse lying on back. Cough with heat attended by soreness in throat and bronchial region. Face will be flushed with tears in eyes from coughing so much.

FEVER: Sweating relieves all symptoms except the headache. Chills between 9pm and 9pm, preceded by a great thirst for liquids. Soreness and aching of the bones attend the fever.

EXTREMITIES: Ache in lumbar region of back. Chills will start in low back and move upward. Arms and wrists ache. Knees and calves painful and stiff. Muscles stiff, generally and person is unable to move or bend very much. Back may have a trembling sensation to it during the fever portion. Arms and legs feel as if they have been badly bruised and severely beaten.

NOTE

Eupatorium Perfoliatum 200 - Can be taken twice daily for three days and subsequently at least two doses a week at the interval of three to four days till the epidemic ends for the prevention of dengue fever.

Ipecac 200C - Can be given twice a day for three days and two doses a week in all the patients those who have already suffered with the dengue fever and are prone for dengue hemorrhagic fever. This remedy can also be used alternately with Eupatorium Perfoliatum 200 to prevent both the types of dengue fever in so far not infected individuals.

Lachesis 30C - Delirium tremens with much trembling and confusion. Very important for patients of a melancholic disposition. Ill effects of suppressed discharges. Cannot bear anything tight anywhere. In fever they are chilly in back; feet icy cold; hot flushes and hot perspiration. Upper part of windpipe very susceptible to touch. Sensation of suffocation and strangulation on lying down, particularly *when anything is around throat*; compels patient to spring from bed and rush for open window. Cough; dry, suffocative fits, tickling. Little secretion and much sensitiveness, Boils, carbuncles, ulcers, with bluish, purple surroundings. Purpura, with intense prostration. There is a bleeding tendency running all through this remedy.

Yellow Fever

Cause - Yellow fever also known as Yellow Jack is a mosquito-borne flavivirus infection endemic in tropical South America and sub-Saharan

Africa. In urban yellow fever the virus is transmitted by the bite of an *Aedes aegypti* mosquito infected about 2 weeks previously by feeding on a infected person. In jungle (sylvatic) yellow fever, the virus is transmitted by *Haemagogus* and other forest canopy mosquitoes that acquire the virus from wild primates. Incidence is highest during months of peak rainfall, humidity, and temperature in South America and during the late rainy and early dry seasons in Africa.

Disease Process - Symptoms may include sudden onset of fever, relative bradycardia, headache, and, if severe, jaundice, hemorrhage, and multiple organ failure. Infection ranges from asymptomatic (in 5 to 50% of cases) to a hemorrhagic fever with 50% mortality. Incubation lasts 3 to 6 days. Yellow fever is an acute highly infectious, epidemic and endemic disease, characterized by an abrupt period of invasion, followed by a remission and that by a relapse. Also by a high fever accompanied by a yellowish discoloration of the skin (often mottled), frequently by oozing hemorrhages from mucous surfaces, and by a black vomit. This disease prevails during the middle and late summer months and is abruptly terminated by frost.

Yellow Fever has three stages:
1. EARLY STAGE - Headache, muscle aches, fever, loss of appetite, vomiting, and jaundice are common. After approximately 3 - 4 days, often symptoms go away briefly (remission).
2. PERIOD OF REMISSION - After 3 -4 days, fever and other symptoms go away. Most people will recover at this stage, but others may move onto the third, most dangerous stage (intoxication stage) within 24 hours.
3. PERIOD OF INTOXICATION - Multi-organ dysfunction occurs. This includes liver and kidney failure, bleeding disorders, hemorrhage, brain dysfunction including delirium, seizures, coma, shock, and death.

Diagnosis - Diagnosis is with viral culture and serologic tests. When an epidemic is declared the sudden onset, the intense backache, the pain in the eyes, and after perhaps forty-eight hours the marked slowing of the pulse while the temperature is yet very high, are characteristic. In the period of remission the jaundice will determine the diagnosis, and later the black vomit, with increased jaundice and suppressed urine, are unmistakable evidences. The facial expression is of great assistance in diagnosis, to those familiar with the disease. The extreme flushing of the face and the intensely injected and jaundiced eyes, are characteristic.

Prevention - Prevention involves vaccination and mosquito control.

Suspected or confirmed cases must be quarantined. To prevent further mosquito transmission, infected patients should be isolated in rooms that are well screened and sprayed with insecticides.

The most effective way to prevent outbreaks is to reduce the number of mosquitoes and limit mosquito bites by using mosquito netting, and protective attire. During jungle outbreaks, people should evacuate the area until they are immunized and mosquitoes are controlled. For people traveling to endemic areas, active immunization with the yellow fever vaccine is indicated and is 95% effective. The vaccine is contraindicated in pregnant women and in those with compromised immunity.

Symptoms - There are usually three distinct stages to this disease. For a few hours only before the abrupt onset of the disease there may be malaise, some lassitude, vertigo and headache. The rigor is sudden and unannounced, and with it there is pallor, severe muscular pains, especially in the back, and with the headache which is usually very severe, there is pain in the eyes, and much distress in the stomach. There is a rapid rise in the temperature to 104.5° or even 106° F within twenty-four hours. This usually persists for two or three days, although in the mild cases there will be a fall of the temperature within a few hours. The pulse, usually rapid initially, by the second day becomes slow for the degree of fever. The face is flushed and the eyes are injected. Nausea, vomiting, constipation, severe prostration, restlessness, and irritability are common. Mild disease may resolve after 1 to 3 days. When the fever persists there are slight morning and evening remissions until the end of the third day, when the remission in the fever is marked and all the phenomena abate, the pulse remaining abnormally slow. There are, however, marked evidences of serious impairment of health, and at this time the characteristic jaundice—the yellow or bronzed condition of the skin and conjunctivae appears. If all conditions are favorable and if the previous course of the disease has not been too severe, the patient may recover from this point.

In moderate or severe cases, however, the fever falls suddenly 2 to 5 days after onset, and a remission of several hours or days ensues. The fever recurs, but the pulse remains slow.

After one day perhaps, or a little less or more, there is a recurrence of all the symptoms in a greatly aggravated form. Exhaustion occurs with signs of collapse, the temperature may rise even beyond its previously highest point (secondary fever), or it may fall below normal and the skin become positively cold, with a rapid and compressible pulse, increased gastric distress, and the vomiting of, at first, a clear liquid in which float reddish or brown flakes which increase in quantity and color until it assumes the character of well-known black vomit. Hemorrhage may occur from the stomach and unchanged blood may appear in the vomit. Or passive hemorrhages may be general from all mucous surfaces or even from the skin. With these serious symptoms an abatement and a change for the better may occur, but this is rare. There is usually a suppression of urine more or less complete, with serious depression and rapidly approaching collapse, hiccough, coma and convulsions, which may be of uremic origin, and death. The urine of yellow fever is often albuminous from the first, and this is considered a positive evidence in the diagnosis. The quantity is lessened at the onset and often decreases to final complete anuria.

There is a wide variation of symptoms in this disease. The course above outlined is most common, the three stages being distinct. But the course may be different in individual cases in a given epidemic. The disease in some cases may last less than 1 week with rapid recovery and no sequelae. In the most severe cases, delirium, intractable hiccups, seizures, coma, and multiple organ failure may occur terminally.

Prognosis - Up to 10% of patients with disease severe enough to be diagnosed die. The mortality varies in different epidemics; some are light, some virulent. In severe cases with no improvement in the second stage, the prognosis is bad, as from thirty to forty per cent die.

Treatment - Treatment is supportive. Total bed rest even through the remission. Use the bed pan all the time so it can be noted if blood is in the urine or bowel. Use a bland and easily digestible diet with hardly any fat so as to take the weight off the liver.

Herbal Treatment

After the virus enters the blood it can then be transported around the body and reproduces itself in a variety of the body's cells, usually the liver, kidneys and blood vessels. In serious cases, these cells may become damaged and begin to fail leading to death. The treatment here is very similar to Dengue but here Echinacea will become very important not just for its immune building Actions but mainly for its Antimicrobial Action on the blood stream for in this disease we really have to attack the virus to get the numbers down along with protecting the liver and kidneys along with the insides of the blood vessels. Read the herbal treatment for Dengue. Here we will do the same with the fever our main herbs will be Peruvian Bark and Boneset and again Lemongrass, Lemon balm and Peppermint as a tea to sip throughout the fever and especially during remission. For the liver we will use Milk Thistle for protection and regeneration of any damage and to that we will add Dandelion for its further help to the liver but also for its Diuretic Action as we want to keep the kidneys passing water to this we will add PauD'Arco because it is a Diuretic and also Antiviral, Alterative, Anodyne and Febrifuge. As a good Stimulant but mainly for its effect on circulation and bleeding we will use Prickly Ash which also has actions of Astringent, Alterative, Anodyne, Diaphoretic and Febrifuge. Another herb that helps with low pulse and the repair of blood vessels is Hawthorn. Other herbs to consider are Barberry especially if the spleen becomes involved, Fenugreek as a background remedy, Goldenrod, Bearberry or Agrimony for blood in the urine, Baptisia for it Antiviral, Alterative and Stimulant properties, Pleurisy Root if we have lung problems. We must work very hard during the remission to get the viral population down.

Homoeopathic Treatment

Aconite 6C to 30C - Nearly all authorities praise this remedy in the early stage of yellow fever where there is high fever, chilliness and dry skin, bounding pulse and the characteristic mental accompaniments which are quite likely to be present in this disease. It will speedily calm the febrile storm in these conditions.

Gelsemium 6C to 30C - Is a remedy for the onset when the patient is apathetic and dull, and Belladonna or Bryonia may also come in during the first stage. Very often, too, Camphora with its coldness and tendency to collapse may be the remedy. The vomiting of the first stage is often controlled by Ipecac.

Arsenicum 6c to 30C - This remedy come in most frequently in the second and third stages, and is one of the most important remedies in the disease. The patient has continued nausea and vomiting, and the vomited matter consist of bile or mucosities filled with blackish or sanguinolent streaks; the face is yellow and the pulse is small, weak and tremulous. There is much burning in the precordial region and intense burning thirst, but, of course for small quantities of water only. No better remedy for these symptoms is to be found than Arsenicum. It sill often alone suffice to cure.

Lachesis 6C to 30C - This remedy has given very satisfactory results in yellow fever, especially when vomiting is present, abdominal tenderness, brown tongue, delirium, slow speech, nausea, offensive discharges and black urine. It corresponds to nerve-poisoning and suits bad looking cases.

Sulphuric Acid 6C to 30C - Is a useful remedy for haemorrhages of black blood, profuse sweat with exhaustion, foetid stools and diminished secretion of urine.

Argentum Nit 6C to 30C - Is also one of the best remedies in the disease. It covers the vomiting; especially is it of use when the patient sinks and the vomiting become worse.

Phosphorous 6c to 30C - Phosphorous with its hemorrhages; jaundice and other symptoms is a close simile to certain forms; it was successfully used in an epidemic occurring in Rio de Janerio.

Crotalus 6C to 30C - This remedy produces a perfect picture of yellow fever, and it corresponds to the stage of black vomit and blood poisoning- there is a low delirium, yellow skin and oozing of blood from every orifice of the body, even bloody sweat is sometimes present. The yellow skin produced by this remedy is characteristic, and denotes blood poisoning rather than jaundice. Cadmium sulphate has also the symptoms of black vomit, and its study in the disease is suggested.

Carbo Veg 6C to30C - This remedy has been considered as a preventive of yellow fever. Hering says this remedy more than any other drug corresponds in the totality of its action to yellow fever. It suits the third stage where collapse, coldness, extremely fetid discharge and great exhaustion of the vital forces are present.

Ross River Fever

Cause - First isolated from *Ochlerotatus vigilax* (previously called *Aedes vigilax*) mosquitoes collected in 1959 near the Ross River in Townsville, the cause of Ross River virus disease was confirmed in 1971 by its isolation from the blood of an Aboriginal boy with the disease. Ross River virus is one of a group of viruses called arboviruses (or arthropod-borne viruses), which are spread mainly by blood-sucking insects. Ross River virus is a germ that infects people, particularly in rural areas, sometimes causing a flu-like illness with joint pains, rash and fever. Ross River virus is not fatal. In 1979, a major outbreak of RRV disease (probably exported from

Australia) occurred in Fiji and spread to other Pacific islands, including Tonga, the Cook Islands and Samoa. RRV is endemic throughout Australia, Papua New Guinea, East Timor, adjacent islands of Indonesia and the Solomon islands

Disease Process - The virus is spread by certain types of female mosquitoes. Female mosquitoes feed on animals and people. If they feed on the blood of an infected animal, the mosquito may become infected. The virus then multiplies within the mosquito and is passed to other animals or people when the mosquito feeds again. The virus is not spread directly from one person to another. Approximately 30 per cent of people infected with the virus will develop symptoms three to eleven days after being infected. The number of infections tends to peak in the summer and autumn months.

Diagnosis - Ross River infection is diagnosed by detection of antibodies against the virus in the blood. Blood test taken early in the illness and again two weeks later may be required to confirm the infection.

Prevention -☐Avoid being bitten by mosquitoes, especially in the summer and autumn months when infections are more common. Follow mosquito eradication plans and use personal repellent. Presently, there is no vaccine available.

Symptoms - Many people who are infected with the virus will never develop symptoms while some will have flu-like symptoms that include fever, chills, headache and aches and pains in the muscles and joints. Some joints can become swollen, and joint stiffness may be particularly noticeable in the morning. Sometimes a rash occurs on the body, arms or legs. The rash usually disappears after seven to 10 days. A general feeling of being unwell, tired or weak may also occur at times during the illness. This may affect work performance. Rheumatic symptoms are present in most patients except for the few who present with the rash alone, these consist of arthritis or arthralgia primarily affecting the wrist, knee, ankle and small joints of the extremities. Prolonged symptoms are common. In some cases, there may be remissions and exacerbations of decreasing intensity for up to a year. Symptoms persisting longer than a year may be due to other reasons. Cervical lymphadenopathy occurs frequently, and tenderness of the palms and soles are present in a small percentage of cases.

Prognosis - The disease can cause incapacity and inability to work for two to three months. About one-quarter of patients have rheumatic symptoms that persist for up to a year but rarely more.

Treatment - There is no specific treatment for Ross River virus infection so treatment generally involves managing the symptoms that develop. Your doctor will advise on treatment for joint and muscle pains. A combination of plenty of rest and gentle exercise are important to keep joints moving and to prevent overtiredness, but medication may sometimes be necessary.

Herbal Treatment

As usual you should of started off with our main Disease Fighting Herbs which have hopefully made this a much milder version of the disease. From there think of Boneset as it will help with the fever and aches and pains. This can turn out to be a long term Chronic Disease so treat the symptoms as they come with the herbs needed while concentrating our main attack on the virus. Cats Claw is a good herb to use, its suitable Actions for use in this disease are Antiviral, Anti-inflammatory, Anti Rheumatic and Immune Stimulant (think of Licorice too). It has also been used for fatigue and depression. Sticking to claws the next one to think about is Devils Claw with its Actions of Alterative, Analgesic, Anti-inflammatory, Anti Rheumatic as well as being a Stimulant though this herb can sometimes take a few weeks to start working. PauD'Arco and Sarsaparilla are similar types of herb worth considering. Willow Bark is a herb to consider for long term pain relief, I think of this herb as Caveman's Aspirin as it has been used for thousands of years and was the main ingredient of the original aspirin. Willow Bark will not taking the lining off the stomach as the long term use of aspirin can do as it is absorbed in the large intestine so it takes a while to get into the body. If the disease turns into a Chronic Fatigue type then we start to use herbs known as Adaptogens, these herbs help you adapt to get the best you can out of your current situation. The main ones to use here which is nearly a specific for this disease is Astragalus which also has the Actions of a Antiviral, Immune Booster and Stimulant. Another one to add to this especially where there is a lot of pain is Withania which is Adaptogen, Analgesic, Anti-inflammatory, Rejuvenative and a Immune Stimulant, this is a good herb to use especially if the patient is female. As a nutritional supplement you could use Glucosamine to help relieve the pain of joint inflammation and if you think the joints are becoming damaged use Glucosamine with Chondroitin and MSM.

Homoeopathic Treatment

Eupatorium Perfoliatium 6C to 30C - Pain in the limbs and muscles with fever. There may be severe bone pain. Swelling of ankles and feet. Aching pain in bones of extremities with soreness of flesh. great thirst, perspiration relieves all symptoms except head ache.200 potency is found to be more effective.

Gelsemium 6C to 30C - Associated with severe headache and coryza. Thirstlessness, slow pulse, muscular pains. There may be drowsiness, dullness and dizziness.

Rhus Tox 6C to 30C - Fever with polyarthritis and maculopapular rashes. Pain and stiffness in joints. worse first motion. Rheumatism in cold seasons. Restlessness. Worse for Cold. Wet, Rainy weather. The 200C potency is most effective.

Bryonia 6C to 30C - Fever with aching in every muscle. Dry mouth with excessive thirst, knees stiff and painful. Joints red, swollen, and hot with stitching and tearing pain. Worse by motion; Bursting, splitting headache as if everything would be pressed out.

Arsenic Alb 6C to 30C - Restlessness and anxiety during fever, severe weakness. Unquenchable thirst, nausea and vomiting. Fever worse mid-day or midnight.

Pulsatilla 6C to 30C - Fever with chilliness, thirstlessness and wandering joint pains

China 6C to 30C - Pain in the limbs and joints as if sprained. worse slight touch.
Better for hard pressure. Swollen joints. Debilitating night sweats.

Belladona 6C to 30C - High fever with burning heat. No thirst with fever. Joints swollen, red, shining with red streaks radiating. Heat, redness, throbbing and burning.

Pyrogen 6C to 30C - Septic fevers, temperature rises rapidly. Great heat with profuse hot sweat. But sweating does not cause a fall in temperature, aching in limb and bones.

Murray Valley Encephalitis

Cause - Murray Valley encephalitis is a mosquito-borne disease caused by the Murray Valley Encephalitis virus. It is also known as Australian Encephalitis. The virus is spread by the bite of an infected mosquito (usually *Culex annulirostris* also known as the "common banded" mosquito). Not all of these mosquitoes carry the virus, and only about 1 person in a 1000 who get bitten by infected mosquitoes will become unwell. The virus is thought to be mainly carried by water birds. Mosquitoes become infected by biting birds or other animals that carry the virus. Spread to south eastern Australia is thought to occur with water bird migration that follows unusually wet conditions in inland Australia.

There have been seven major outbreaks in Australia since 1917. The last was in 1974 when 58 cases were reported from all mainland states. Since 1974 nearly all cases have occurred in the north of Western Australia and the Northern Territory, with occasional cases in Queensland, Central Australia and central regions of Western Australia.

Disease Process - Murray Valley encephalitis virus is a flavivirus. It has the capacity to cause severe human disease, with encephalitis being the most notable clinical feature. It can commonly infect humans without producing apparent disease (subclinical infection), or it may cause a comparatively mild disease with features such as fever, headache, nausea and vomiting. In a small percentage of all people infected, mild disease may be a prodrome to disease progression and involvement of the central nervous system, causing meningitis, or in the worst scenario, encephalitis of variable severity. Signs of brain dysfunction, such as drowsiness, confusion, fitting, weakness, or ataxia, indicate the onset of encephalitis.

Diagnosis - MVE is diagnosed when a blood test or test of the spinal fluid shows evidence of the virus (through nucleic acid testing or a rise in antibodies). A diagnosis of MVE disease should be considered in any patient who presents with encephalitis or central nervous system symptoms and who has been in the MVE endemic area within the incubation period of the disease, especially in the period between November and July.

Prevention - There is no specific treatment or vaccine available for MVE. The only protection from is to avoid being bitten by mosquitoes. This is particularly important to travelers and visitors to areas where the disease might be active.

Symptoms - The disease takes about 5 to 15 days (normally 7 to 12 days) between getting bitten and becoming sick. The majority of people infected will have no symptoms. Of those who do, symptoms can include high fever, severe headache, seizures or fits (especially in young children), tremors, neck stiffness, lethargy, irritability, drowsiness, vomiting, nausea, diarrhea, dizziness, confusion, coma in severe cases. When encephalitis develops, brain dysfunction may be experienced after a few days with lethargy, irritability, drowsiness, confusion, convulsions and fits; neck stiffness can be expected, and both coma and death may ensue.

Prognosis - People most at risk are babies, young children and newcomers to the region. The disease is fatal in about 20 per cent of those who become sick, and a further 25 per cent can develop major neurological complications. About 40 per cent of cases will make a complete recovery.

Treatment - Patients with MVE will usually require extensive support sometimes in an intensive care unit in hospital. There is no specific treatment for MVE.

Herbal Treatment

As usual you should of started off with our main Disease Fighting Herbs which have hopefully made this a much milder version of the disease. For this disease you really don't want to get a bad case. Treat the symptoms as they come using the Actions needed. For the fever think of Peruvian Bark for it has a affinity with mozzie caused fevers (quinine was made from this herb) and our main herb will be Baptizia which is not only Anti-Viral but has been used in the treatment of meningitis. To this think of adding St Johns Wort as this is a Nervine Antiviral (especially for the Herpes Virus) that we can use for any virus attacking the nervous system. Instead of using Licorice to force the formula into the body use Ginkgo Biloba as this opens the arteries in the neck and is good for getting the herbs you want into the brain as it increases the blood flow to the head and also has a strong Antioxidant Action which might tone down the damage. Think of our Lemongrass and Lemon balm tea not just for the fever but because it is also good for headaches and is Antiviral. In Japan they tested Astragalus for use in Japanese Encephalitis which is another mozzie bourne encephalitis, the results were 60 to 80% of infected mice treated survived compared to a 10% survival rate for the untreated. So think of giving Astragalus early.

Homoeopathic Treatment

Aconite 6C to 30C - Nearly all authorities praise this remedy in the early stage especially with a sudden onset where there is high fever, chilliness and dry skin, bounding pulse, thirst, delirium and vertigo to a point. Any noise or light will aggravate the condition.

Belladonna 6c to 30C - Corresponds to the initial stages, where there is intense heat of the body, strong pulse, bright red face and delirium, where the cerebral irritation is marked by intense pain in the head, starting out of sleep crying out, grinding teeth. There are shooting pains in the head which make the patient cringe. These pains are stabbing and come on suddenly and may be accompanied by vomiting. Great irritability.

Hyoscyamus 6C to 30C - Is Suitable for cerebral inflammation with pulsating waves through the head relieved by shaking the head or sitting with the head bent forward. Muscular twitching, vertigo, brain feels loose, worse at night better stooping.

Stramonium 6C to 30C - This remedy suits inflammatory conditions of the brain with violent delirium. Vertigo is a prominent symptom and also a transient blindness.

Typhus

Cause - Epidemic typhus is caused by Rickettsia prowazekii. Typhus is caused by one of two types of bacteria: *Rickettsia typhi* or *Rickettsia prowazekii*. The form of typhus depends on which type of bacteria causes the infection.

Rickettsia typhi causes murine or endemic typhus. It is usually seen in areas where hygiene is poor and the temperature is cold. Endemic typhus is sometimes called Jail Fever and also used to be known as Ship Fever. *Rickettsia prowazekii* causes epidemic typhus and Brill-Zinsser disease. Brill-Zinsser disease is a mild form of epidemic typhus that occurs when the disease re-activates in a person who was previously infected. It is more common in the elderly.

Typhus is a bacterial disease spread by lice or fleas. Humans are the natural reservoir for R. prowazekii, which is prevalent worldwide and transmitted by body lice when louse faces are scratched or rubbed into a bite or other wounds (or sometimes the mucous membranes of the eyes or mouth). Scrub typhus occurs in the western Pacific region, northern Australia, and the Indian subcontinent. The incidence of scrub typhus is largely unknown. Many cases are undiagnosed because of its non-specific manifestations and the lack of laboratory diagnostic testing in endemic areas.

Epidemic typhus occurs in Central and South America, Africa, northern China, and certain regions of the Himalayas. Outbreaks may occur when conditions arise that favor the propagation and transmission of lice. Brill-

Zinsser disease develops in approximately 15% of people with a history of primary epidemic typhus.

Murine typhus occurs in most parts of the world, particularly in subtropical and temperate coastal regions. Murine typhus occurs mainly in sporadic cases, and incidence is probably greatly underestimated in the more endemic regions. Rats, mice, and cats, which are hosts for the disease, are particularly common along coastal port regions. Populations of the flea vector may rise during the summer months in temperate climates, subsequently increasing the incidence of murine typhus.

Diagnosis - Louse infestation is usually obvious and strongly suggests typhus if history (eg, living in or visiting an endemic area) suggests possible exposure. The early rash is a light rose color and fades when you press on it. Later, the rash becomes dull and red and does not fade. People with severe typhus may also develop small areas of bleeding into the skin

Prevention - Immunization and louse control are highly effective for prevention. Lice may be eliminated by dusting infested people with malathion or lindane. Avoid areas where you might encounter rat fleas. Good sanitation and public health measures reduce the rat population. Measures to get rid of lice when an infection has been found include, Bathing, Boiling clothes or avoiding infested clothing for at least 5 days (lice will die without feeding on blood), Using insecticides (10% DDT, 1% malathion, or 1% permethrin)

Symptoms of Rickettsia prowazekii (epidemic typhus) The vector is the body louse - Symptoms are prolonged high fever, intractable headache, joint and muscle pains and a maculopapular rash. After an incubation period of 7 to 14 days, fever, headache, anorexia and prostration suddenly occur. Temperature reaches 40° C in several days and remains high, with slight morning remission, for about 2 weeks. Headache is generalized and intense. Small, pink macules, which appear on the 4th to 6th day, rapidly cover the body, usually in the axillae and on the upper trunk and not on the palms, soles, and face. Later, the rash becomes dark and maculopapular. In severe cases, the rash becomes petechial and hemorrhagic. Hypotension occurs in most seriously ill patients. Vascular collapse, renal insufficiency, encephalitic signs, ecchymosis with gangrene, and pneumonia are poor prognostic signs. Further developments may include enlargement of the spleen, neurological problems, delirium and prostration. The mortality rate is 6 to 35% with death often the result of secondary infection and usually coming at about the second week of infection. Re-infection is not uncommon in endemic areas.

Symptoms of Murine typhus (*Rickettsia typhi*) may include - Abdominal pain, backache, dull red rash that begins on the middle of the body and spreads, extremely high fever (105 - 106 degrees Fahrenheit), which may last up to 2 weeks, hacking, dry cough, headache, joint pain, nausea and vomiting

Symptoms of Scrub typhus is caused by *O tsutsugamushi* (formerly *Rickettsia tsutsugamushi*) via the mite *Leptotrombidium akamushi* and possibly *Leptotrombidium deliense*. Symptoms and signs are almost always mild and resemble those of epidemic typhus, with similar circulatory disturbances and hepatic, renal, and CNS changes. The remittent febrile course lasts about 7 to 10 days. The rash is often evanescent or absent. Mortality is nil. Scrub typhus may be difficult to recognize and diagnose because the symptoms and signs of the illness are often non-specific. A painless papule develops at the site of the chigger bite and subsequently undergoes central necrosis. It starts as a painless papule, and the lesion becomes indurated and enlarged. The centre of the lesion becomes necrotic and develops into a black scab.

Prognosis - Fatalities are rare in children under 10 years, but mortality increases with aging and may reach 60% in untreated patients over 50 years of age. Less than 2% of untreated patients with murine typhus may die. Prompt antibiotic treatment will cure nearly all patients.

Treatment - The disease responds well to tetracyclines, which must be taken until three days after the fever subsides. Primary treatment is doxycycline until the patient improves and has been afebrile for 24 to 48 hours but continued for at least 7 days. Chloramphenicol is 2nd-line treatment. The disease can affect many organs, so a wide range of supportive measures may be needed, e.g. analgesics, maintenance of blood pressure, supporting of breathing must be kept ready. Intravenous prednisolone and cold-sponging of patients with high fevers (>40°C, 104°F) are often used in the treatment of rickettsial disease.

Herbal Treatment

Follow the directions given in The Acute Treatment Of Disease. If this has been done hopefully this will now be a milder form of the disease. The specifics for this disease are Echinacea and Baptisia and I would add to that

Myrrh. For the fever as it is fairly fierce think of Peruvian Bark and Boneset (to help with the pains) or if you haven't any of these pick a couple from the list of Febrifuges. To begin this disease we want a very strong Antibiotic Action focused on the blood stream so as to kill as much of the attacking bacteria as we can at the beginning of the disease before it starts doing damage to the body especially the blood vessels. I feel the symptoms described so far are fairly bland so let's take a dose of reality, here is a description of Epidemic Typhus by **Herbalist Finley Ellingwood, M.D. 1910**

Symptomatology:— The disease requires ten days for its incubation, during the last two of which there is usually general malaise, indisposition and loss of appetite. The occurrence of a severe chill, or a series of light chills, is suddenly followed by immediate prostration, severe muscular pains, headache, tinnitus and vertigo and an almost immediate high temperature, which reaches 104° F. on the first day, and 105° F. on the second day, and persists with no regular remission. There is nausea and vomiting, sometimes most persistent. The tongue is coated with a thick, dirty, yellowish white coat; there is great thirst, but scanty urine of a high specific gravity.

The Nervous Symptoms are often pronounced from the first. With the appearance of the fever there is delirium, which may quickly become active, and as quickly, later on, assume a violent maniacal form, or assume the form of a typhomania. **Coma** and coma vigil quickly follow, the patient profoundly unconscious, yet staring into space with widely opened eyes. There are tremors, carphologia and subsultus tendinum. The face then assumes a dull, expressionless, even stupid appearance, the bright flush assumes a dull, dusky purplish hue, and evidences of the most extreme prostration, tending to complete exhaustion, are plainly apparent, the patient sinking down in the bed in the dorsal position.

About the third day of this serious disease, but often delayed twenty-four or thirty-six hours, a rash, which is characteristic of the disease, appears upon the abdomen first, and then extends to the chest and extremities, seldom appearing upon the face. This quickly assumes the form of a rose-colored eruption. There is no abatement of the temperature, but frequently an increase of the febrile phenomena. The pulse becomes rapid, feeble and irregular. The red spots become darker in hue, are hemorrhagic or petechial, and they coalesce, causing the skin to assume a spotted or mottled appearance. The tongue becomes brown and is dry, fissured and tremulous, and the teeth are covered with sordes.

On the fourteenth day there is usually a sudden rise of the temperature, and the crisis occurs. The decline of the fever is quite rapid, although marked with some exacerbations and irregularities.

The above is a truly great description by **Herbalist Finley Ellingwood, M.D. 1910** a obvious teacher of his profession. To help with the Nervous System and the Circulatory System Rosemary, Prickly Ash, Gravel Root and Angelica have been used in the past, they also add a Stimulant Action as well. Try to avoid the Sedative Nervines especially if the patient is going into a coma. Have a good read up of the herbs above to see how they fit into the picture especially the Nervine Stimulants, other than that treat the symptoms with the Actions needed as they arise.

Homoeopathic Treatment

One of the earliest tests of the homeopathic system was in the treatment of Typhus Fever in an 1813 epidemic which followed the devastation of Napoleon's army marching through Germany to attack Russia, followed by their retreat. When the epidemic came through Leipzig as the army pulled back from the east, Samuel Hahnemann, the founder of Homeopathy, was able to treat 180 cases of Typhus losing but two. This, at a time when the conventional treatments were having a mortality rate of over 30%. The main two remedies he was using were Bryonia and Rhus Tox which are below. Hahnemann would of used 6C to 30C Potencies. You only really use the 200C potency when you are positive the symptoms match especially the Mental Symptoms which are listed below as Mind and Emotions. Read through the symptoms below and imagine them as two different people, individuals each having a different experience of the disease Typhus. You must always try to prescribe holistically to the patient as we are all different. This is very important in Homoeopathy and I always try to do the same with my herbal formulas.

Bryonia 30C to 200C

MIND/EMOTIONS: person wants to lie still, in a dark, quiet room and remain undisturbed. If bothered, becomes extremely irritated and angry. A 'grump.' Fears he's going to die.

HEAD: Has a red face after being angry. Faint feeling upon rising. Pain is bursting, splitting feeling in rear (occiput) of head. Feels as if hammers were being struck inside his head. Worse with any motion. Headache comes on upon waking and as soon as he opens his eyes. Left-sided over eye, brow and across top of head to back of the skull (occiput).

MOUTH: Very dry feeling with urgent sense of thirstiness. Everything in mouth is dry, including tongue, throat region. Tongue has a thick, white coating or a dirty yellow one. Burning blisters on sides of tongue. Wants to drink large amounts of water.

STOMACH: Vomiting after drinking water. Worse: warm drinks, which are vomited even more quickly. Sore stomach. Pressure in stomach after eating. Knife-like pains felt in stomach.

EXTREMITIES: Stiff neck, red spots on the sides of the neck. Shooting, tearing pains all over the back, especially under left shoulder blade. All symptoms worse around 9pm. Worse: any kind of movement, better: lying still. Feels better lying on something very hard. Worse cold of any kind and better for heat of any kind.

FEVER: Pulse is full and hard. Chill, worse in evening. Cold and shivering all over, even under covers of bed. And then, followed by heat with sweat and thirst. Dry, burning heat felt throughout body. Always needs cold drinks. Unique symptoms: chill and heal alternate., and then heat and shuddering alternate.

Rhus Toxicodendron 30C to 200C

MIND/EMOTIONS: Feeling of extreme restlessness, will change position constantly. Senses become muddled. Apprehensive about nightfall and will refuse to stay in bed. A feeling of great helplessness coupled with deep sadness. Mental perceptions are dulled. With high fever there can be delirium and delusions.

HEAD: Feels heavy and scalp is super sensitive. Pain in the rear of the skull (occiput) and painful upon touch. Pain in forehead and headache moves up and over head to the rear of it. Worse with motion, better: morning, heat (cloth) and lying down. A sensation as if someone were pushing down on your forehead and driving head into the pillow.

MOUTH: Gums sore. Tongue has a red triangle at the tip of it/ Fever blisters around mouth. Pain in jaws. Bitter taste.

STOMACH: Unquenchable thirst. Desire for cold milk. Mouth and throat feel very dry. Feeling of stone in stomach.

EXTREMITIES: Hot, swollen, painful joints that are better with motion. If sitting or lying down, stiffness sets in along with pain. Neck very stiff, but feels better with warm cloth applied to area. Better: heat of shower or bath.

Tearing pains in joints. Worse: cold air, cold cloth on affected parts. Limbs become so stiff person may feel partly paralysed until they can begin to move and "loosen" up.

FEVER: Chilled but later, feels hot and wants to stretch limbs. Skin is cold and clammy feeling to it. Shivering or shaking in open air along with a great thirst for liquids. Pulse weak and very soft; cannot be felt sometimes. Odd sensation of chill and cold on the back, but a feeling of heat on chest and torso. Fever in evening, first shivering, then heat and thirst, with sweating, and then followed by diarrhoea. Fever strikes every 3rd or 4th day.

Plague
(Black Death)

Cause - Plague is caused by Yersinia pestis. Yersinia pestis is a short bacillus that may resemble a safety pin. Plague occurs primarily in wild rodents (eg, rats, mice, squirrels, prairie dogs) and is transmitted from rodent to human by the bite of an infected flea. Human-to-human transmission occurs by inhaling droplet nuclei from patients with pulmonary infection (primary pneumonic plague), which is highly contagious. The disease has an incubation period of 1 to 3 days pneumonic form or 2 to 6 days bubonic form.

Massive human epidemics have occurred (eg, the Black Death of the Middle Ages). More recently, plague has occurred sporadically or in limited outbreaks. Yersinia is considered a possible agent of bioterrorism.

Disease Process - *Yersinia pestis* is primarily a rodent pathogen, with humans being an accidental host when bitten by an infected rat flea. The flea draws viable *Y. pestis* organisms into its intestinal tract. These organisms multiply in the flea and block the flea's proventriculus. Some *Y. pestis* in the flea are then regurgitated when the flea gets its next blood meal thus transferring the infection to a new host. While growing in the flea, *Y. pestis* loses its capsular layer. Most of the organisms are phagocytosed and killed by the by the immune system in the human host but a few bacilli are taken up by tissue macrophages. The macrophages are unable to kill *Y. pestis* and provide a protected environment for the organisms to synthesize their virulence factors.

The organisms then kill the macrophages and are released into the extracellular environment, where they resist phagocytosis and quickly spread to the draining lymph nodes, which become hot, swollen, tender, and hemorrhagic. This gives rise to the characteristic bubo responsible for the name of this disease.

Within hours of the initial flea bite, the infection spills out into the bloodstream, leading to involvement of the liver, spleen, and lungs. The patient develops a severe bacterial pneumonia, exhaling large numbers of viable organisms into the air during coughing fits. 50 to 60 percent of untreated patients will die if. As the epidemic of bubonic plague develops (especially under conditions of severe overcrowding, malnutrition, and heavy flea infestation), it eventually shifts into a predominately pneumonic form, which is far more difficult to control.

Diagnosis - Diagnosis is epidemiologic and clinical, confirmed by culture and serology. Diagnosis is made by stain and culture of the organism, typically by needle aspiration of a bubo (surgical drainage may disseminate the organism); blood and sputum cultures should also be obtained.

Prevention - Transmission from cats can be by bite, or if the cat has pneumonic plague, by inhalation of infected droplets. Those with primary or secondary pneumonic plague require strict respiratory isolation. Rodents should be controlled and repellents used to minimize flea bites. Travelers should consider prophylaxis with doxycycline

Symptoms - Symptoms are either severe pneumonia or massive lymphadenopathy with high fever, often progressing to septicaemia. In bubonic plague, the most common form, the incubation period is usually 2 to 5 days but varies from a few hours to 12 days. Onset of a fever of 39.5 to 41° C is abrupt, often with chills. The pulse may be rapid and thready; hypotension may occur. Enlarged lymph nodes (buboes) appear with or shortly before the fever. The femoral or inguinal lymph nodes are most commonly involved, followed by axillary, cervical, or multiple nodes. Typically, the nodes are extremely tender and firm, surrounded by considerable oedema and can be excruciatingly painful. They may suppurate in the second week. The overlying skin is smooth and reddened but often not warm. A primary cutaneous lesion, varying from a small vesicle with slight local lymphangitis to an eschar, occasionally appears at the bite. The patient may be restless, delirious, confused, and uncoordinated. The liver and spleen may be enlarged.

Primary pneumonic plague has a 2 to 3 day incubation period, followed by abrupt onset of high fever, chills, tachycardia, and headache, often severe. Cough, not prominent initially, develops within 24 hours. Sputum is mucoid at first, rapidly develops blood specks, and then becomes uniformly pink or bright red (resembling raspberry syrup) and foamy. Tachypnea and dyspnea are present, but pleurisy is not. Signs of consolidation are rare, and rales may be absent.

Septicemic plague usually occurs with the bubonic form as an acute, fast coming illness. Abdominal pain, presumably due to mesenteric lymphadenopathy, occurs in 40% of patients. Pharyngeal plague and plague meningitis are less common forms.

Pestis minor, a more benign form of bubonic plague, usually occurs only in endemic areas. Lymphadenitis, fever, headache, and prostration subside within a week.

Prognosis - The mortality rate for untreated patients with bubonic plague is about 60%, with most deaths occurring from sepsis in 3 to 5 days. Most untreated patients with pneumonic plague die within 48 hours of symptom onset. Septicemic plague may be fatal before bubonic or pulmonary manifestations predominate.

Patients with pulmonary symptoms or signs should have a chest x-ray, which shows a rapidly progressing pneumonia in pneumonic plague. Immediate treatment reduces mortality to less than 5%. In septicemic or pneumonic plague, treatment must begin within 24 hours with streptomycin.

Treatment - The main antibiotics Streptomycin, tetracycline and Chloramphenicol however there has been found antibiotic resistance so Fluoroquinolone or Doxycycline should be tried. All pneumonic plague contacts should be under medical surveillance. Temperature should be taken every 4 hours for 6 days.

Herbal Treatment

Follow the directions given in The Acute Treatment Of Disease. If this has been done hopefully this will now be a milder form of the disease. The specifics for this disease in the past are Echinacea, Baptisia Poke Root and Berberis. Baptisia and Berberis are both Febrifuges and Antibacterials, so along with Echinacea these would be good herbs for starting treatment. Poke Root is our main Lymphatic herb and here we will use it internally and externally. Externally use it in a half and half mix with Echinacea as a lotion mixed 1 to 10 for the buboes, even saturate a cloth and leave it there.

Cleavers is another herb that can be used for the Lymphatic System. If the disease is becoming the Pneumonic form our main herb then becomes Pleurisy Root which will help with the fever and to reduce inflammation. Garlic is very important here for it exits the body via the lungs putting its Antibiotic Action right where we need it. Elecampane is another good respiratory herb which is Antibacterial, Expectorant and Diaphoretic. Looking back through history herbal treatment has not done much to help the victims of plague mainly because the disease moves to fast to its fatal end. This disease is a good example of why treatment should begin as soon as a person recognizes that they are getting sick. Another thing to bear in mind about this disease is that when it gets to the lungs it is highly contagious so you would have to do your treatment in a quarantined area wearing a mask a the least.

Homoeopathic Treatment

BUBONIC PLAGUE -- Anthrac., Ant. t., *Ars.*, Bapt., Bell., Bubon., Carbo v., Cinch., *Crot.*, Ign., Iod., *Lach.*, Naja, Operc., *Phos.*, *Pyr.*, Rhus t., *Tar. c.*

The above are the main remedies for the plague taken from Boerickes Materia Medica.

Arsenicum 6c to 30C - For high temperature septic fevers, complete exhaustion, great restlessness. The patient has continued nausea and vomiting, the face is yellow and the pulse is small, weak and tremulous. There is much burning in the precordial region and intense burning thirst, but, of course for small quantities of water only. Suffocative catarrh, worse lying on back, coughing blood with pain between shoulders, burning heat all over. Gangrenous inflammations.

Baptisia 6C - Use from 6C and upward in potency. Baptisia suits poisoned blood conditions, a dull, dark besotted countenance. Has a drowsy, stupid state, has a black or brownish coated tongue, patient falls asleep while answering questions, bed feels too hard, seems as if intoxicated this is very characteristic. The patient feels tired and bruised all over; is restless, and tosses about the bed to find a soft spot, but his restlessness is rather due to the mental rather than to the physical condition. Delirium is often present, profound prostration; the breath is fetid, and all exhalations and discharges from the patient are exceedingly offensive. The temperature is high, and so is the pulse, and there is tenderness in the ileo-caecal region. Lungs feel compressed, breathing is difficult, sense of suffocation, seeks open windows

Lachesis 30C - Delirium tremens with much trembling and confusion. Very important for patients of a melancholic disposition. Ill effects of suppressed discharges. Cannot bear anything tight anywhere. In fever they are chilly in back; feet icy cold; hot flushes and hot perspiration. Upper part of windpipe very susceptible to touch. Sensation of suffocation and strangulation on lying down, particularly *when anything is around throat*; compels patient to spring from bed and rush for open window. Cough; dry, suffocative fits, tickling. Little secretion and much sensitiveness, Boils, carbuncles, ulcers, with bluish, purple surroundings. Purpura, with intense prostration. There is a bleeding tendency running all through this remedy.

Pyrogen 30C to 200C - Pyrogen is the great remedy for *septic states*, with intense restlessness. "In septic fevers, especially puerperal, . *All discharges are horribly offensive* diarrheal, vomit, sweat, breath, etc. Great pain and violent burning in abscesses ,*Septic fevers*. Latent pyogenic condition. Chill begins in back. Temperature rises rapidly. Great heat with profuse hot sweat, but *sweating does not cause a fall in temperature*. Coldness and chilliness.

Man Made And Natural Disasters
Nuclear Weapons And Radiation

As there has only been two nuclear weapons detonated over cities the best place to start would be here. Hiroshima was the first city to be attacked with a nuclear weapon. This 26 square mile city had a population at the time of 225,000 which was less than normal due to an evacuation ordered by the Japanese Government because of conventional air raids. Three quarters of the population lived in a densely built up area in the center of the city.

On August the 6th at 2 am the Superfortress named Enola Gay took off from the airfield at Tinian Island. Around 7.15 am the air raid sirens begun at Hiroshima, at 8am local radar reported that only 3 aircraft were involved in the raid and the radio broadcasts warned civilians that no raid was expected as these were probably reconnaissance planes. At 8.16 am the weapon named little boy was released from the bomb bay. Little boy exploded with the explosive force of 15,000 tons or TNT in a airburst 1,900 feet above the city. 66,000 people were killed instantly in the fireball, and their bodies were vaporized in temperatures hotter than the sun. The blast wave destroyed or severely damaged more than 60,000 of the city's 90,000 buildings although some reinforced concrete buildings built to withstand earthquake shocks remained standing but were burnt out in the firestorm that raged in a 6,000 feet radius from the detonation. The total death toll was 118,661. A further 79,130 people were injured. The survivors suffered appalling injuries, burns from the bombs thermal radiation peeling the skin in scorched and charred tatters from their bodies. There was no treatment available as 90% of the Doctors and Nurses were killed or injured and only 3 of the city's 55 hospitals were usable.

Sometime after the attack a reporter Peter Burchett of the London Daily Mail wrote in an article the following. In the hospitals I found people who when the bomb fell suffered absolutely no injuries but are now dying from the uncanny side effects. For no apparent reason their health begun to fail. They lost their appetite, their hair fell out, bluish spots appeared on their bodies and then bleeding begun to form in their ears, nose and mouth. At first the Doctors thought that these were symptoms of general debility so they gave the patients Vitamin A injections. The results were horrible, the flesh started rotting away from the hole caused by the injection and in every case the victim died. Burchett was describing the symptoms of radiation sickness. Tens of thousands of people returned to Hiroshima after the blast and got radiation poisoning. It is estimated that 97,000 people died of cancers caused by the bomb in the three decades from 1950 to 1980.

On August the 9th three days after the attack on Hiroshima another Atom Bomb was dropped this time on the city of Nagasaki with a population of 173,000 which was a major ship building port. The bomb was more sophisticated and named Fat Man with a 21KT yield. The Japanese picked up two bombers on the radar but presumed it was just a observation flight and did not issue an air raid warning. The bomb was released a 11.02 am and exploded at a height of 1660 ft. The effects were similar to Hiroshima although the local terrain provided protection from the heat and blast to some areas it made it worse in others. An area of 4.5 square miles was leveled by the blast, 11,574 homes were burnt down and a further 2,652 completely destroyed in the blast. A total of 73,884 people were killed and another 74,909 injured. The radiation sickness afterwards mirrored that experienced at Hiroshima. About 24 hours after the Hiroshima blast relief workers from outside the city began to arrive and the situation stabilized somewhat. Power in undamaged areas of the city was even restored on August 7th, with a limited rail service resuming the following day. Several days after the blast, however, medical staff began to recognize the first symptoms of radiation sickness among the survivors. Soon the death rate began to climb again as patients who had appeared to be recovering began suffering from this strange new illness. Deaths from radiation sickness did not peak until three to four weeks after the attacks and did not taper off until seven to eight weeks after the attack. No one really knows the dose of radiation that the relief workers received for their efforts. Long-range health dangers associated with radiation exposure, such as an increased danger of cancer, would linger for the rest of the victims' lives, as would the psychological effects of the attack.

The casualty rate due to radiation was higher in Hiroshima, because although Fat Man (the bomb used at Nagasaki) had a higher yield than Little Boy (the bomb used at Hiroshima), Fat Man was a plutonium weapon, which is actually much less radioactive than a uranium weapon of equal yield.

Signs and Symptoms Of Radiation Poisoning

With acute radiation sickness, the amount of radiation is what decides how severe the radiation sickness will be. A dosage of 100 roentgens is sufficient to cause sickness. A dosage of 400 Roentgens will cause death 50% of the time and a dosage of 100,000 rads will cause death within an hour. Symptoms of radiation sickness do not usually develop immediately, rather over a period of time since it takes time for the mutated DNA to produce enough proteins to make an obvious change in body chemistry and structure. The faster the symptoms come on the higher the dose the patient has taken.

The symptoms of radiation sickness are vomiting (may include vomiting blood), diarrhea, skin burns, fatigue (can include fainting and weakness), dehydration, bleeding (from the nose, mouth, gums and rectum), open skin sores, ulceration (peeling and/or disintegration) of oral mucous membranes, the esophagus and internal tissues, inflammation, and hair loss. The tissues most affected by ionisation are those where the cells are rapidly reproducing with the best example being the mucous membranes especially those of the intestines. These tissues include blood forming tissues, the gonads, the skin, and tissues of the digestive tract.

During the atomic bombing of Hiroshima, thousands of Japanese were subjected to unprecedented amounts of radiation, resulting in a horrific situation. It is said that more people died from radiation sickness than the actual atomic blast, because the radiation spread throughout the region. Not surprisingly, the people who survived the radiation ended up having badly mutated children since they were being constructed with mutated DNA. Studies conducted on mice during the 1960s have showed that young children and babies are the most susceptible to severe radiation sickness complications since they are still growing and need pure DNA to ensure that their bodies grow in a normal. Once their DNA is mutated, their body grows in strange ways, often resulting in death or disability. Doctors can't do much about radiation sickness since they have no way of repairing the DNA. They can, however, treat the symptoms using medication and basic comfort care. Even if you survive radiation sickness, you will likely die early and experience complications in the future.

Natural Treatment For Radiation Poisoning

Trying to restore the immune system or at least keeping it going the best it can is the main objective. Other than that all you can do is try to relieve the symptoms as and when they come for example Peppermint and Ginger for the nausea and vomiting and Astringents for diarrhea. Other than that our treatment is the same as we use for people undergoing Radiation Treatment for Cancer which is the use of Adaptogens with one of the best for this condition being Astragalus which will help in building up the immune system along with helping with the fatigue and lack of energy.

Biological And Germ Warfare

This form of warfare is probably as old as humanity. Since the earliest of times wells have been poisoned, diseased bodies have been catapulted over fortress walls into cities and from one case of this the plague spread into Europe and only God knows how many political assassinations have been done this way through time. But unfortunately things look as if they may become worse even though so many treaties have now been signed and it is mainly because of cost and money.

To make a biological weapon compared to the other weapons of mass destruction is cheap, easy and you don't even need a scientist. To give you an idea of cost, $10 million would allow a country to develop a large arsenal. A similar arsenal of nuclear weapons would cost 200 million. Evidence presented to a UN panel in 1969 estimated that for a large scale operation against a civilian population casualties might cost about $2000 per square kilometer with conventional weapons $800 with nuclear weapons, $600 with nerve gas and just a $1 with biological weapons. Don't forget these figures are in 1969 currency. Modern technology is bringing the price down even more as laboratory and manufacturing equipment gets cheaper. The next step for biological warfare is genetics where they could program the germs genes to attack only certain races or to become more or less deadly or eventually to do whatever they wish.

The diseases listed below are the ones that are most commonly considered to be used as biological warfare agents, we will divide them up into viruses and bacteria etc and have a look at them.

Viruses - Colonize other cells forcing them to produce more viruses. Spread through the air by coughs and sneezes, others spread by blood and body fluids.

Diseases - Colds, AIDS, herpes, chicken pox, flu, polio, hepatitis, yellow fever, small pox, dengue fever, and the various sorts of encephalitis.

Animal Diseases - Foot and Mouth, canine distemper, rabies, African swine fever, Newcastle's disease (poultry), Rift Valley fever in cattle, sheep and goats.

Plant Diseases - Mosaic diseases in tobacco, tomatoes and soybeans, Curly top in sugar beat

Bacteria - In general bacteria causes illness by invading tissues or by producing toxins or both.

Bacterial Toxins - Botulism, ricin, tetanus, diphtheria, shiga (causes dysentery) and staphylococcus enterotoxin (food poisoning).

Bacterial Diseases - Anthrax, brucellosis, cholera, glanders, melioidosis, pneumonic plague, tularemia and typhoid. These are considered antipersonnel weapons rather than actual biological weapons with the possible exception of Russia's last batch of Anthrax which they reckon defeats all antibiotics.

Plant Diseases - Rice and corn blight.

Rickettisia - Sort of a cross between bacteria and a virus. They are bacteria but they can only live in host cells. They like insects such as lice, ticks and fleas.

Diseases - Typhus, Q fever, psittacosis and Rocky Mountain spotted fever.

Animal Diseases - Heart water in sheep and goats.

Fungi - Larger and more complex then bacteria and they reproduce by spores.

Diseases - Coccidioidomycosis a lung infection.

Animal Diseases - Aspergillosis in poultry.

Plant Diseases - Late blight in potatoes (caused the Irish potato famine), black stem rust in cereals and rice blast.

The only Army to have really practiced biological warfare and probably the first one to begin a in depth study of it was the Imperil Japanese Army. In 1935 under the command of General Shiri Ishii the secret research unit 731 started work in China at a place called Harbin in Manchuria. Three divisions of this unit were concerned with bacteriological research, warfare research and field experiments and the mass production and storage of bacteria. They investigated the effects of plague, anthrax, botulism, brucellosis, cholera, smallpox and typhus along with their vectors especially insects. They also looked for antidotes tested drugs, chemical toxins and plant and animal diseases. The remote location of this unit was chosen so that the scientists could experiment on humans without observation from others. Over 3000 Chinese prisoners were believed to have been killed from these experiments. The unit went on to design and produce delivery vehicles one being called the Ha, a steel bomb containing 1500 cylindrical pellets which had been immersed in anthrax or tetanus emulsions. For use against civilians the Uji was made which was a 25kg porcelain bomb that could contain up to 30,000 plague infested fleas or a large number of dysentery ,typhoid or anthrax bacteria. They also produced anthrax infected chocolates. The Uji was detonated by a small internal charge which made it explode in the air above the ground. During the 1942 Chekiang campaign against Chinese forces the Japanese tested their new weapons by pouring huge quantities of microbes into wells, reservoirs and rivers as well as using their Uji bombs in aerial attacks. Chinese losses were said to be incalculable and the Japanese lost 10,000 of their own men when by mistake they were sent to a contaminated area. The above mentioned is only a small part of what this unit got up to, it is well worth looking into them more as there is a few good books out on them now and it is a good example of how low humanity can go if given free rein. At the end of WW2 the USA gave the Japanese scientists from Unit 731 immunity from prosecution for war crimes in return for their expertise and silence. In this way the US received valuable information from the human experiments that they did not have.

To end this section the Americans in July 2001 staged a exercise code named Dark Winter simulating a attack on America using the smallpox virus. It was reported that by the end of the simulation the disease had spread to 25 states and 15 other countries. A biological warfare expert from the Center for Strategic and International Studies said to a Congressional hearing afterwards "No city, no state is capable of dealing with a incident like this".

The Russian Anthrax Accident

In the Russian city of Sverdlovsk in 1979 66 people died from a anthrax infection. Early in April 1979 patients began turning up at the hospitals complaining of flu like symptoms. Doctors were confused when these people started to die. The official reports said the victims had been infected by contaminated meat despite the autopsies showing airborne infection. Shortly after the victims began to die special emergency squads were brought in to shoot stray dogs, wash down houses and hospitals with chlorine and to pave roads. Medical records were seized by the KGB and the bodies were buried together in lime under guard at the states expense. Unknown to the authorities some tissue samples along with hand written notes and photos were hidden away.

In 1992 Boris Yeltsin head of the communist party in Sverdlovst at the time admitted that the anthrax outbreak was indeed caused by the military. The leak is thought to have happened by a technician removing a air filter and not replacing it right away. Eventually the tissue samples were examined at the Los Alamos Laboratories and were found to contain a mixture of 4 different strains of anthrax. Such a multi strain of anthrax would not occur naturally in nature but the 4 strains together in a bio-weapon would not give the average person much of a chance to avoid infection.

The Scottish Island Of Gruinard

During WW2 the British tested an anthrax bomb on the Island of Gruinard and within a few days the sheep on the island began to die. Because anthrax spores can survive in the soil the island was quarantined. It took 48 years before the government declared the island anthrax free. In 1990 the quarantine was lifted.

US Biological Weapons Fully Developed By 1969

Disease	Incubation Period	Effects	Period Survivors	Military Considerations
Anthrax		Lethal		
Bubonic Plague	2 - 3 Days	Lethal	Incapacitated	May contaminate the ground
Yellow Fever	2 - 6 Days	40 to 100% mortality	4 to 5 weeks	Potentially uncontrollable
Brucellosis	3 to 6 Days	Incapacitating 2% Mortality	1 to 5 weeks	Devastating to non-immune populations
Tularemia	7 - 60 Days	30 to 40% mortality	1 - 2 weeks	Recurrent fever over a month, may last 12 months.
Q-fever	2 - 10 Days	1% mortality	8 to 12 weeks	Illness lasts a month. Hardy bacteria can survive in soil for long periods

Global Warming

No one can deny the existence of global Warming any more. In late February 2009 I was in country Victoria just outside Bendigo prospecting and it was very hot about 45 degrees, so much for my idea of having a cool summer in Victoria especially when you are living in Van. As the heat wave was to continue for a few weeks I decided it was time to slowly head back home to Queensland with the first stop being the Murray River on the NSW border where I spent a few days cooling off in the river. While I was cooling down in the river fire raged through the country towns taking over 200 lives and causing mass destruction. It was the worst Natural Disaster in Australia's History. At the same time as this was happening Northern Queensland was flooding with the main highways under water causing towns to be isolated and people, animals and crops trapped where they were till the waters go down. But the waters can't go down till it stops raining which it didn't for a few weeks. While the fires were burning and the flood flooding a old disease started heading south to claim new lands as the temperature had changed and the disease could feel comfortable in more places now, that disease is Dengue Fever with its four different strains thanks to modern air travel. Then along comes a cyclone that keeps gaining strength becoming as strong as you can be but thank goodness it stayed 200ks off the coast but unfortunately it damaged a large ship that released over 200 tonnes of oil onto some of the most beautiful coast in the world and that's not mentioning the 31 containers loaded with chemicals that went overboard that they are still trying to find. All this has happened in only 5 weeks. These few weeks are similar to what's happening all round the world now. This is the beginning of where the effects of Global Warming are becoming really noticeable to the person on the street. From here on its only going to get worse. As you would of noticed a lot of our cyclones, hurricanes and typhoons are getting stronger than normal, in the future add to this the rising sea levels form the melting poles and the king tides caused by the storms and you can start to imagine the potential coastal damage that is going to happen in the future. Let's look at part of the economic side as well. In parts of Australia such as the Gold Coast a lot of wealthy have brought what is called canal homes in other words a home that backs up to canal that exits out to sea. This allows the owners to moor their yachts and power boats to a pier at the back of their homes. Local insurance companies are now getting worried because they could be up for massive repetitive claims and may one day decide not to insure these homes. If you cannot insure your house its value is not worth much anymore. The yearly fires in Australia are also becoming more common in other countries around the world especially in California, Greece and other places in Europe along with the heat waves that cause them. The heat waves especially take a toll on the elderly more so when they are in places which are not set up for hot summers such as institutions without air conditioning. This leads to another question what happens when everyone in these countries turn on their new air conditioners at once, will the power grid collapse? There are lots of problems that we will have to deal with in the future from the disasters that come on fast and the ones that come on slow such as rising sea levels, drought, hotter temperatures, the great rivers drying up along with massive displacement of populations but let's now concentrate on disease. Time has moved on now and since then I have been evacuated from Brisbane City in the 2011 floods only to go home and get cut off by flood waters and loose power for seven days, as I am writing this in October 2013 a 300 kilometer fire front is burning outside Sydney in the mountains destroying houses in its path and it's only the beginning of spring!

Surviving Natural Disasters

Surviving different types of disasters requires different types of plans but there are some constants such as a good First Aid Kit, a basic survival kit of pocket knife, torch, radio, batteries, maybe with all your old still working mobile phones along with a wind up charger for the phones as you can still usually access the emergency number without a card. Another constant is a food and water stash in some easily accessed place in your home. Another two very important ones are medications taken and official documents.

It is always good to give copies of important documents and computer backups to a good friend or family member who does not live with you for safe keeping maybe do a swap so you are both safe.

Many disasters are difficult or impossible to predict and even the expected ones can happen so fast that you do not have much time to react; fate and chance play a very big role in determining the outcome. You must have at least the basics ready to maximize your chances of survival. It is vital to understand the disasters that the area in which you live is prone to whether it be Cyclones, Fires or Floods. One very important thing to have in a family plan is where you will all meet up again if and when you are separated. Ensure that at least one member of the family knows First Aid and that you have a good manual. You may need specialized equipment for your Disaster Plan such as water pumps for fire and flooding so make sure you know what you need and get them and even more important make sure you know how to use them and that they will work when needed.

Study carefully the plans and procedures that your local authorities have put in place and make sure that you and your family know what to do. If you have to evacuate make sure you know the shortest and safest routes to use and always obey the commands of the civil authorities and emergency services for they have trained for this and generally have a better all-round knowledge of what is happening and going on, remember time is of the essence in a disaster so don't argue just keep on moving as fast as you can to safety remember they are trained to save lives not property. Don't become a victim become a survivor. A few steps now and a check on equipment and supplies just once a year maybe just before the Cyclone season to replace batteries and water etc can make you a survivor. Survive with confidence.

Tsunami

A Tsunami is a chain of fast moving waves known as a train that is generated when water in the ocean or even in a lake is suddenly displaced either by an earthquake, volcanic eruption, massive landslide or meteorite impact. Tsunamis are nearly undetectable out in the open sea and their waves can travel up to 600mph. Many a fisherman has returned home only to find ruin and wonder at the cause. As the wave approaches land the shallow water acts as brake on the front of the wave slowing it down to about 200mph, while the back of the wave continues at full speed. Then the back catches up to the front to form a massive wall of water. The separation of the waves in a Tsunami train can be in excess of 60 mile apart and are sometimes separated by as much as a hour. Tsunamis don't all make their final approach as massive waves some may be more like a rapidly rising tide with a considerable underwater turbulence sucking people under and tossing heavy objects around. The Tsunami has the force of the whole sea behind it hence the power to throw massive weights miles inland while a normal wave only has the force of the wind and tide. Often the only warning of a Tsunami is the sight of the tide suddenly going out as far as the horizon; experts say when you see this you have about five minutes to get to high ground. Animals seem to have a sixth sense that danger is imminent and flee to high ground, this has reportedly happened through history. We have all seen the results of Japan where not only did they suffer from the wave but are still suffering from the radiation fall out, you could not have made a worse disaster even if you had tried.

What To Do In The Event Of A Tsunami

1. Pay Attention To The Warning Signs. A strong earthquake or unusual rapid changes in sea level can be signs of an imminent Tsunami. On some prone coast lines people will run immediately for the high ground. Fisherman should take their boats out to deep water so as to avoid there destruction. Animals seem to instinctively know if a tsunami is on the way so if they run for the hills, follow them.

2. Act Quickly. A few minutes can be the difference between life and death.

3. **Move To High Ground.** Or to the strongest and highest structure you can find if you can't make it to high ground.

4. **Avoid The Initial Surge.** If caught in the current don't fight it but head to the nearest suitable floating object.

5. **If you are caught by the first wave and survive** seek higher ground immediately as the water does more damage heading back out to sea then in.

6. **Be Aware Of Further Waves.** The second and third waves are often far bigger than the first wave so stay somewhere safe or go to even higher ground.

Recent Tsunamis

17th of July 1998 Papua New Guinea - An offshore earthquake triggered a 40ft Tsunami which hit the coast killing 2200 people and left thousands more homeless.

26th of December 2004 Banda Aceh - There was a magnitude 9 earthquake off the coast of Aceh resulting in a Tsunami hitting Banda Aceh 15 minutes latter causing destruction to 60% of the city. Some local villages and towns where virtually wiped out. The end result was about 250,000 killed and 800,000 homeless. 90 minutes latter Thailand was hit, Two hours latter Sri Lanka was hit. Three and a half hours later the Maldives were hit. Seven hours later Somalia was hit. The chain of Tsunamis from off the coast of Aceh was a major multinational disaster affecting many millions of people by its death and destruction.

March 2011 The Japanese Tsunami - Huge earthquake, towns and Nuclear Plants wiped out the worst case scenario for a tsunami.

After The Waves

Banda Aceh after the waves was close to the worst case scenario, bodies everywhere, no power, no water, ruined sewerage system, no shelter, stagnating salt waters pools everywhere with who knows what's in them, damaged roads, bridges down and cut off from the outside world. Some people had to wait 11 days till the first help arrived; people were still being picked up out at sea clinging to trees 8 days after the disaster.

Looking at all the countries hit the long term problems were massive unemployment, loss of trades and industries especially the fishing industry which had most of its fleet destroyed, damage to the coast and agricultural land which became salt laden, loss of homes, long term refugee camps and having to rebuild the infrastructure again which comes with great cost.

The main diseases the authorities were most concerned about were cholera, diphtheria, diarrhea, hepatitis, dengue, malaria and respiratory tract infections especially from those who had inhaled water. One of the main problems after the disaster was getting fresh water to the people.

Japan was saved from the ravages of disease but had to pay the price Nuclear Power, some of the reactors were so old and so poorly designed that it was a disaster waiting to happen.

Floods

With the weather patterns changing and storms becoming stronger than normal we can expect a lot more flooding especially in the areas that are prone to flooding. Rising sea levels and stronger storm surges will no doubt in the future lead to the abandoning of some areas especially when the insurance companies stop insuring properties. The most dangerous floods are the flash floods which come and go fast but catch everyone unexpected. Unlike the flash flood a broad scale flood can last for weeks especially if the affected area is flat and the water can only disperse slowly. In the case of a long river the flood peak can take over a month to travel down the river system. If the flood destroys bridges and roads as they do frequently then you will have isolated pockets of population trapped without food or water living in unsanitary conditions. People who live in flood prone areas should have a disaster plan already prepared along with what they need to survive and know where the safe high ground is without having to cross streams, rivers or bridges.

What To Do During A Flood

1. Monitor the news and weather for any new warnings or developments. Be prepared to evacuate if the need arises.
2. Take your car to high ground or a safe area; maybe load it with some supplies and delicate electrical equipment.
3. Block the space under the doors and ventilator holes of your house with sandbags. Tie curtains away from the floor and store electrical gear and furniture as high up as possible.
4. Store food water and warm clothing in a high part of the house also

have torch, batteries, candles and a transistor radio ready in case of power failure.
5. Store valuable documents and any medications in a safe and dry place.
6. Turn off power and gas.
7. Prepare as much as you can in the daylight hours in case of power failure at night.
8. Do not walk or drive through flood water.
9. Stay clear of watercourses and drains.

Floods cause people and animals to seek high ground especially rodents whose burrows flood, which in turn causes them all to live very close together for a while allowing for diseases and parasites to cross to humans. A good example of a flood disease in a warm climate is Leptospirosis. Outbreaks are caused by exposure to water contaminated with the urine of infected animals, including rodents, cattle, pigs, horses, dogs and wild animals. Flooding can increase the risk of disease in animals and humans. Humans become infected through contact with urine or tissues of infected animals. The infection can enter the body through a cut or abrasion or through the mucous membranes of the eyes or nose as well as drinking and eating contaminated food and water. People wading or immersed in flood waters in contaminated areas are susceptible especially if they have cuts and abrasions. This is just one of the many waterborne diseases a flood victim has to deal with for the others see the section on Waterborne Diseases.

Earthquake

For many people Earthquakes are a common occurrence, small tremors are felt on an almost daily basis in certain parts of the world and people live with a resigned fear of the next big one. During a strong Earthquake many people's lives are going to depend on a few unpredictable factors such as which part of the world they are in and is it day or night.

You could be driving in a car, working in a factory or shop or asleep in your bed in a multi-story apartment building. Earthquakes occur unexpectedly and if you live in an Earthquake prone area you should have a Disaster Plan already made with everyone knowing what to do and especially stating where you will all meet up if you are separated when a disaster happens.

What To Do During A Earthquake

1. If Outside move quickly away from buildings and power lines and get into the open if you can. If there is no open space watch for falling masonry and glass and dodge them if you can while making your way to get under a table, car, truck or the best structure you can see that can protect you. Hold on to the structure tight and move with it. Stay there till the ground stops shaking. After the shaking stops make your way to open ground avoiding hazards as you go.

2. If Indoors do not try to run outside or you will be injured by falling debris. Collapses of substandard buildings can happen in seconds which is a insufficient time to make it to anywhere safe. Quickly drop to the floor and take cover under a sturdy piece of furniture such as a desk or table. Hold on to it tight and move with it. Stay there till the ground stops shaking then make your way to a safe area avoiding hazards on the way.

3. If Driving stop as soon as it is safe to do so but not under trees, power poles or power lines. Stay in the car, keep clear of structures that may collapse such as bridges, overpasses and tunnels. Do not block the road and if you have to leave your car leave the keys in it so it can be moved by others if necessary.

4. If In The Mountains watch out for falling rocks and landslides, get out of areas downstream from dams.

5. If At The Beach beware of the possibilities of Tsunami's and that they could arrive in minutes and move to higher ground or as far inland as possible.

6. After The Earthquake assist others who have been injured. Check your home and if it has been damaged turn off the gas, electricity and water. Fires caused by earthquakes have wiped out many cities in the past.

7. Beware Of Aftershocks use extreme caution when entering buildings even if they look safe. Already damaged buildings can collapse during aftershocks.

If you live in an Earthquake prone area it would be an idea to buy some whistles on chains or even use some string to replace the chain because whistles can save your life if you become trapped in a collapsed building. You can only shout for a few hours then you lose your voice but you can blow a whistle for as long as you are breathing. I've been using whistles for years, give them to your kids and you can never lose them in the bush. I use them when I go Gold prospecting in remote areas because when I get to engrossed in my metal detector I never know where I might end up and have been lost a few times.

Hurricanes, Typhoons And Cyclones

A Hurricane is in the Atlantic Ocean, a Typhoon is in the Northwest Pacific Ocean while a Cyclone is in the Southwest Pacific and North Indian Oceans other than that they are the same storm except that the winds move clockwise in the southern hemisphere and anticlockwise in the northern hemisphere. Cyclones generally move away from the equator and then either hit land or cooler ocean waters, when this happens in both cases the Cyclone weakens. When Cyclones start moving across land they form rapidly into rain depressions which can cause extensive flooding especially if they hang around. If the Cyclone moves out to sea again it can reintensify and get its strength back and start moving in a highly unpredictable course. As the Cyclone approaches a coast it creates a storm surge which occurs when strong and persistent winds blow towards the coast from the sea pushing the water toward and then across the shoreline and then further inland. The central pressure at the center of the Cyclone also lifts the water a bit like sucking through a straw which adds to the storm surge and coastal flooding. Sometimes the storm surge causes more damage than the Cyclone. Unfortunately for us Global Warming with its increasing temperatures is making Cyclones stronger than what they were and increasing the number of them as well.

Hurricane Classifications

1. **Category 1** - Winds between 74 and 95 miles per hour (119 to 153 ks). Minor Damage to housing and infrastructure.
2. **Category 2** - Winds between 96 and 110 miles per hour (154 to 177 ks). Roofing is peeled off houses and small trees blown down. Small water craft are torn from their moorings.
3. **Category 3 -** Winds between 111 and 130 miles per hour (179 to 209 ks) significant damage to housing and infrastructure occurs plus a increasing storm surge in coastal areas. Large trees are blown down.
4. **Category 4** - Winds between 131 to 155 miles per hour (211 to 249 ks) Major damage inflicted to housing and infrastructure. Extensive flooding

occurs in coastal areas through a rising storm surge. Wide spread destruction of forested areas.

5.   **Category 5** - Winds greater than 155 miles per hour (249 ks) Catastrophic damage occurs to buildings and infrastructure. Massive storm surge generates wide spread flooding on the coast and most trees and shrubs are destroyed. Loss of life is likely in populated areas.

What To Do During A Cyclone

1.   **Monitor The Media** and listen for the storm warnings. Be ready to evacuate if the need arises.
2.   **Have A Battery Operated Radio** and torch ready in case of power failure. Have your disaster kit in a secure place.
3.   **If You Are In A House Stay In The House** and shelter in the most secure part of the building away from the windows. Small rooms are usually the strongest so head to the bathroom even the bath an put a mattress on top of you.
4.   **If The Wind Drops** don't go outside because you could be in the eye of the storm and it will start again at full force in about 10 minutes or so depending on the size of the eye of the cyclone.
5.   **If You Are Caught In A Car** park well away from the sea or any watercourses, power lines and trees. Stay inside the vehicle.
6.   **After The Cyclone Has Passed** help your neighbors, don't go sightseeing, clear the area for emergency vehicles.

Volcanoes

Volcano Alert Systems

The United States Geological Survey has developed a color coded warning system to describe the current state of active volcanoes.

Green Alert - Volcano displaying above background levels of activity through to a moderate levels of unrest.

Yellow Alert - Intense unrest. Seismic activity is elevated. Potential for eruptive activity is increased. A plume of gas, steam, and minor amounts of ash may arise several thousand feet above the volcano.

Orange Alert - Accelerating and intense unrest. A eruption is likely within hours to days. Small ash eruptions are expected or confirmed. Seismic disturbance has been recorded on local seismic stations, but not at more distant stations.

Red Alert - Eruption is in progress. A plume is likely to rise to 25,000 feet or more. Strong seismic disturbance is recorded on all local and commonly on more distant stations.

What To Do During A Volcanic Eruption

1. **Be Aware Of The Volcanic Alert Status** - Organizations such as the Smithsonian Institute and the United States Geological Survey maintain a active list of global volcanoes with their status being updated regularly available online. If you live in a high volcanic risk area or are visiting one on high alert, prepare an evacuation plan and a emergency communication plan and have disaster supplies on hand and readily accessed. Torch, battery operated radio, emergency food and water, first aid kit, dust masks and goggles.

2. **Evacuate Quickly** - Accounts of historic eruptions show that people and even civil authorities were reluctant to leave despite extremely dangerous signs of volcanic activity often to their peril. To leave one's home and comfortable surrounding is not an easy decision but make it well before the disaster strikes.

3. **Be Aware Of All The Dangers** - Close to the volcano you may be affected by the blasts from the explosion. Lava flows; mud flows and floods will travel down the river valleys and cover low lying areas so avoid these while moving away from the volcano.

4. **Be Prepared For Ash Falls** - Ash poses a threat as it can travel hundreds of miles from a erupting volcano blanketing downwind towns and cities.

5. **In The Event Of A Ash Fall** - It is best to remain inside and seal all doors, windows and vents. The sharp jagged ash particles are extremely abrasive so it is necessary to wear goggles and a dust mask out doors and to avoid using the car or any other motors as the ash will damage them. Where there is a adequate warning of an eruption cover all motors and appliances.

6. **Keep The Roof Of Your Home Clear From Ash** - Wet ash is extremely heavy and even a buildup of only a few inches can cause the roof to collapse.

Fire

Check with your local Fire Station about the fire dangers in your local community, they always have lots of information for you to take away. In summer during the fire danger season keep the radio on and listen to the media for any problems that may be happening. Have your own fire plan ready and always prepare your house and property for the worst at the beginning of every fire season especially now as the weather patterns are changing.

Fire Danger Classifications

Fire dangers are calculated by taking into account past rainfall, air temperature, humidity and wind speed. Present and forecasted weather is also taken into consideration. Fire danger is usually expressed by the following ratings - Low, Moderate, High, Very High and Extreme. Various fire restrictions or bans are usually attached to these ratings. Always listen to the local radio or media for current bans and warnings.

When Approaching Fire Catches You At Home

1. Shelter inside the house away from the windows
2. Close all doors and windows to prevent the entry of embers and block any gaps from inside using wet towels.
3. Take furniture away from the windows and remove the curtains.
4. Keep everyone and pets inside the house and make sure there is plenty to drink. Ensure everyone stays together. Make sure everyone is wearing long pants and shirts and has adequate footwear to avoid burns to unprotected skin.
5. Turn off the gas supply at the mains.
6. Plug down pipes with tennis balls and rags and fill the gutters with water.
7. Assemble a emergency water supply by filling the bath and all basins with water and place fill buckets in areas they will be needed.
8. Drink plenty of water and avoid dehydration from heat stress.
9. Pack any items you may need to take away with you in the event of a evacuation.
10. Park your car in a clear area and close all the doors and windows and put some blankets in the car as well as water.
11. After the fire front has passed exit the house and check for spot fires.
12. If fires have started that cannot be extinguished evacuate the house,

First Aid Naturally

Here we will mainly concentrate on wounds and their treatment which is very important because if you do not deal with wounds properly they could lead on to the three diseases that we lead the First Aid Section with, they are Tetanus, Septicemia and Gangrene. In this section we give you both Herbal and Homoeopathic Treatment.

One of the best ways to learn Homoeopathy and prove to yourself its worth is by getting to know and using some of the main First Aid Remedies. For First Aid we will most of the time use the low potencies usually from 6C to 30C. An example is Arnica 6C which is a Low potency while Arnica 30C is the highest of the low potencies. Paradoxically the higher the potency the stronger the action, this is the opposite of Allopathic Medicine which is our modern medicine. Low potencies of about 6C can be given every half hour while 30C can be 4 to 5 hourly or sometimes daily. With Homoeopathy you try to match the intensity of the symptom to the potency eg the more intense the pain the higher the potency. If you want to learn more about Homoeopathic First Aid one of the best books about the subject was written by Dr Dorothy Shepherd who used most of the remedies you will soon be learning during the Nazi Blitz of London, and she gives you good examples from her patients.

Tetanus

Cause - Tetanus is an acute poisoning from a neurotoxin produced by Clostridium tetani. These bacteria form durable spores that can be found in soil and animal faeces and remain viable for years. The cause is from a contaminated wound especially puncture wounds that force dirt deep inside the body. In the past this disease was a lot more common with horse manure all over the streets and was known as lock jaw. Worldwide, tetanus is estimated to cause over half a million deaths annually, mostly in newborns and young children, but the disease is so rarely reported that figures are only rough estimates.

Disease Process - The disease attacks new-born infants, especially in hot climates. It is at times epidemic in camps of laborers. It occurs most frequently among men and barefooted boys. It is common to workers of the soil, gardeners, laborers and to those who work around barns and stables. Tetanus is an acute infectious disease, characterized by tonic spasm of the muscles, first of the jaw and neck; later of the trunk and limbs. The toxin enters the CNS along the peripheral motor nerves or through the blood from a contaminated wound to nervous tissue. Tetanospasmin binds irreversibly to the membranes of nerve synapses, blocking release of inhibitory transmitters from nerve terminals and causing a generalized tonic spasticity. Once bound the toxin cannot be neutralized.

Diagnosis -A history of a recent wound in a patient with muscle stiffness or spasms is a clue. In the end it is the fixed smile and raised eyebrows that give the diagnosis but by then it's usually too late.

Prevention - Vaccination. Because dirt and dead tissue promote C. tetani growth, prompt and thorough debridement of especially deep puncture wounds is essential. See treatment of wounds. St Johns Wort is the specific in tetanus prevention.

Symptoms - The average incubation period is 5 to 10 days. The most frequent symptom is jaw stiffness. Other symptoms include difficulty swallowing, restlessness, irritability; stiff neck, arms, or legs, headache, fever, sore throat, chills and tonic spasms. Later, the patient has difficulty opening their jaw. Facial muscle spasm produces a characteristic expression with a fixed smile and elevated eyebrows. Rigidity or spasm of abdominal, neck, and back muscles may occur. Sphincter spasm may cause urinary retention or constipation. Difficulty in swallowing may interfere with nutrition. Mental state is usually clear, but coma may follow repeated spasms. During generalized spasms, the patient is unable to speak or cry out because of chest wall rigidity or glottal spasm. Spasms also interfere with respiration, causing cyanosis or fatal asphyxia. The immediate cause of death may not be apparent.

Prognosis - Tetanus has a worldwide mortality rate of about 50%. Mortality is highest at the extremes of age and in drug abusers. The prognosis is poorer if the incubation period is short and symptoms progress rapidly or if treatment is delayed. Death may occur on the second day in the more acute cases, or life may be prolonged in agony until the fifth or sixth.

Treatment - Treatment is immune globulin to neutralize the toxin and intensive support.

Herbal Treatment

All wounds must be thoroughly cleaned with Calendula and St Johns Wort (specific) lotion mixed 1 to 10, especially puncture wounds where dirt has been pushed deep into the wound. Clostridium tetani is anaerobic so it lives and thrives without oxygen, so deep inside puncture wounds is its ideal home. Echinacea is another specific, internal and external and if I was worried I would even use Garlic oil in a deep wound probably Tea Tree oil too. Also consider giving Passion Flower. This is a very nasty way to die so every ounce of prevention is worth it.

Homoeopathic Treatment

Nux Vom 6C to 30C - The leading remedy. It has tetanic convulsions with distortion of eyes and face, with dyspnoea excited by any external impression. Strychnia, the alkaloid of Nux-vomica, produces a perfect picture of tetanus, with its convulsion of muscles renewed by the slightest external impression, its "risus sardonicus," its respiratory spasm, with blue cyanosed face and clear mind. The value of Strychnia in tetanus is recognized by Trousseau and Stille, and it is a striking example of Homoeopathy.

Hydrocyanic Acid 6C to 30C - This is a remedy very homoeopathic to tetanus. It produces a persistent tonic spasm from its direct action on the spinal cord. It shows itself in the muscles of the face, jaws and back. There is trismus or locked jaw, risus sardonicus and impeded respiration, with lividity and frothing at the mouth; the rigidity is firm, the body is bent backwards, the attack is sudden, and there is less reflex excitability than with the Strychnia case. Angustura produces a tetanic rigidity of the muscles, a painful stiffness and stretching of the limbs. The lips are drawn back showing the teeth and the jaws are locked.

Cicuta Virosa 6C to 30C - A useful remedy in tetanoid convulsions, with sudden rigidity and jerkings followed by prostration. There is great oppression of breathing, locked jaw, opisthotonos renewed by touch. There are oesophageal spasms and a marked symptom is fixed eyes staring at one point.

Physostigma 6C to 30C - Here the sensory nerves are irritable; there are tetanic spasms stiffness of spine and legs alternate dilation and contraction of the pupils. This seems to be characteristic. Carbolic acid has been used with success in tetanus. Phenol has been found to work better than antitetanic serum, which is preserved by phenol. There is no question but that it is a powerful remedy.

Hypericum 6C to 30C - Trismus from injury to nerves; it is considered prophylactic in cases of wounds of palms or soles. Especially useful in spinal injuries. It has a growing clinical record in this disease. Dr. Zopfy corroborates the use of Hypericum in tetanus in a practice of sixty years.

Septicaemia

Cause - It is commonly referred to as blood poisoning. Septicaemia, sometimes referred to as bacteremia, is a syndrome resulting from an acute invasion of the bloodstream by certain microorganisms or their toxic products from an infection elsewhere in the body. Any pathogenic organism can cause septicemia and septic shock. Septic shock is most commonly caused by gram-negative bacteria. Staphylococci, streptococci and other gram-positive organisms are less frequent, as are fungi and certain rare viruses. Any person with an impaired immunity, the newborn and the elderly are at the greatest risk. Infections can be hidden and hard to find with good examples being an infected wisdom tooth or a bone abscess.

Disease Process - In this condition it is generally the toxins made by the bacteria that are causing the damage that's why identifying the toxin or toxins are important.

Diagnosis - Is from blood tests and cultures.

Symptoms - Fever, chills which can have a fast onset, rapid heartbeat, and rapid breathing are common acute symptoms of septicemia. When hypotension and signs of inadequate organ function develop, the condition is termed septic shock. The symptoms vary in septicemia with the cause of the infection. The period of incubation may be very short if the infection is virulent, or it may last ten to fourteen days when the intoxication is from the products of germs in development. There is malaise and headache, disordered digestion and perhaps nausea, vomiting and diarrhea, with perhaps dullness and tendency to sleep, these would be the symptoms of a slow build up.

Prognosis - Septic shock has a 40 to 60 percent death rate.

Treatment - The stopping and reversal of septicemia especially when it gets to the septic shock stage depends upon aggressive treatment of the underlying infection. The treatment will vary according to how severe the septicemia is to the general health of the patient and the cause. If possible, the surgical removal or drainage of the source of the infections should be done. Antibiotics should be started as soon as the diagnosis is suspected.

Intravenous fluids and blood pressure medications may be necessary if hypotension or shock develops.

Herbal Treatment

Here we have to find the cause, sometimes this will be easy and at other times we will not be able to, but treatment must be started immediately. In a cases where you are desperate and can't find any answers take the patients clothes off and get them to lie on the bed. What you are going to do is check the lymphatics mainly where the main glands are. Start at the neck under the jaw and see if those glands are swollen then move on to the arm pits and then to the inside top of each thigh. For example if you find the glands at the left thigh are swollen check out the whole of the left leg and see if you can find the source of the infection causing the glands to swell. Heat can sometimes lead the way. The main Actions we shall use are those of the Antibacterials and Alteratives. With Echinacea being one of the main ones and Garlic of course. If you can find the cause try to match your herbs to the cause and parts or organs affected. If the patient goes into shock and the blood pressure starts to drop give Hawthorn to raise it again. If the lymphatic glands are swollen especially at the throat think of Poke Root and other lymphatic herbs such as Baptisia.

Homoeopathic Treatment

Lachesis 6C to 30C - This remedy does its best work in localized pyaemia, traumatic gangrene, and carbuncles. The indications are blue skin, sensitive parts, great prostration and scanty discharges. It has the prostration of Arsenicum but lacks its restlessness.

Rhus Tox 6C to 30C - Produces a perfect picture of septicemia, with redness and soreness at the point of infection. Chilliness, dry tongue, diarrhoea, restlessness.

Echinacea 6C to 30C - Pyaemia, dull aching in head and extremities. Infections spreading from uterus, tympanitis, sensitive abdomen, foul discharges. It seems to overcome to toxaemia of absorption.

Carbolic Acid 6C to 30C - This, internally, is a neglected remedy in septicaemia. Prostration, exhaustion to the point of collapse are indications. The patient falls asleep from weariness and wakens unrefreshed.

Arnica 6C to 30C - Anaemia and pyaemia, sore bruised sensations, loose stools, foul odours. **Baptisia** offensive exudates, is antistreptococcic, Arnica, quiet, mental restlessness. **Arsenicum**. A frequently indicated remedy in septic conditions. Restlessness, anguish, local and general burning, vomiting and prostration. Pyrogen has a good clinical record. We cannot give its special indications, it is evidently a "mixed vaccine."Boericke speaks well of both Streptoccin and Staphyloccin as to be compared with this remedy.

Gangrene

Cause - Two major types of gangrene exist. Dry gangrene is caused by a reduction of blood flow or blockage of an artery. It appears gradually and progresses slowly. In most people the affected part does not become infected. In this type of gangrene, the tissue becomes cold and black, begins to dry. Dry gangrene is most often seen in people with blocked arteries. Wet or moist gangrene develops as a complication of an untreated infected wound. Swelling resulting from the bacterial infection causes a sudden stoppage of blood flow. Cessation of blood flow allows invasion of the muscles by the bacteria where they multiply because disease-fighting cells cannot reach the affected parts. Gas gangrene is a type of wet gangrene caused by the bacteria known as *Clostridia*. *Clostridia* are a type of bacteria that grow only in the absence of oxygen. As the *Clostridia* grows they produce poisonous toxins and gas causing the condition known as gas gangrene. Gangrene can involve any part of the body but the most common sites include the toes, fingers, feet, and hands.

Disease Process - The following conditions are risk factors for the development of gangrene, Injury or trauma, such as a crush injury, a severe burn or frostbite, diseases that affect the circulation of blood, such as arteriosclerosis, diabetes, smoking, or Raynaud disease and untreated wound developing an infection.

Symptoms - For dry Gangrene the symptoms are the affected area becomes cold and numb after being initially red, then it develops a brown discoloration and finally it becomes black and shriveled. For Wet Gangrene the affected area becomes swollen and decays and is extremely painful. Local oozing occurs producing a foul odor and the part becomes black, the affected person develops a fever. In Gas Gangrene when the wound becomes infected a brown-red or bloody discharge may ooze from the affected tissues. Gas produced by Clostridia may produce a crackling sensation when the affected area is pressed. The part becomes swollen and the pain is severe. The affected person develops a fever, increased heart rate, and rapid breathing when the toxins spread into the bloodstream.

Treatment - For dry gangrene because the cause is a lack of blood flow, restoring the blood supply is vital. Assessment by a vascular surgeon can help determine whether surgical intervention can restore blood supply. For wet gangrene surgical debridement (removal of dead tissue) of the wound is performed, and intravenous antibiotics are administered to control the infection. For gas gangrene the condition needs to be treated aggressively because of the threat of the infection rapidly spreading via the bloodstream and damaging vital organs. The wound requires immediate debridement and usually IV antibiotics are administered.

Herbal Treatment

Some specifics for this condition are Echinacea, Garlic, Figwort and Baptisia. The main actions we need are those of Antibiotics and Alteratives. If the condition is brought on by a vascular condition or clot think of Ginkgo Biloba as this herb is a peripheral vasodilator and may improve blood flow.

Homoeopathic Treatment

Arnica 6C – Low doses of Arinca can sometime dissolve clots.

Arsenicum 6C to 30C - Dry gangrene in old people, soreness and burning relieved by warmth, restlessness. It is often indicated in gangrene of the lungs. Secale is aggravated by warmth, thus differing from Arsenicum. Arsenicum has a fetid diarrhea, great weakness, emaciation, and coldness and heat alternately. **Lachesis.** Traumatic gangrene. Franklin recommends this remedy highly in gangrene following wounds, saying that it is eminently curative of gangrenous affections. **Crotalus** has hot, bluish, moist gangrene, the limb being covered with black blisters and much swollen, emitting a foul odor.

Secale 6C to 30C - Corresponds to senile gangrene with tingling and formication. Dry gangrene of toes; a number of cases of cure of this condition by Secale are on record. The skin in wrinkled and dry, shrivelled and cold, no sensibility, black and free from fetor. Large ecchymoses and blood blisters, which become gangrenous, will indicate the remedy.

Carbo Veg 6C to 30C - Carbuncles and boils, becoming gangrenous. There is no restlessness, as in Arsenicum, but the parts have a livid purple look, and they are icy cold. It also suits moist gangrenous in cachectic persons whose vitality is weak. The secretions are foul and there is great prostration. Arnica may be useful in gangrene following contusions.

Foreword To First Aid

This does not replace your First Aid manual but complements its use and allows you to take the best from both worlds. The main purposes of this book is to empower you and give you options that previously you had not, as well as to speed up the healing processes and help relieve pain, stress and trauma. Modern medicine seems to concentrate more on antiseptics and sterile environments especially for wound care but not much on the actual healing processes of the wound especially when you consider that some antiseptics can burn the wound while doing its germ killing. Anyone like me who has had straight iodine poured into deep puncture wounds can vouch for that.

We will concentrate on the healing and closing of wounds along with the knitting together of bones with remedies that concentrate on healing as well as having germicide and antibacterial properties. A lot of the emphasis is on finding the cause or causes of the problem and removing them as prevention is the best way to go for good health and a long life. This book gives you the options of Herbal or Homoeopathic remedies or of using them together.

Most of the Remedies mentioned can be acquired fairly easily and locally with the exception being the tinctures and the Homoeopathics but this will vary from country to country.

Natural First Aid
Abscesses - Boils and Carbuncles

These are typically caused by a bacterial infection usually starting in a hair follicle. The first stage is characterized by a painful red swelling after which pus begins to form; this will usually discharge itself in a few days. Do not squeeze as this usually causes internal damage and a spread of the wound and infection. Lots of boils or recurring boils need professional help so as to remove the cause. Diabetes is a condition that causes boils.

Herbal Treatment

The easiest and fasted method would be to use Tea Tree Oil as this tends to draw out infections and bring them to a head. Start as soon as possible, the earlier the better and apply frequently. Use more diluted if using frequently especially if you have sensitive skin. Hot poultices are very effective at drawing the core out of boils so here we shall use a hot poultice of Slippery Elm (half a tea spoon full) with about 4 drops of Castor Oil which is also good at drawing out unwanted matter and mix this with a bit of boiling water to form a hot paste. Alternative poultices are Linseed or Fenugreek, these need to be ground and boiled first before being applied. Apply to the area and leave on for 20 minutes and repeat several times till suppuration occurs.

After suppuration you can mix together a bit of Calendula and Comfrey creams and apply them to the area. These two herbs working together will speed up the healing time, disinfect and reduce or prevent scaring.

For internal treatment think of the herbs Echinacea and Burdock as these are both blood cleansers that will start to work on the causes of the problem and help to prevent more.

Homoeopathic Treatment

A boil is an infected, reddened, swollen area of the skin usually in a hair follicle or some other pit in the skin. Boils can be very painful while they develop until they come to a head and burst.

Arnica 6C - For crops of boils with a bluish area around them.

Tarantula Cubenis 6C - For painful hard feeling boils that develop rapidly after a slow start especially on the back of the neck or on boils where the skin turns red blue or purple. Give this remedy 3 or 4 times daily along with a Hypericum Lotion compress taped over the area.

Bites and Stings

I will cover here just bites from pets and bee and wasp stings. Snakes spiders and jellyfish stings require prompt medical attention. With snake and spider bites apply a pressure bandage to the area and keep the limb still and transport to hospital or better still ring a Ambulance. (You can give rescue remedy).

Animal bites can be treated the same as wounds as they are usually a mixture of puncture, bruising and maybe scratches, treat shock with rescue remedy especially in children. With wounds from animals you should always get a tetanus shot or a booster and always treat with lots of Calendula Lotion so as to prevent infection which is common after animal bites especially from cats. If there is a lot of pain add Hypericum to the lotion.

Herbal Treatment

For insect bites and stings Rescue Remedy taken internally and applied to the sting can bring relief especially in children. Witch hazel cream is good for insect bites and stings.

Wasp stings and Ant bites - apply vinegar or lemon juice

Bee stings - Dab on bicarbonate of soda mixed with water. This can also bring relief to sand fly and sometimes mosquito bites as well. Baking Soda works in two ways, firstly it buffers the acid and then the sodium part draws the poison out. On all stings ice can reduce pain and swelling. Aloe vera may sometimes help.

Homoeopathic Treatment

Can be painful in varying degrees; always follow the normal first aid procedures especially from bites from venomous creatures. After a bite or a sting from a animal or insect take one dose of **Ledum 6C** immediately. If you get no relief try one of the following.

Apis 6C - If the injury swells, burns, stings and looks very red, angry and puffy with swelling, worse for warmth , better for cold applications. This remedy is made from the bee and should always be considered for bee stings.

Arnica 6C - Shock, bruising like pain, soreness and does not want area touched.

Cantharis 6C - Violent burning and smarting pain, blisters may develop.

Staphysagria 6C - Large bites that itch violently with smarting, stinging pain.

Bruises

Arnica is the main remedy that is used for bruising mainly as a lotion or a cream but it must not be used where the skin is broken. If used on broken skin it will cause a bad reaction. Arnica is good for the bruised like pain in limbs and joints which have been over used or sprained as well as your everyday type of bruises. For accidents where you hit your finger with the hammer especially when the fingernail is involved put your finger under the cold water tap and leave it there till it nearly feels numb with the cold, this if done fast enough can save you from a bruised nail and a lot of pain.

Herbal Treatment

For bruises where there are open wounds such as cuts and grazes use Witch hazel and Calendula together in a lotion and later you could mix the creams together and apply as healing resumes. For your normal everyday bruises rub Arnica cream gently on the area. If a nerve rich area such as the elbow is bruised add Hypericum to the lotion.

For internal treatment take a Vitamin C powder with hesperidin, rutin and the bioflavonoids as this will help to repair the damaged capillaries. If you bruise easily consider taking this powder regularly as you may be deficient.

Homoeopathic Treatment

The black and blue appearance of a bruise are caused from blood vessels that have ruptured under the skin as a result of trauma, as the blood from the broken vessels is slowly absorbed the color becomes paler then red or yellow.

Arnica 6C - For bruised soft tissues, muscles and connective tissue. Rapidly aids in the absorption of effused blood. The swelling which usually accompany bruising reduces fairly quickly but if there is little reaction use Ledum 6C. Arnica cream can be used on the external area of the wound.

Caution - Arnica lotion or cream must not be used on or near broken skin only use Calendula or Hypericm cream on wounds.

Ledum 6C - Helps in blood reabsorbing, may be needed if swelling remains after taking Arnica. Affected parts are cold and worse for warmth.

Hypericum 6C - For bruised nerves, use where there is sharp shooting pains in punctured or penetrating wounds, for bruises of nerve rich areas such as the fingers, tail bone, lips and nose. Hypercal cream can be applied to the site externally.

Ruta 6C - Bruises of the bone or the bone covering the periosteum, good for shin bone injuries.

Note - Hypercal cream can be used externally on bruises where the skin is broken as Arnica cream or lotion cannot be used on broken skin.

Bleeding

The main rule for bleeding is to apply pressure to the wound so as to stop the bleeding. For a normal type of slow blood flow from a wound that is persistent Calendula tincture applied with pressure on a pad will usually stop the bleeding, make sure you hold it there for a few minutes.

For the more scary type of bleeding Witch hazel tincture can be used on a pad and applied with pressure to the wound as this herb is much more astringent then Calendula, this extra astringency should cause the ends of the blood vessels to spasm and close off the injured vessels.

Herbal Treatment

Calendula for slow bleeding wounds.

Witch hazel for the fast bleeding wounds.

I would be inclined here to mix the tincture half water half tincture as this would still work and be less painful as the alcohol in the tincture is much more reduced.

See also Cuts and Wounds and consider using Hypercal (Hypericum and Calendula mixed together)

Homoeopathic Treatment

Use normal first aid procedures, apply pressure to the wound, if there is a lot of blood loss seek medical help and be on the lookout for shock.

Arnica 6C - For bleeding after injury, helps with the shock and bruising.

Bone Injuries and Fractures

The main remedy here is Comfrey or to use its old fashioned name knitbone. This is good to use on the injured area when the cast is removed as it will help to strengthen the mend. For areas that cannot have casts on or for fine fractures Comfrey is ideal and will speed up the healing process.

Comfrey has a chemical in it that speeds up cell division it is also astringent and mucilage which gives it soothing and protecting qualities and has been used for hundreds of years in the healing of bones and wounds. Some people grow this herb and then turn it into liquid manure as it is one of the most mineral rich herbs around.

Herbal Treatment

Apply cream to affected area regularly, if you grow comfrey in your garden you can make a poultice out of the leaves and apply it to the affected area.

Homoeopathic Treatment

Follow normal first aid procedures, if the bone is obviously broken it is best to call a ambulance. If you do have to move the patient make sure the injured limb is supported or a sharp piece of bone may cut an internal artery. Most bone injuries need x-rays to determine the extent of the damage.

Arnica 6C - Can be given straight away for the shock and will help ease the pain from the bruising and swelling.

Ledum 6C - Take after Arnica 4 hourly or 3 times a day to assist in the absorption of the extravasation of blood after a fracture so as to reduce the swelling which may take up to 3 to 4 days. (Helps to absorb the internal bleeding after a fracture)

After the bones have been set properly use these two remedies

Calc Phos 6X - Helps in nutrition especially of the bones and promotes the knitting together of the bones. Helps fractures heal much faster. Can be used in alternation with Symphytum 6C.

Symphytum 6C - More commonly known as Comfrey or knitbone or bone set. The name says it all. Promotes fast healing of bones, use with Calc Phos 6X. Take both 3 times daily till recovered.

Burns

The usual rule is to place the burnt area under cold water as soon as possible. I usually leave it under there till it's nearly numb from the cold. The point to remember here is that when you take let's say your hand away from whatever burnt it the heat from the burn is still traveling inward and will continue to do so for about 15 seconds so this is why you must get to the cold water fast so you can reduce the severity and the depth of the burn. For minor burns and scolds Aloe Vera gel straight from the plants leaf can give quick relief and speed up the healing. In Herbal Medicine we use astringents for burns (with the exception being for burns that cover a very large area) as the tannins in the herbs will seal and protect the burned surface. Tannins also have a antibacterial action so this should help in the prevention of infections. Deep burns always require prompt medical attention.

Herbal Treatment

Aloe Vera - apply to burn straight from the plant.

Witch Hazel - Use as a lotion at about 1 to 20 strength and apply to the burn, this herb is a strong astringent and should seal and protect the surface.

Hypericum - This can be added to the above lotion as it has some similar actions but for burns we are mainly using it to reduce the pain.

Once the healing has begun you can continue applying aloe vera especially if there is still pain. Another good herb for around the edges of the burn as it heals is Calendula Cream.

Homoeopathic Treatment

On first degree burns the skin becomes red only. 2nd degree the burn begins to destroy living tissue, blisters develop, 3rd degree the burns are deep and involve all layers of the skin, these are life threatening depending on the size of the area mainly through the loss of fluids and the risk of infections.

Urtica Urens 6C - For first degree burns take as needed internally for the pain with Hypericum lotion used externally.

Causticum 6C - For 2nd degree burns take as needed for the pain with Hypericum lotion used externally on the burn and Calendula cream on the edges.

Cantharis 6C - For 3rd degree burns taken as needed. This time wait for the healing to begin before using Hypericum and Calendula.

Hypericum Tincture - To be used as a lotion 20 drops of tincture to 1 cup of water.

Calendula Cream - Use this on the edges of the burn.

Cuts and Wounds

The first consideration is to stop the bleeding, rule out any deeper internal damage and clean and disinfect the wound. To stop the bleeding refer to bleeding section. Calendula is one of the main lotions used for cleaning wounds as it is gentle, soothing, astringent, healing and anti-microbial so it kills the germs as well. Calendula has a tendency of sometimes welding the skin together (handy for closing knife cuts) this is more noticeable on wounds with clean cut edges. Because of this tendency it is very important to make sure that all wounds are very clean and no dirt remains inside.

Now we will introduce you to Hypericum (St Johns Wort) I use Hypericum lotion on wounds that are in very nerve rich areas, a good example is crush injuries to the finger as we all know how painful and sensitive a wound is to this area. As well as being used for nerve damage Hypericm is also astringent so it will help in stopping the bleeding and its anti-inflammatory action should help to reduce the swelling. I usually get a separate bottle and fill it up with half Hypericum and half Calendula tincture and call this bottle Hypercal. I use this bottle for making my lotions for wounds on nervy areas. Consider also that these are both astringents so our power to stop bleeding has been increased.

Tea Tree Oil is good for small wounds and has a strong antibacterial action but can sometimes hurt in open wounds. The oil is good where there is infection as it draws pus to a head. And now for something completely different. If you have a clean cut wound fairly deep but on the border line of getting stitches and have managed to stop the bleeding here's a way of putting a kind of skin graft on it which will hold the wound shut while you decide what to do. Break and empty an egg. On the inside of the egg shell you will see a plastic like skin, peel this off and lay across the wound wet side down. The skin is also meant to have an antibiotic action which protects the egg. If you are going to try to get away without stitches try to immobilize the area for a couple of days so you don't accidentally rip the wound open again and use plenty of Calendula to close the wound.

Herbal Treatment

1. Deal with bleeding and clean wound under running tap water if possible.
2. Do the final cleaning with Calendula or Hypercal lotion mixed 1 to 20 parts water.
3. Cover and protect the wound if you think it is necessary.
4. When wound is dry and healing (if weeping use Hypercal lotion) you can use Calendula cream with maybe Comfrey cream as well for scar prevention or if the wound is healing slowly. You can also medicate a little bit of Calendula cream with Hypericum to make a Hypercal cream for a healing wound giving off nervy pain.

Homoeopathic Treatment

Use normal first aid techniques, control bleeding etc. When you have everything under control and are ready to see to the wound the best way to start is usually to clean the area with water running from a tap washing everything away from the wound. Calendula lotion is our main treatment for wounds as it is gentle, encourages healing, stops bleeding and no germs can survive in its presence. Use plenty of lotion on the wound and in deep ones let it get into all the cavities. Calendula can make wounds close up very fast especially if they have clean sharp edges so great care must be taken to ensure the wound is clean. Calendula is a great help to old and infected wounds and can usually turn the condition around in a few days. (See Tea Tree oil)

Hypericum is the next most well used lotion, its main calling is for wounds of the very nervy parts of the body such as the fingers, tail bone, lips or for any part that really hurts and is nervy. One of the leading symptoms for Hypericum is shooting pains along the nerve pathways from the injured area. Hypericum is good for infections and septic conditions in nervy areas and I would use it with Calendula for any infection in a wound especially deep wounds. In the past Hypericum was used to prevent Tetanus in deep puncture wounds especially from rusty metal objects. Remember infections are trying to get the rubbish out of the body so when they begin to discharge do not try to stop the discharge let the body get rid of its rubbish.

Hypercal - Which is a half and half mixture of Hypericum and Calendula tinctures, you can use this to make lotions when you want the effects of both Calendula and Hypericum together. A example would be an infected crushed finger.

Creams - Calendula and Hypericum creams can be used when the healing begins and are applied for the same reasons as the lotions but always remember the lotion gets in better. Creams are more for the latter stages of healing.

Arnica 6C - For shock, bruised sore pain of the wound, doesn't like effected area being touched.

Ledum 6C - Used for puncture wounds, prevents tetanus.

Puncture Wounds

Splinters and accidents from stepping on pins, rusty nails, barbed wire or from tools can be dealt with very effectively with homoeopathic remedies.

Arnica 6C - Can help bring splinters to the surface and deal with any shock.

Hypericum 6C - Intense pain shoots up from injured parts especially from those in nerve rich areas, if given immediately with the lotion it can prevent tetanus from developing but it is always best to get a booster shot.

Ledum 6C - This remedy also helps to prevent tetanus and can be used for the same injuries as Hypericum but with Ledum the part feels cold and is relieved by cold, there is puffiness and a pale mottled appearance.

Hypercal Lotion - Externally use a lotion of Hypercal making sure plenty gets inside the wound.

After Surgery

Homoeopathic remedies used before and immediately after surgery will speed up the healing process considerably. Not only does this get you over the problem sooner but it also helps in the prevention of post-operative complications such as hemorrhage, inflammation, and infection. Will also help with the internal healing and bruising.

Aconite 6C - Great fear and anguish with restlessness. Possible fear of death, great suddenness of symptoms. This is a good one to think of before surgery.

Arnica 6C - Bruised sore pain with fear of being touched. Take this immediately before and straight after a operation.

Bellis Perennis 6C - Follows after and is similar to Arnica but is used for the deeper internal bruising while Arnica is more external. Good for trauma and wounds of the pelvic and abdominal organs.

Hypericum 6C - For damage to tissue rich in nerves or the nerves themselves, pains shoot along nerve pathways.

Staphysagria 6C - Stinging, cutting, smarting pains after surgery, good for knife cut like wounds. This remedy has strong mental symptoms of Feels as if the body has been invaded, or a sense of humiliation after a physical exam, resentment and anger to hospital staff may be present.

Calendula Lotion - This is our main lotion and cream used for wounds. Apply the lotion to the wound and surrounding area as Calendula is very soothing and healing. Latter when the wound is healing Calendula cream can be used.

Hypercal Lotion - Is a mixture of Calendula and Hypericum tinctures that are used as a lotion. The Calendula is used for its healing, anti-microbial, anti-hemorrhagic and soothing properties while the Hypericum is used for the nervy type of pain from the wounds in nerve rich areas.

The lotion is mixed at a strength of 1 to 20 parts water or stronger if needed.

Diarrhea

Diarrhea is a natural bodily process that is used to rid the body of toxins, infections or irritants of any kind so unless it continues for too long it should not be suppressed. Lots of fluids should be taken and in some cases it may be wise to stay off food for 24 hours. Always try to find the cause; it may be from stress, viruses, bacterial infection or maybe a food allergy.

Herbal Treatment

Chamomile tea can be given if the symptoms match as this is calming, soothing, and antispasmodic and will help to heal the irritation and if you put a pinch of ginger in the tea this would also help to relieve nausea if it is present. Always think of Chamomile if nerves or worry are the cause. Slippery elm powder in water also soothes the irritation and relieves the diarrhea as well as being nourishing. Agrimony is our specific for diarrhea especially in children. Witch Hazel due to it astringency helps in the control of diarrhea and may help in reducing dysentery but like agrimony it is better to give in tea form as this allows maximum contact with the intestines as it travel through so it can medicate a far wider area.

The aim of treatment is to help the body rid itself of the toxins rather than suppressing the problem. Garlic oil capsules may be taken if you are reasonably sure that the problem is caused from a virus or bacterial infection. (See herb list at back for more information on this). If the problem continues longer than it should seek medical advice.

Dysentery

Dysentery is when the above problem continues and there is colicky like pains with maybe wind and gurgling with the motions becoming more water like. Herbal treatment of this condition mainly concentrates on the actions of the astringent herbs which contract the tissue and slow down the motions, the main one to think of here is Agrimony with maybe Witch Hazel added so as to increase the astringency. To the astringents you can add herbs like Peppermint, Ginger and Chamomile which will help with the tummy cramps, colic, wind and pain. Slippery Elm is a very gentle astringent and also provides the body with nutrition and if you add a bit of unprocessed honey to it your giving extra energy and an antibacterial action as well. When dealing with the intestines always use the remedies in tea form as tis allows the tea to spread through a large area medicating as it goes.

Emergency Rehydration Fluid
1 litre of boiled water
2 tea spoonful's of salt
2 tablespoons of sugar
Mix together and sip regularly throughout the day

Ear Ache

Try to find the cause, is it an acute infection, tooth ache, from sinus problems etc. Recurring ear infections need professional help so as to build up the immune system to cope. Seek medical help if the pain is excessive or there is pain in the mastoid bone (behind the ear) or any discharge.

The juice of garlic or alternatively onion in olive oil warmed to body temperature but no more can be put in the ear but only if the drum is not perforated. If the drum is perforated they will be in great pain and there may be a discharge. To get the juice from a onion slice it thinly into circles and lay flat in a saucer and sprinkle a bit of sugar on it then put another layer of onion more sugar etc and keep building it up. When finished leave for at least a hour and the sugar will draw out the juice.

Herbal Treatment
Garlic or onion juice in olive oil warmed to body temperature.

Eczema and Dermatitis

Is an irritating skin inflammation that may be due to a allergy caused by certain foods or from repeated contact to certain chemicals (dermatitis) or just inherited. This condition can be made worse from stress. This is more of a problem needing professional help except for contact dermatitis which can be cured by removing the cause or to a certain degree through the use of a barrier cream.

Weeping eczema requires a wet dressing of Chamomile (anti-inflammatory) and Witch hazel (astringent) which should start to dry the area out. Once the weeping has stopped you can use Calendula and Comfrey creams which will start healing and give some relief. Chickweed lotion can be used as a wet dressing as well, the leading symptoms for this is itching and irritation with the main emphasis on itching. You can if you want medicate some cream with a few drops of Chickweed tincture and can use this cream to relieve any itching that may happen when healing is in progress. A good mix for this cream would be Calendula.

Herbal Treatment

For weeping eczema Chamomile tea used as a lotion mixed with Witch hazel lotion made at 1 to 10 parts water. This mixed lotion is applied as a wet bandage to the area (moisten bandage frequently) or you can wet a pad with the lotion and bandage that to the area till weeping has stopped.

Replace Chamomile with Chickweed lotion if symptoms are very itchy with irritation. For dry eczema Comfrey and Calendula cream used together will speed up the healing if itching is a problem you can medicate some Calendula cream with a few drops of Chickweed tincture.

Eye Problems

See also conjunctivitis. Eyebright as you can guess is the main herb for the eye and is used for most eye problems and even for just sore or strained eyes it can be soothing. For a little splinter in the eye or a hard to remove foreign body a few drops of Castor oil can be used for its drawing power as it has a good reputation for removing embedded objects and it will sooth the irritation at the same time. If the eye is irritated and you have suspicion there is something in put a few drops of Castor oil in before you go to sleep and leave overnight and the problem will usually be gone by the morning.

Herbal Treatment

Eyebright lotion at 1 to 20 parts water in a eyebath (always try in a very diluted form first, 2 drops to a eyebath) for sore red eyes or better still as a compress especially with hay fever symptoms.

Castor oil 2 or 3 drops into the eye to draw out foreign bodies and relieve irritation. Best left overnight.

Conjunctivitis

The conjunctiva is a delicate membrane which covers the whites of the eyes. This may become inflamed due to irritation, infection or allergic reaction. Try to avoid touching and rubbing the eye as this usually irritates it more and if it is an infection there is a chance that it may spread to the other eye. The herbs to use here are Calendula and Eyebright used as lotions in the strength of 1 to 20 parts water. Eyebright is a very astringent herb so you would use it if the eye was very watery and inflamed while Calendula is soothing and anti-infective. If the eye was watery and infected you could mix both the herbs together for a more effective treatment.

Herbal Treatment

Calendula lotion 1 to 20 in a eyebath (healing and soothing).

Eyebright Lotion 1 to 20 in a eyebath (astringents will help in stopping watering and help with the inflammation).

Homoeopathic Treatment

Here I will cover mainly blows to the eyes and the simple removal of foreign objects and will also give you one of the main eye remedies. For a blow to the eye you can give Arnica 6C or Aconite 6C which has been called the Arnica of the eye, a leading symptom for Aconite 6C is if the eye feels gritty or as if something is in the eye. If pain is felt in the eyeball give Symphytum 6C.

Arnica 6C is more suited for a black eye (see bruising).

After removal of a foreign object from the eye Aconite 6C can be given and if the eye is still sensitive and sore an eye bath of water with 2 drops of Euphrasia (Eye Bright) tincture can be tried.

Arnica 6C - For shock and bruising.

Acconite 6C - For the suddenness of the condition and shock, pain feels like a piece of grit in the eye, eye looks red and inflamed.

Euphrasia Lotion - Conjunctivitis after injury, eyes are hot, burning and watering, soreness, eye strain. 2 drops of tincture into a eye bath full of water gives relief to sore and wind burnt eyes. You can also use Euphrasia 6C internally at the same time.

Symphytum 6C - for blows to the eyeball itself, blunt injury trauma such as a tennis or squash ball.

Gastritis and Gastroenteritis

Gastritis or inflammation of the stomach can often be from overindulgence or upsetting foods and can lead to nausea, vomiting, diarrhea and heartburn. Symptoms are usually short lived. Gastroenteritis is usually more serious it can have the above symptoms with abdominal cramps added. In children the commonest cause is a virus but it can be caused by bacteria from contaminated food. This can be serous in children and small babies since the constant vomiting and diarrhea can lead to dehydration. Always consider a fast for 24 hours so the system has a chance to recover.

Peppermint or Chamomile infusion every hour for the first day, you could even take them alternately if you think the symptoms call for this. After this one cup 3 or 4 times daily for a week before breakfast, between meals and before bed. These infusions should bring relief to pain, fever and spasms in the digestive tract. Slippery elm powder taken with a lot of water will soothe, help heal and reduce irritation and over active peristalsis. A little bit of Cardamom could be put in the infusions and this might help with any vomiting and help to settle the stomach. In digestive problems always use the tea form (infusion) of the herb for treatment as this allows a far greater volume area to be medicated.

Herbal Treatment

Agrimony -Iinflammation, mucous colitis, indigestion, appendicitis and diarrhea.

Chamomile tea - anti-inflammatory, anti-spasmodic, carminative and pain killer.

Peppermint tea - anti spasmodic, carminative, diaphoretic, anti-emetic (prevents vomiting), anti-septic, pain killing.

Cardamom - Carminative, stomach tonic, digestive tonic.

Slippery elm powder in water - soothing, astringent, nutritive.

For gastroenteritis stop all foods and avoid milk and milk based products for a least 24 hours. Refer to other sections for vomiting, nausea and diarrhea.

Hay Fever

This is more a deep seated type of problem that needs Professional help. Before the season begins start preparing the body, consider a non-mucous forming diet, start taking Vit C daily for it is a natural anti histamine and one of the main anti-oxidants for the lungs. Start taking Garlic daily as this will start clearing out the system with its anti-bacterial and anti-viral actions along with its high content of sulphur. Before the season and throughout the season take the formula below about 3 times a day.

Elder Flowers 2 parts
Chamomile 1 part
Eyebright 1 Part
Golden Seal 1 part

For relief of the eyes you can try a Euphraisa eye bath. Add 2 drops of tincture to the water in the eye bath and mix well. (See eye problems)

Homoeopathic Treatment

Hay fever is a allergic condition affecting the mucous membranes of the eyes, nose and air passages in people who are sensitive to pollens and grasses. Typical symptoms are running nose or eyes with a stuffed up sensation with may be itching of the eyes, nose or throat.

Allium Cepa 6C - Frequent sneezing with heavy burning nasal discharge and bland watery discharge from the eyes. The smell of flowers aggravates.

Euphrasia 6C - Red, burning, itching, watering eyes, water from the eyes burns the skin while the nasal discharge is bland. (Opposite to Allium Cepa).

Hemorrhoids or Piles

Hemorrhoids are a painful condition that really needs Professional help so as to remove the cause. For self-help treatment Witch hazel, Calendula and Hypericum creams can be used with Witch hazel being the main remedy as its strong astringency will stop any bleeding and help reduce the size of the pile a lot faster. If you have a feeling this condition is coming on attack the area straight away with Witch hazel cream and keep at it, if you are prone to piles you will find that this is a good and effective treatment that may sometimes prevent the condition from occurring. If you keep the cream in the fridge you will find that it is more relieving.

Herbal Treatment

Witch hazel cream - Apply immediately even on suspicion.
Calendula cream - Healing, soothing and antiseptic.

Hypericum cream - Will help with itching and pain. Also consider Chickweed for the itching.

All of the above can be used in lotion form to clean the area.

Indigestion

Indigestion or dyspepsia can have many symptoms varying from heart burn to bloating with maybe nausea and abdominal discomfort somewhere in the middle. There can be many causes some of which are not chewing food properly, eating too fast, too much rich or fatty foods, or if you are finding that this is getting to be a common problem the cause may be from low levels of stomach acid, stress or poor pancreas or liver function so it would be wise to seek professional help. You can mix and make your individual formula from the herbs below or just use one at a time.

Herbal Treatment

Slippery elm for heart burn or acidy symptoms mix with water.

Agrimony -Inflammation, mucous colitis, indigestion, appendicitis and diarrhea.

Licorice is a strong demulcent and can sooth areas hurt from excess acid.

Ginger capsules or in a mixed tea for flatulence, dyspepsia, colic and nausea.

Peppermint tea stimulates bile and digestive juices, flatulence, nausea.

Chamomile tea for indigestion, inflammations and colic and cramping like sensations.

Cardamom added to any of these will help.

In digestive problems always use the tea form (infusion) of the herb for treatment as this allows a far greater volume area to be medicated.

Itching

Itching can have many different causes some are from fungal infections, hemorrhoids, intestinal worms (itchy anus), liver problems, allergies, bites, stings etc. Treating the cause should relieve the problem but for temporary relief for the skin you could try a baking powder paste (good for sand flies etc) or some Chickweed cream or lotion.

Herbal Treatment

Chickweed cream or lotion - Apply to itchy areas.

Baking powder - Mix with water to make a paste and apply to itchy area. Usually draws out the toxin causing the itch and if the toxin is acid it will alkalize it.

Motion Sickness

This can be car sickness, air sickness and sea sickness the remedy to take here is ginger.

Herbal Treatment

Ginger - Take a few capsules just before the trip.
Peppermint.-. Take as a tea or you can buy peppermint oil capsules from a chemist.

Nose Bleed

The usual rule for this is to lean your head right back and pinch the top of your nose and stay this way till the bleeding is stopped. If you are still having problems after that you can get a small piece of cotton wool and soak it in a strong lotion of witch hazel and insert it in the nose (make sure it is a long piece so you can get it out easily) and pinch your nose gently, the idea is for the lotion to make contact with the wound and the astringency of the lotion should close the blood vessels.

Herbal Treatment

Witch hazel lotion at about 4 to 10 parts water strength applied as described above.

Nausea

Try to find the cause, common ones are digestive upsets, nerves, motion, migraines, liver problems and pregnancy. The main herbs to use here are chamomile, peppermint and ginger.
Refer to the herbal at the back and try to match your symptoms to the herbs you may have to mix a few herbs together to cover everything or maybe even all three.

Herbal Treatment

Chamomile tea - Colic, cramps, nervy.
Peppermint tea - Stimulates bile and digestive juices, good if cause is from

food

Ginger tea or capsules - Good for nausea and vomiting and gentle for those who are pregnant.

Cardamom added to any of these will help.

In digestive problems always use the tea form (infusion) of the herb for treatment as this allows a far greater volume area to be medicated.

Ringworm

Ringworm is a fungal infection which usually attacks when the immune system is weakened by stress or exhaustion. Fungi thrive in damp, dark and confined places. If you think your immune system is run down you can take Echinacea, Zinc, and Vitamin C and you might as well take Garlic as this has an anti-fungal action. Externally treatment can be a lotion of Calendula 1 to 5 strength for cleaning the area and around it. Stronger anti fungals may be necessary as this can sometimes be a very stubborn condition to get rid of. Garlic is a stronger anti-fungal and you can use this externally (break open a Garlic oil capsule) and internally at the same time.

Herbal Treatment

Raise immunity if needed refer to influenza for the method.

Calendula lotion 1 to 5 strength on and around the affected area.

Tea tree oil - strong anti-fungal dab on to the affected area neat.

Garlic externally on effected area and latter if problem is not resolving take internally.

Sunburn

A lotion of Witch hazel and Hypericum would help the burn and relieve the pain. If you have a Aloe Vera plant you could rub the gel on the burn. Be sure to rehydrate. Refer to the burns section.

Herbal Treatment

A mixture of Witch hazel and Hypericum lotion 1 to 20 parts water.

Sprains

Severe sprains usually need a supporting bandage and a medical checkup to see if there has been any other damage. A lot of damage and trauma can be prevented if the injured area was put under cold water or ice immediately after the injury the quicker the less the damage. For a bad sprain I would use lots of Arnica cream to start with and at night apply Arnica and Comfrey mixed creams along with a support bandage for the area so as to keep the cream there and also for the extra heat to the area that would create. If you grow Comfrey in your garden then you could put on a Comfrey poultice at night. Ginger is another herb that could be used in a poultice at night. In the past they also used what was known as Hot and Cold Treatment especially for ankles. It works like this put the swollen ankle in a bucket of hot water as hot as they can bear leave for about 5 minutes then put in a bucket of very cold water for 5 minutes, keep repeating the process, this probably works like a mechanical pump eg hot expands cold contracts so you may be pumping the inflammatory swelling out and fresh blood in leading to decongestion and fast healing.

A very fast method of treating strains and sprains is with Glucosamine, Chondroitin and MSM in the powdered form, you should be able to find this at most chemists. Glucosamine is an anti-inflammatory while the chondroitin helps rebuild cartilage and heal joints and attachments. You use this in the powdered form dissolved in water as it is rapidly absorbed by the intestine and enters the blood which takes it to the injury. A lot of athletes and horses use this frequently during the day along with the hot and cold treatment to force heal their injuries so they can compete again as soon as possible. Three times a day is good enough for the rest of us.

Herbal Treatment
Cold water or ice immediately.
Arnica cream (do not apply on open wounds).
Comfrey Cream mixed with Arnica cream overnight.
Ginger poultice overnight.

Homoeopathic Treatment
Joint problems due to twisting, wrenching or over use. A sprain is damaged tendons or ligaments while a strain happens when the connecting tissues around a joint are over stretched. Use your normal first aid procedures and support the joint with supporting bandage and give the appropriate remedies with the first one being Arnica. If there is no sign of improvement in 24 to 36 hours get checked for a fracture.

Arnica 6C - For the shock and bruised sore pains. Arnica cream can also be applied as long as the skin is not broken.

Bellis Perennis 6C - Deeper acting then Arnica, intense soreness of the muscles, where swellings and lumps remain after the injury.

Ledum 6C - Injuries where the swollen part is cold or numb, sometimes looks purple and puffy, feels better for cold applications.

Ruta 6C - If the bones inside or near the joint feel bruised

Splinters

This is here for splinters so deep you can't remove or those really annoying ones that you can feel but can't see. To get these out we will use a poultice. There are two to choose from, the first is a Slippery elm poultice made by adding hot water and turning into a paste and applying to the wound site, cover and secure with a bandage and renew every 2 hours till drawn out.

The other is Castor oil, with this one it is easier to put it on cotton wool and apply it to the wound at night so it can work while you are sleeping.

Herbal Treatment
Slippery elm poultice
Castor oil compress

Shock

All accidents and emergencies cause a certain degree of emotional shock sometimes very noticeable in children. Shock should always be treated along with any other injuries. Signs of shock can be they look pale, cold and sweaty skin, restless, rapid pulse and there may be shallow and fast breathing. Lay them down and get them comfortable keep them warm and calm and reassure them. Loosen tight clothing. Rescue Remedy is a effective remedy for this condition and can be used for any type of shock physical or emotional. Emotionally it will relieve that uptight feeling or apprehension before a certain event. Rescue Remedy is a mixture of five Bach Flower Remedies and has been used since the late 30s so it has been well proved and is easily found in most health shops and chemists.

Herbal Treatment
Rescue Remedy - For physical and emotional shock in any circumstances.

Homoeopathic Treatment
As you would of noticed by now Arnica is our main remedy for shock with

Aconite being a very good second remedy if the symptoms match. Don't forget to follow all your normal first aid procedures and keep the patient warm and calm.

Acconite 6C - Severe shock with great fear and restlessness. Fear is so great, person may scream, or say they will die, useful after surgical shock.

Arnica 6C - Reduces shock and hemorrhage and helps relieve the pain.

Notes

Our Two Main Wound Herbs
Calendula

Medicinal Actions - Anti-inflammatory, astringent, vulnerary, anti-fungal, germicide, demulcent.

Part Used - The Flowers

Used For.-. Minor skin problems, cuts, abrasions, rashes, spots, acne, sore nipples Slow healing wounds, skin ulcers and to improve post-operative healing Fungal skin infections such as thrush, athletes foot and ring worm. Used to stop bleeding, heal bruises and sprains, skin ulcers, minor burns and scolds, healing, soothing, anti-microbial. As a douche or bath to treat vaginal thrush, Gargle for sore throat and tonsillitis It can be applied as a lotion, ointment, wash, gargle, compress, poultice, bath and douche as required. . Use as a lotion (1 to 20) to clean wounds, one of our main germicides for wounds and if Hypericum is added to the lotion you may prevent tetanus as well

Caution - Calendula closes wounds rapidly so make sure they are very clean and no foreign bodies remain.

How To Use – For very serious wound bleeding medicate cloth with tincture and apply with pressure to the area till bleeding stops. Use as a Lotion one part tincture to twenty parts water to wash out wounds or medicate affected area, make at 1 to 10 for bleeding or fungal infections. Use a teaspoon of tincture to medicate a small jar of cream then stir rapidly for 5 minutes or less if it mixes in fast, usually they don't. I usually get a cheap Vitamin E cream from one of the big cheap wholesalers and medicate the cream with Calendula. Use Tincture for medicating creams.

Hypericum
(St Johns Wort)

Medicinal Actions - Anti-inflammatory, astringent, anti-viral, anti-spasmodic, nervine, vulnerary, antibacterial.

Part Used - Aerial parts

Uses – For First Aid we are concentrating on external use only. Used for wounds with pains that shoot along the nerves, in nerve rich areas such as the fingers, lips, tail bone and toes. As a lotion it will speed the healing of wounds and bruises and is used where there is nerve damage and the possibility of tetanus. The main remedy for puncture wounds. Good for, varicose veins especially the painful kind and mild burns. Patients recovering from surgery where the nerves have been damaged often recover faster with Hypericum. For inflamed joints and rheumatic pain, painful abscesses, bad insect stings, damaged nerves from impact injuries, sprains and ulcers. Eases the pain in conditions such as lumbago, sciatica and Shingles where a cream can be used on the sore and the oil applied along the affected nerve path. As a lotion it is commonly mixed with Calendula, Homoeopaths call this lotion Hypercal.

How To Use - Use as a Lotion one part tincture to twenty parts water to wash out wounds or medicate affected area, make at 1 to 10 for painful and dirty wounds. Mix with Calendula in large painful bleeding wounds with a chance of tetanus. Use Tincture for medicating creams.

Hypercal

Hypercal is a 50 50 mixture of Hypericum and Calendula Tinctures. This is a combination of two of the best wound healing herbs mixed together. Calendula is more for dealing with the blood vessels and bleeding along with the rapid closure of the wound so care must be taken to ensure the wound is clean and no foreign bodies are there to be sealed in. Hypericums work is more on the damaged nerves and pain as well as infections in and of the nervous system especially those caused by deep and painful puncture wounds which could harbor tetanus if not properly cleaned and dealt with. By using these two herbs together you are doubling their main actions of anti-inflammatory and astringents with the last action being good for stopping bleeding and also infection. Wounds calling for Hypercal are usually bloody and painful. Works well on long and extensive grazes and cleaning gravel rash and wounds but is mainly called for impact injuries to the lips, fingers or toes. Ideal for closing clean incisions fast and after surgical operations. So the leading symptoms for Hypercal are painful wounds.

Use as a lotion at one part to ten or 1 to 20 depending on your judgment of pain and infection. In emergency bleeding use the tincture as this will spasm the arterioles but be aware that the high alcohol content will cause pain in its raw state. Use Tincture for medicating creams.

First Aid Herbal

Aloe Vera

Actions - External demulcent, healing, soothing,

Use for sunburn, thermal burns, cuts, sores, inflamed skin, eczema, insect bites.

I suggest you buy a couple of these plants and put them in a handy place.

Part Used - The fresh juice from the leaves

Agrimony

Actions – Astringent, cholagogue, tonic, diuretic.

This is the specific for childhood diarrhea. Used for a number of gastrointestinal problems such as inflammation, mucous colitis, indigestion, appendicitis and diarrhea. Acts as a tonic due to it bitter stimulation. Best given in tea form so it can spread along the intestines and do its job. Consider mixing with licorice for extra soothing and anti-inflammatory action or peppermint but mainly to make it taste better.

Arnica

Actions - Anti-inflammatory, vulnerary.

For external use only Homoeopathic preparations can be used internally. For the treatment of shock and pains from accidents, bruises, joint stiffness and wounds, swellings, paralysis, sprains, rheumatic conditions or where ever there is inflammation on the skin.

Part Used - The flowers

Caution - Do not apply to open wounds or broken skin.

Calendula

Actions - Anti-inflammatory, astringent, vulnerary, anti-fungal.

Used for cuts, grazes, infected sores, fungal infections, any skin inflammations, regulates the oil production of the skin so is good for acne, to stop bleeding, bruises and sprains, skin ulcers, minor burns and scolds, healing, soothing, anti-microbial. Use as a lotion (1 to 20) to clean wounds, one of our main germicides for wounds and if Hypericum is added to the lotion you may prevent tetanus as well.

Part Used - The Flowers

Caution - Calendula closes wounds rapidly so make sure they are very clean and no foreign bodies remain.

Cardamom

Actions - Antispasmodic, carminative, digestive tonic, stomach tonic, appetizer.

Use for anorexia, bloating, bronchitis, celiacs disease, colic, cramps, depression, fatigue, flatulence, indigestion and vomiting, best used mixed with another herb. Cardamom belongs to the ginger family and shares a lot of common properties with ginger and could be looked upon in use as a milder form of ginger.

Part Used - Ripe seed.

Dose - 1 Teaspoon of powder infused. Three cups a day.

Castor Oil

Castor oils main claim to fame is from its purgative action. It is one of the main purgative remedies from the past and still does well today because it is one of the few purgatives that clears the bowels effectively with one dose and has no unpleasant side effects (besides taste) like gripping pain, spasms etc which made it safe to use for pregnant women to use. Castor oil was used in the hospitals of the past for decades. Castor oil is not the cure for constipation but it can be used for relief of this now and again. Castor oil used in a poultice has good drawing out power on foreign objects imbedded in the body such as splinters in the fingers and especially in the eye where it soothes the irritation at the same time.

Chamomile

Actions - Carminative, sedative, anti-spasmodic, anti-inflammatory, analgesic and anti-septic.

Use for indigestion, colic, diarrhea, teething children, anxiety, insomnia, nervous upsets, slowing down hyperactive children, flatulence. It is a famed blood cleanser and pain reducer, reduces tumors (poultice), remedy for female ailments, inflamed gums, use for blood and skin disorders, aches and pains, external and internal inflammations, cleanser and toner of the digestive tract, improves and helps appetite. This herb is also anti-allergy.

Good all round tonic for the nervous system.
Part Used - Flowers
Dose - 2 to 4mls 3 times daily of the Tincture, in the tea form 3 to 4 cups per day.

Chickweed

Actions - Healing, anti-inflammatory, astringent, emollient.
One of the main uses of this herb is for itching skin conditions whether from insect bites or eczema like conditions. Has wound healing and demulcent properties.
Part Used - Aerial parts
Dose - Usually given in infusions (tea form) or used as a lotion or cream.

Comfrey

Actions - Demulcent, astringent, healing, expectorant.
Once widely cultivated as a fodder plant, sheep and cows eat it greedily, the impressive wound healing powers of comfrey are partially due to allantoin which stimulates cell proliferation and speeds the healing process inside and out.

Uses - Its old name is knit bone and that describes well what it does. Comfrey also guards against scar tissue from developing incorrectly, all internal hemorrhages, reunion of wound and fractures, internal ulcers, ruptures, pulmonary problems, bronchitis, irritable cough, ulcerative colitis, skin ulcers and varicose veins.
Part Used - Root, rhizome and leaf.

Echinacea

Actions - Immune stimulant, anti-microbial, anti-inflammatory, alterative, healing.
Is a infection fighter active against strep bacteria (abscesses and boils), a blood cleanser, (blood poisons, snake bites, poisonous insects) and a glandular and lymphatic system cleanser. Use it particularly for respiratory infections and for any disease above the waist. This is one of our main immune boosters for the acute diseases.
Uses - All infections, depressed immune function, inflammatory

conditions, allergies, effective against both bacteria and viruses.

Part Used - Root

Dose - 1 to 4mls of tincture three times daily, In the tea form 3 to 4 cups per day.

Warning - Do not use continually as you will burn out the immune system use month on month off.

Eye Bright

Actions - Anti-inflammatory, astringent, anti-catarrhal.

As the name says this is one of the main herbs in the treatment of eye problems. The whole plant is also nervine, tonic and astringent. Its use is both internal and external strengthening greatly the eyes nerves when used so. The high potassium and sulphur content of the plant make it also of value in treatment of gastric ailments especially insufficiency of gastric juices. Acts as a internal medicine for the constitutional tendency to eye weakness.

Uses- Best known for its use in the eye where it is helpful in acute or chronic inflammations, stinging and weeping eyes, over sensitivity to light, conjunctivitis, allergies, sinusitis, ulcers and general eye weakness.

Part Used - Dried aerial parts.

Garlic

Actions - Immune stimulant, anti-bacterial, anti-viral, anti-fungal, anti-septic, anti-oxidant, diaphoretic, cholagogue, hypotensive, anti-spasmodic, vermifuge and many more. The plant is rich in volatile oil and sulphur and because of its remarkable penetrating, disinfecting and mucous expelling powers garlic is a valuable basic remedy for the treatment of all ailments in which the cleansing of the blood stream and expulsion of mucous accumulations is required. Garlic is extremely effective in dissolving and cleansing cholesterol from the blood stream, it stimulates the digestive tract, kills worms, parasites and harmful bacteria, normalizes blood pressure, reduces fever, gas and cramps.

Uses- All infections, coughs, colds, flu, bronchitis, all fevers, pulmonary conditions, gastric and skin complaints, rheumatism, all worms, ringworm, ticks and lice. Acts on Bacteria, Viruses and Internal Parasites.

Dose - 1 clove 3 times a day. Garlic oil capsules are good.

Externally - You can use garlic for ring worm and ear ache, to disinfect wounds and sores, parasitical infections.

Ginger

Actions- Carminative, anti-inflammatory, vasodilator, circulatory stimulant, diaphoretic.

Aids in fighting colds, colitis, digestive disorders, wind, increases saliva, is excellent for the circulatory system and helps increase stamina.

Uses- Indigestion, nausea, feverish conditions especially when chills are present, travel sickness especially sea sickness, dyspepsia, colic, flatulence.

Part Used - Root

Dose - Weak tincture 1.5 to 3mls 3 times daily. Can be found in tablets. Teas may also be made.

Caution - Dont use large doses on an empty stomach..

Hypericum (St Johns Wort)

Actions - Anti-inflammatory, astringent, anti-viral, anti-spasmodic, nervine, vulnerary, antibacterial.

Uses - Taken internally has a sedative and pain reducing effect, neuralgic pain, anxiety, tension, rheumatic pain, sciatica, for pains that shoot along the nerves, as a lotion it will speed the healing of wounds and bruises and is used where there is damage to the nerve rich areas, varicose veins and mild burns. Good for inflamed joints and rheumatic pain. Recently the herb has become popular to use as a antidepressant especially for cases of anxiety. Use as a lotion on wounds especially in the nerve rich areas such as the lips and fingers. As a lotion it is commonly mixed with Calendula, Homoeopaths call this lotion Hypercal.

Part Used - Aerial parts

Dose - 1 to 4mls of tincture 3 times a day. In the tea form 3 to 4 cups per day.

Peppermint

Actions - Carminative, diaphoretic, anti-spasmodic, anti-emetic, nervine, analgesic, anti-septic.

Uses- Nausea, heartburn, indigestion, colic, flatulence, dyspepsia, vomiting, fevers, migraine headaches and irritable bowel syndrome (IBS).

Part Used - Leaf.

Dose - 1 to 2mls of tincture 3 times a day. In the tea form 3 to 4 cups per day.

Caution - May reduce milk flow if breast feeding.

Rescue Remedy

For First Aid use, emergencies and associated stress, use for any type of shock physical or emotional. Emotionally it will relieve that uptight feeling or apprehension before a certain event.

Rescue Remedy is a mixture of five Bach Flower Remedies and has been used since the late 30s so it has been well proved.

Dose - 4 drops in a little water and sipped.

Slippery Elm Bark Powder

Actions - Demulcent, emollient, nutrient, astringent.

Slippery elm bark provides a nutritious gruel which also possesses remarkable medicinal properties acting as a poultice both internally and externally. A nutrient and food for very old or young or weak, coats and heals all inflamed tissues internally and externally and is used for the stomach, intestines, ulcers, ulcerative colitis, enteritis, dysentery, constipation and internal bleeding of the digestive tract.

Uses - Treatment of all digestive complaints especially ulcers for which it is a specific, dysentery, all pectoral disorders including TB, lung and bronchial hemorrhage, wasting diseases, rickets, stunted growth.

Externally - A poultice for all skin ailments especially old ailments and hard swellings.

Part Used - Inner Bark.

Dose - 1 part powder to 8 parts water.

Tea Tree Oil

Australian Tea Tree Oil is one of the world's best antiseptics and is also anti-bacterial, anti-fungal and anti-viral which means you can use it with good results on virtually any wound on the skin. The oil is good for drawing out infections, once they have been drawn out use Calendula to finish the healing.

Witch Hazel

Actions - Astringent one of the most widely used ones. Anti-septic.

As with all astringents this herb may be used wherever there is bleeding both externally and internally, commonly used for piles, bruises and inflamed swellings, varicose veins, diarrhea.

Uses - Internally to heal ulcerated and burnt tissues in cases of poisoning, stomach and intestinal ulcers, Externally - wounds, sores, bruises, ulcers, sore eyes and inflamed ears.

Part Used - Bark or leaves

Dose - Used mainly as a lotion 1 to 10 or as a cream.

Glossary Of Herbal Terms For First Aid

Anti-microbial - Helps the body destroy or resist pathogenic micro-organisms.
Herbs - Aniseed, Cayenne, Calendula, Echinacea, Garlic, Peppermint, Rosemary, Sage, Thyme, Wormwood.

Antispasmodic - Prevents or eases spasms and cramps.
Herbs - Aniseed, Chamomile, Fennel, Lemon Balm, Passion Flower, Rosemary, Sage, Skullcap, St Johns Wort, Thyme, Valerian.

Astringent - Contracts tissue which in turn reduces discharges, these herbs contain tannins and usually have a antibacterial action.
Herbs - Agrimony, Calendula, Chickweed, Comfrey, Eyebright, Raspberry, Sage, Rosemary, St Johns Wort, Slippery Elm, Thyme, Witch Hazel.

Carminative - Stimulates peristalsis of the digestive system and relaxes the stomach and helps remove gas and wind from the system.

Herbs - Aniseed, Chamomile, Fennel, Garlic, Ginger, Lemon Balm, Parsley, Peppermint, Sage, Rosemary, Thyme, Valerian.

Demulcent - Soothes and protects irritated or inflamed internal tissues.
Herbs - Corn Silk, Comfrey, Fenugreek, Licorice, Marshmallow, Oats, Plantain, Slippery Elm.

Diaphoretic - Aids the skin in the elimination of toxins and produces sweat.
Herbs - Chamomile, Fennel, Garlic, Ginger, Lemon Balm, Peppermint, Sarsaparilla, Thyme.

Emetic - Causes vomiting.

Emollient - Acts externally the way demulcents do internally.
Herbs - Chickweed, Comfrey, Fenugreek, Slippery Elm.

Infusion - Is like how you make a cup of tea but when you make herb teas you don't use milk. The teas you will be making here are mainly Peppermint and Chamomile tea. Pour boiling water onto the tea bag in the cup and cover the cup (to stop the essential oils from evaporating) and leave for about 5 minutes. To sweeten add honey.

Lotion - A water and tincture mixture example 2 parts tincture to 20 parts water.

Nervine - Has a beneficial effect on the nervous system.
Herbs - Chamomile, Oats, Peppermint, Rosemary, Skullcap, St Johns Wort, Thyme, Valerian.

Tincture - Herbal tinctures are made from herbs mixed with a water and alcohol mix of about half and half and are usually of the strength of 1 part herb to 5 parts solvent.

Homoeopathy

Homoeopathy is one of the hardest of the Natural Therapies to master and requires a lot of work and effort to do the job as it is meant to be done. The main principle and rule is that like cures like. So you have to match the symptoms of the <u>dis - ease</u> with the known symptoms that a remedy causes. The closer the match with the known symptoms of a disorder with those of the remedy the higher the Potency (strength) you use. With this First Aid Kit I am using all the remedies in a Low Potency mainly the 6C Potency because I know they will generally cover most of the symptoms but will not be exact all the time. So instead of using the remedies like a sniper concentrating on exactness we will be using them in the shot gun approach, in other words we are aiming to hit a very wide and broad area. This book is meant as a introduction into Homoeopathy and in using it you shall learn that it works and is very effective and once you have proven its worth to yourself you may wish to study it further. Homoeopathy is a very complex science and I could go for pages and pages in just explaining how it works but I feel that the best way for you to learn is to try it for yourself and take it from there. Read the list of remedies below and become familiar with what they can do and what they treat and above all always follow the normal First Aid procedures and use your common sense and you shouldn't have many problems.

A Warning About Potencies And Handling Homoeopathic Remedies.

1. Remedies should be touched as little as possible as the heat and moisture of your hands can spoil them.
2. Do not transfer remedies from one container to another as the potencies are easily contaminated by another remedy.
3. Keep potencies away from strong smelling products such as perfume, soap, incense, essential oils, peppermints, coffee and anything containing peppermint or menthol. Menthol is used in homoeopathy to antidote any remedies that is giving a bad reaction.
4. Keep away from heat and light; try to keep them under 40 degrees Celsius.

Taking The Potencies

1. Dissolve under the tongue.

2. Do not swallow with a drink; the potencies are absorbed through the membranes in the mouth.

3. Do not eat, drink, smoke or clean teeth for about 15 minutes before or after taking a remedy.

Dosage For The Potencies

1. For minor problems take one twice daily up to 7 to 10 days.
2. For acute problems take one every 2 to 4 hours up till 2 days. Reduce to 3 times daily for a further 3 to 5 days.
3. For very serious problems one every 5 to 15 minutes for 6 to 8 doses or until relief is obtained.

Homoeopathic First Aid Remedies

Aconite

Aconite is best used in the first stages of a illness, especially when fear and anxiety are present.

Symptoms appear suddenly, without warning and they may be caused by exposure to cold winds or draughts or by a severe fright. Symptoms are a marked restlessness, extreme anxiety or fear, high fever with a burning skin, extreme sweating and a burning thirst, a hoarse dry painful cough, bright light noises stress and cold worsen the symptoms, rest and quiet relieves the symptoms. The pains of Acconite are unbearable, sharp, shooting, burning pains, tingling and numbness.

Allium Cepa

Characteristic symptoms of this remedy are increased secretions from the eyes and nose, like those of the common cold. Frequent sneezing with watery discharge which burns the nose and upper lip, but the eye discharge is bland and doesn't burn (the opposite of Euphrasia). Tickling in the throat with incessant cough (feels as if larynx is split) holds throat when coughing. Being in cool open air relieves the symptoms.

Apis

Apis is used for various types of swelling and inflammation such as that from animal bites and bites and stings from insects; it is also used for measles, mumps, sore throats, sore red eyes and fever. Apis is a quick acting remedy for inflammations especially those ones with edema and lots of swelling which is its main use. Symptoms are swelling with edema which makes the effected parts look shiny, red and puffy, the swollen parts feel soggy and waterlogged, a fever that develops rapidly but without thirst, extreme restlessness and fidgeting, an irritable nature and perhaps jealous, cool air and cold compresses relieve the symptoms. Pains are burning and stinging.

Arnica

Bruises and similar injuries where the skin is unbroken and there is mental or emotional shock. Symptoms are any type of bruising or similar injury caused by crushing, squeezing or wrenching, muscles strains which feel sore and bruised, shock after accidents, there is a fear of being touched because of the pain, good for the soreness after birth and medical operations.

The kit contains Arnica in potency and also as a cream. The cream must not be used on broken skin or wounds.

Bellis Perennis

Trauma to abdomen and pelvic organs especially after surgery and child birth if Arnica does not give relief. Injuries to the nerves with intense soreness, back ache from hard physical work such as gardening, pain is bruised sore and aching, better cold presses, worse touch, after getting wet.

Calendula

We use this in the tincture form and make lotions from the tincture. The part used is the Flowers and it is used for wounds and skin irritations, it is healing, soothing, anti-inflammatory, astringent, anti-fungal and anti-microbial.

Use For - Cuts, grazes, infected sores, fungal infections, any skin inflammations, regulates the oil production of the skin so is good for acne, to stop bleeding, for bruises and sprains, skin ulcers and minor burns and scolds.

Cantharis
Important first aid remedy for minor burns and for other pains that feel burning and fiery, also has a healing effect on the bladder, urethra and other parts of the urinary tract where burning pain is the key symptom., burns and scalds especially where blistering and inflammation occur, sunburn, insect bites that feel hot and burn, cystitis. Pains are violent burning, cutting, stabbing or smarting, rawness. Better from warmth rest and rubbing.

Causticum
Burns and burning pains such as cystitis also used for coughs, burns to the skin especially with marked inflammation and blistering, coughs, laryngitis and hoarseness from straining and over using voice, cystitis especially with involuntary passing of urine when coughing, exposure to cold dry air may make symptoms worse.

Euphrasia
Affects the mucous membranes of the eyes, nose and chest producing copious watery secretions, eye secretions cause smarting of the skin while the nose discharge is bland. used for conjunctivitis, eye strain generally but especially from computers, eyes that feel sore and inflamed and look red, hay fever symptoms including a tickly throat, sneezing, a runny nose, and itchy red watering eyes. Sunlight wind and warmth worsen the symptoms.

Hypericum
Used for bruises and other injuries especially to nerve rich areas like the fingers, lips, ears, eyes ,tail bone, good for the pain of puncture wounds of any cause eg animal or insect. Helps with the pains after operations especially amputations. Pains are violent shooting pains along a nerve path, burning, tingling and numbness. Worse from shock and touch and better from rubbing

Ledum
Has a action on the capillaries and is useful for cleaning up bruises especially around the eyes, mainly used for puncture wounds made by sharp points such as nails and wood splinters and insect bites and stings

especially ones that don't heal properly and look purple and puffy. Wounds that feel cold to the touch, septic conditions, sprains, pains are throbbing, tearing ,prickling, they shoot upwards, stiff and sore. Better cold, cold bathing.

Ruta

Has effects on the joints, tendons, cartilages, and the periosteum which is a fine membrane that covers bones and gives the shiny look it is also used for eye strain where the vision goes dim. Used for painful bruises affecting the bones, strains to the tendons or joints, aching with restlessness, pains are gnawing, digging, burning, bruised, sore as if beaten, banes as if broken, pain deep in the bones. Worse from over exertion, touch, cold wet weather. Better from lying and warmth.

Rescue Remedy

Is one of the Bach Flower remedies or to be more exact is a mixture of four Bach Flower remedies. Rescue remedy is used for shock of any kind physical or emotional and has been well proven to be effective over the years.

Staphysagria

Suits sensitive people who suppress their feelings and suffer in silence or who boil over with indignation, remedy for cut and wounds especially those that are from medical procedures and have the mentioned feelings. The pains are stinging, stitching, smarting, squeezing, as if stabbed by a knife. Worse from touch, emotions and suppressed anger.

Symphytum

Causes bone to grow and promotes fast healing. Used for injuries to the hard parts of the body while Arnica is for the soft parts. Also used for eye injuries caused from blows.
Caution - do not use if a pin has been placed in the bone as the pin has to be removed latter.

Tarentula Cubensis

For abscesses, boils, carbuncles, swellings of any kind but especially on the back of the neck where the skin turns black, red/blue or purple. with great pain. Deep septic conditions with hardening of the effected part, condition comes on fast, pains are burning, stinging, throbbing, pricking like a needle.

Pandemic Flu

The Big One

A Naturopaths Story

Foreword

I am a Naturopath who prefers to be on the front line of medicine instead of sitting in an office waiting for people to come to me. I found that the best way to do this was to work in markets doing Iridology and in large Pharmacies as a Naturopath. Working in Pharmacies was a win win situation for me because I could treat everyone for free and all parties were happy and word of mouth always brought in more people. Eventually I found myself in one of the biggest Pharmacies joined to a Doctors surgery in the State Capital in the heart of the City working with not only the locals but helping my Chinese customers to look after their Grandparents and family back home along with doing the same for my Vietnamese customers and helping tourists from all round the world. The Pharmacy had Korean, Japanese, Chinese and Vietnamese translators, today it is truly a very small world. The story starts here as it is the best setting for the start because a Pharmacy especially a large one will always figure out if theirs is something wrong first because they deal with the most people and get a very broad view of what is happening in the community. It is also easier and faster to write from what you know and about yourself so what you read about my work and me is very close to how I do really work and deal with people and what it is like working in a big pharmacy. So far I have seen Bird Flu 1, SARS, and Swine flu come and go with our intern getting Swine Flu. This story is fiction based on my reality but is mainly about how a situation can get out of hand without really anyone seeing the big picture till it's far too late and how people who have had to survive in the past can rise to the occasion and survive again. At the back of the book is a reference section that allows you to see and understand what I am doing in the novel and is your own personal survival manual for the pandemic flu.

The Beginning Of The End
Day 1

It was just a normal work day at the beginning of the week, I parked the car in the Coles Supermarket car park and walked the short distance to the Rail Station and caught the train to the city. I took my usual shortcuts through the city to the big Pharmacy with the attached Doctors Surgery where I worked as a Naturopath. As I am usually half an hour early I headed to the lunch room and put my feet up, relaxed and read for a while till it was time to start. I started work in the usual way by walking around the shop seeing what was out of place then went to my section taking note of what was full and empty on the shelves and looking at the back of the shelves for the empty packets that the shoplifters leave behind, one of the problems of working in the big city. The day started quietly with me pulling forward all the stock on the shelves so there would be a nice flat face at the front with no gaps, this also gives me a chance to sit down for a while which I try to do as much as possible now so as to reduce the pains that would come on latter and get worse as the week went on. As I sat I thought about the chain of events that had brought me to here. Life had not been kind to this beaten and battered body of 48 with the last year being the worst.

Twelve years before I was working in a large woodworking factory breathing in all the dust for years, mainly from MDF particle board which filled the air from the work of the routers. On what was to be my last day I managed to get myself half buried in MDF dust after emptying a silo went wrong. At about 11.30 that night I started coughing up mouthfuls of blood so I took myself to the hospital. The hospital x-rayed my chest but got no answers so I was sent to another hospital by ambulance with a nurse because of the uncontrolled internal bleeding. Arriving about 3 in the morning they promptly rang the cancer specialist who said he would be there at 6 am. The main diseases for coughing up large amounts of blood are TB or Cancer. All through my working life as a Naturopath I have always applied the theory of mechanics and logic to my medical training so this is what I did while waiting for the Specialist, I laid on my side with a pillow under my hips so as to put my lungs on a downward angle so gravity would drain the blood from them. This would also only allow one lung to be flooded and due to the angle it could only become half full. As I was plugged into the pulse and blood pressure machine and could see the readout I concentrated on lowering the blood pressure working on the assumption less pressure less bleeding. There I was on the trolley in emergency with my neck bent towards my chest with a kidney bowel tucked under my jaw catching the blood waiting for the specialist to arrive feeling the loneliest person in the world. The Doctor came and the first order was put a Bronchoscope into the lungs and see what's happening. What they saw from the scope was blood foaming up from the smaller pipelines. Now a CAT scan was ordered to see what was going on. The machine showed the lungs had a ground glass like appearance all the way through meaning that the alveoli were bleeding through the entire lungs. Next came all the blood tests especially for all the rare diseases such as Farmer Lung Disease because of my Farming background. I was sent to an isolation room in the Respiratory Ward as they didn't want to chance me killing off all the others in the Ward until they had the results of all the blood tests which were in a few days. Meanwhile the bleeding had stopped. For the next 36 hours they tried to get me to cough out the blood clots in the pipes of my lungs but there was no way I was going to cough and start the bleeding all over again. Finally they made me cough up and I did not bleed. They found no cause for the condition; apparently MDF dust is only listed as a Carcinogen in Europe and doesn't kill Australians. So after another week and only just passing the lung function test after watching the poor old Gentleman before me being wheeled out on a trolley they told me that if I could walk and feed myself there was no place for me in the Queensland Health System

The first 2 years were the worst but I developed a good system and didn't get any infection for about 3 years. This is what I did. At the first hint that I might be coming down with something I would start taking Vitamin C in 1000 mg doses every hour and start on the Garlic Oil capsules as they are anti-viral, antibiotic, anti-fungal and lots more but the main and important reason is that they exit the body via the lungs which concentrates their actions just where I wanted, sometimes when I was really scared I used to take up to 36 capsules a day so I would be nearly sweating garlic. Echinacea was the next main one that I would take in tincture form so as to stimulate the bone marrow to make an army of more white blood cells as well as to take care of anything wandering around the blood stream. My other main weapon was Tea Tree Oil which I used with water as a gargle especially when you feel the dry pain beginning in the top of your throat in the nasal passage area that usually precedes a cold. What you do is gargle and try to wash a bit of gargle in this area without choking yourself. The whole idea is that if you take out the scouting parties the main force won't follow. Some of these doses were extreme for example the Vitamin C dose would have been on the border of making the bowels loose while the Garlic dose would be close and probably past the dose you would use for worming purposes but I lived and didn't cough for three years.

Following my lung problem I always had a pain under the bottom left rib which I spent a decade guarding with my arm in case anything banged into the area, it was a strange pain because you could not touch the rib to relieve it, it felt as though you had to touch it from inside the chest wall to get any relief. From that time on the mist of spray paint, constant smoke like the sugar cane fires of Nambour and dust storms would always bring on chest pains and make me go and hide. Then along came the Brisbane floods. The boss was fairly sure the Pharmacy was going to go under so he hired a room in the 30 story hotel above us and we moved all the stock up to the 5th floor. Next day when I turned up for work the Police were evacuating the area block by block and it was only about an hour before we were told to evacuate. There was a constant flow of people leaving the city and I was very impressed with the smoothness of the evacuation. I walked to the Central Station and when I got there all the gates were open, you didn't have to pay and were to go straight to your platform as there were extra trains on and get out of the city. I remember sitting on the train and seeing some suburbs going under and watching the wheelie bins start to float away down the street.

A few days later the streets around our home were flooded and we virtually became an Island and then the power was turned off to save blowing all the transformers. I decided that all the meat in the freezer would not die in vain so I feasted for about three days. On the fourth day it felt as if I was going to have a heart attack with severe pains in the heart and chest so I walked down the now draining road and waded to the Medical Center where they promptly put me on the Cardiograph which told them that everything was fine. So then they did a chest x-ray and figured out what was happening. Where the ribs joined the spine and sternum they were all damaged. The diagnosis was Intercostal Rheumatism aggravated by excessive uric acid from the protein breakdown of all the meat in my freezer. Unfortunately the Rheumatism had decided to stay and do its daily lap starting from my old sore rib and then going round the front and then back of my heart leaving my back feeling like a broken compressed shock absorber by the end of each week. But what can you do life must go on.

Most of the people coming in and seeing me today were all coming down with respiratory problems, so in general I told them what I used to do. If the symptoms where just beginning I put them on a Tea Tree Oil gargle of about 3 to 6 drops of oil to a wine glass of warm water to be gargled, trying to get some of the gargle into the nasopharyanx area so as to kill off the rapidly dividing germ cells. Usually a cold or flu starts in the nasopharynx area and from there after it has got its numbers up invades the rest of the system. The way I look at it is if you kill the scouting parties the main force won't follow or if it does it won't be as strong. When you feel a cold or flu coming on you only have about 24 hours to kill it, if you don't succeed it will follow its normal course but maybe a little milder due to the effort you put in at the beginning. I wondered how many of my customers had the flu jab recently as we have had the flu vaccine nurse here twice in the last month though thinking about it they usually tell me because they are usually annoyed. A few of the people who had respiratory problems also had a long history of sinus problems so for these I usual used Iridology because most of the time I see what I expect to see in the eye. After doing Iridology for over 20 years you seem to become slightly psychic especially if you are like me and have done most of your work in Markets and Chemists which are the frontline of health care. People who have sinus usually have what is called a Lymphatic Rosary on the edge of the colored part of the eye. It is made up of little dots, hence the name, in other words it looks like Rosary Beads on the inside edge of the iris. On the Iridology chart this area represents the lymphatic system and when you see this sign it tells you that the lymphatic system is so full of rubbish that it's blocked off. One of my favorite herbs for this condition is Fenugreek for it is a lymphatic cleanser that works by thinning the mucous which allows it to start moving again through the system. I usually explain it this way. When you have sinus the mucous doesn't move but gets thicker, in an acute episode it gets bigger and expands which give you the deep bone pains as the sinus is put under internal pressure. As the sinus has only a small hole the thick mucus can't get out, so to cure you have to thin the mucous which then allows it to exit the small hole. It's always fun to show people in this case a picture of a Lymphatic Rosary and then get them to have a look at their own eye through my magnified mirror and see the same thing reflected back to them from their eye, I then usually tell them one of the basic laws of healing which goes for every year you have had the condition it takes a least one month's treatment to cure. So if you've had sinus for twenty years it's going to take at least 20 months of treatment to cure. The other joy of Iridology is that it makes the day go fast and as it's the beginning of the week time goes fast anyway, Friday always seems to be the longest day. Well it's time to pack up and go home; thank goodness it's been a fast day.

Day 2

I started my work day in my normal way by putting my feet up for half an hour and then went through my usual start of the day's routine. I noticed that the cold and flu remedy shelves had taken a beating especially the Olive Leaf Extract which seems to be a favorite these days. So the first job of the day was to get the shelves full and looking pretty again. There seemed to be something happening at the back of the shop in the pharmacy area so I went to take a look and saw what must have been an Asthmatic having breathing problems with the pharmacist watching her as she used her puffer, he then lead her to a chair so she could sit down, get her breath back and calm down a little. I left them to it as no one likes strangers looking at them when they are unwell and vulnerable. Going back a customer greeted me with ah just the man I want to see, I am coming down with something, what's the difference between a cold and the flu. Colds usually start with sneezing then lead on to a scratchy throat followed by nasal congestion and the symptoms are usually focused in the head. It usually gets to its worst about the 3rd day and is usually over by about the 7th day.

Flu's can start violently with fever, chills, headache and maybe a cough. With flu's you also get muscle aches and pains throughout the body but especially in the back and the neck, you can get most of the symptoms of a cold with the flu but it's the fever, muscle pains along with the malaise and weakness, in other words the feeling of really being sick that makes it easy to distinguish between a cold and flu, also flu's can go on for weeks. So he said I won't know which one it is for a while. Not unless you come down with a fever I replied. What's your worst symptoms I asked, he replied it's mainly a sore throat that seems to be getting worse. As my shelves were taking a beating I took him a couple of isles over where we had the Ease A Cold day and night range and selected the one for him that contained Licorice which I told him has a demulcent soothing action along with an anti-inflammatory action which I thought would suit him better for his throat. Other than that it had its usual ingredients of Echinacea, Zinc and Valerian for the night sleeping part. The Strepcils for sore throats were in the same area so I showed him the new one with the throat numbing action telling him that the Strepcils and the Licorice would help him with the throat now and the rest of the ingredients would probably help to minimize a cold or flu if it followed. I also told him to take a high dose of Vitamin C maybe up to 5000mg a day so as to slow down and help fight the infection. After helping the customer I went to have a look at the Pharmacy at the back for there seemed to be a lot of people there already as it was the beginning of our lunchtime rush for the next couple of hours. There looked like two more Asthmatics having trouble breathing with two of the pharmacists dealing with them leaving just the intern and the Pharmacy Assistant behind the counter, but they seemed to be dealing with the situation alright so I left them to it and walked out to the front of the shop and went outside on to the street to see if there was smoke or anything else in the air that could be upsetting the Asthmatics. The sky was clear and there was no wind so I shrugged my shoulders and went back into the shop. We had about three or four more Asthmatics come in with problems during the rush which kind of threw a spanner in the works on top of that it was very strange as this had never happened before. When the rush was over I went up to the Pharmacist and asked what the hell's going on, we've never had that happen before, he shook his head and said don't know, must be something in the air. Latter I was talking to the young Pharmacist to see what he thought but he didn't have any ideas either, but it had been a very strange day with lots of people coming in who thought they were coming down with a cold or flu and it looked as though the Asthmatics were getting the worst of it. There was definitely something out there that was attacking the respiratory system so I spent the afternoon thinking what's the difference between those getting sick and the Asthmatics who are in trouble. The best answer I could think of was that lots of Asthmatics are on steroids which after long term use would lower the strength of the immune system, maybe the ones in trouble are heavy steroid users, and maybe this bug likes the immune-compromised people while the others have the strength to fight it off. I'll have to watch the news tonight because at this rate all the hospitals are going to be filled with asthmatics, but still that's what all the emergency rooms are designed for now days. All of my Vitamin C, Echinacea, Cold Combat and most of the other types of cold supplements were all getting low on the shelves again and most of my under the shelf boxes of spares were all empty. I went over to the pharmacy and told the young pharmacist and checked out his cold and flu drugs and they were all fairly low as well. He said not to worry as we have 6 pallets of stock arriving in the morning along with extra staff to help put them away. While I was in the pharmacy I went into my own draw full of freshly out of date supplements and grabbed a glucosamine and chondrotin tablet for my back and thought while I am here I'll grab 1000mg of Vitamin C and a couple of Garlic Oil capsules as I don't want to get diseased again, I usually take Garlic Oil every day just to save myself from the customers but I think I'll wack up the dose for a while. Our second rush hour started at 4pm as they all started to go home was not as busy as before and there was only one more asthma incident and that was a lot milder than the others were. Spent the last of the day wondering around the shop yakking and gossiping with the girls and then giving my section a bit of a cleanup. Finished at 6pm and then did my usual dash to the rail station so as not to miss the train. While I was walking I was thinking that I should check the people out at the station and see how many look sick or are coughing. Walking down the platform it was hard to tell, there were a few but it was the first time I had ever done this, usually you just ignore most people and get to where you've got to go but there weren't any collapsed asthmatic around anywhere. Even in the carriage I didn't notice any difference. At home there was nothing on the news about hospitals full with Asthmatics as I was sure there would have been, well I'll just have to watch the news in the morning.

Day 3

There was no mention on the early morning TV news of Asthmatics filling up the hospitals; it was just the usual political bickering. No doubt the hospitals have their bad days especially when there are pollens in the air or dust storms. Most of the people on the train looked fairly healthy on the way to work so maybe things might have calmed down and it will be an easy day. I walked from the station to work via all the other chemists taking there catalogues to read for when I got to work so I could see what they were all getting up to. Arriving at work I walked down my isle and saw that the stock had arrived and I had about thirteen boxes to put away so it was going to be a busy day for me but looking on the bright side I would be able to sit down a lot while putting the stock away which would save my back and being busy makes the day go fast. I did my usual lap around the store when I started and checked the stock bins outside. Before I started with the shelves I went to my draw of supplements and took my usual back pill and then decided that I might as well dose myself up as I got the flu twice last year and I don't want to get this new bug going around. So I took two Echinacea, Garlic, Zinc and C caps, a 1000mg of Vitamin C and two Garlic Oil capsules and decided to dose myself three times a day. As I closed the draw I remembered seeing lots of packets of Eucalyptus cough sweets that had just gone out of date in the lunch room so I headed there to claim them and added them to my draw along with the rest of my stash. Eucalyptus used to be the old remedy for flu in Australia in about the turn of the 18th century; they used to medicate a sugar cube with 1 drop of Eucalyptus oil. Eucalyptus has an anti-viral action along with its main action as a bronchodilator. I figured that if I keep taking these sweets throughout the day it would be nearly as good as gargling with the Tea Tree solution. I better start being careful now as a chest infection is the last thing I need with my damaged lungs and intercostal rheumatism. I started filling the shelves starting with the most empty and it wasn't long till the first customer needed help. She told me that a couple of days ago her son had caught something at school and had brought it home and now most of the family except for her were starting to get sick. I asked her what sort of symptoms her son was showing. She told me he had started with a sore throat which I thought was his usual tonsillitis, but now it's turning into a cough. What type of cough and how old is he I asked. He's six and it's a dry cough and he's not bringing anything up. I want something natural not pharmacy stuff. The only one that I have got is called Prospan (English Ivy) and you can give it to children from 6 months onwards, Blackmores have just copied it and I think it's the only liquid cough mixture they have. You can also use the Homoeopathic cough mixtures as well. What's happening to the rest of the family, are they getting the same symptoms as well. I showed and told her about just what I had taken and stressed the importance of zinc and Vitamin C for the immune system. I also showed her the new Strepcils throat numbing lozenge which would be useful if it turned into a hacking cough. As it was in the same area I showed her the Ease A Cold with the Licorice and said she should think of them if things start getting worse for the rest of the family.

I started filling the shelves again starting with the biggest gaps so it would look all nice and neat fast, The Vitamin C had taken a massive hit and in the cheap brands was nearly empty. Even as I was loading the shelf someone came in after some. Just as I was starting to fill another shelf I heard ah just the man I wanted to see a saying I recognized and had heard for years now, I turned and said how are you? He replied I am getting worse, the throats turned into a cough I turned and looked up at him and saw that he did not look well at all and was perspiring on the forehead, what's the cough like, It's alright it doesn't hurt its just annoying as its not bringing anything up but it's kind of persistent. I stood up and felt his forehead and saw that he was hot and running a temperature and then said let's have a look at your neck. The glands weren't all that swollen so I asked if it hurts when you swallow and the reply was no. You've got a temperature and look a bit feverish. Yeah now that you mention it I do feel a bit feverish. You're coming down with something and it looks as if it's only going to get worse, I reckon it's going to travel down to your chest as that's where most of the flus favorite hangout is, if your fever gets worse then you know you've got the flu If your fever gets worse just pack up and go home, working with a fever is like working stoned or drunk, so remember that when you drive home. Well thank you he said sarcastically. Keep going with the Ease a Cold I gave you yesterday, if you get really bad double the dose of it. Take heaps of Vitamin C at least 5000mg per day. To add to what you are taking I am going to give you Garlic Oil capsules take a least six of them 3 times a day. Garlic is anti-bacterial and antiviral. Garlic exits the body via the lungs hence the garlic breath so we have it exactly where we want it. Vitamin C has an anti-viral action as well. Licorice that you got yesterday is also an antiviral along with being an expectorant which will help with the cough. On your way home go into the Health Shop and buy their Licorice sweets as all our sweets are synthetic Licorice. You don't have problems with your blood pressure? No. That's good because Licorice whacks up the blood pressure. Licorice is a strong anti-inflammatory so it will help tone down the pain and inflammation for you as well.

I kept loading the shelves during the rush hour and helping those who needed it mostly with cold supplements and multivitamins with most saying they were feeling run down. When the rush hour was over I went to the back of the shop where the pharmacy is and asked whether they have had anymore Asthmatics with the reply being not yet, I told them that I was still getting a run on the cold supplements and that it looks as though they are all getting a cough after the sore throat to which they agreed and said same here. While I was there I dosed myself up again with my mid-day dosage of cold and flu supplements and grabbed a handful of the Eucalyptus cough drops and put them in my pocket and went back to finishing the shelves. When the shelves where done I still had some big gaps so I went a few isles over to the Ease A Cold range and took four packets of each of them and made all my little gaps into one big gap and filled the hole with Ease A Cold. Latter in the afternoon a man who looked really sick approached me and asked what have you got to help with the flu. I asked him what was happening and he replied I just feel like shit. How did it start I asked. With a sore throat, then a cough along with a headache and now I am feeling feverish and my chest is congested and I am beginning to cough up clear stuff. He looked so sick that I doubted if any of my supplements would help him fast and he also looked very impatient and in a hurry. I told him that I doubted that any of the products here would give him fast relief and told him to come with me and see the pharmacist as they had strong suppressants behind the counter. I caught the pharmacist's eye and he came over. I told him that this gentleman had started with a sore throat, cough, headache and now fever along with his chest now becoming congested and coughing up clear mucous and left him to the pharmacist as there were people waiting for me in my section. Latter I went back to the pharmacist and asked him what he did. He said I tried to get him to see the Doctor next door as he looked really bad but he refused so I gave him the congested cough medicine and the usual cold and flu.

Have you had any Asthmatics in today to which he replied only a couple and they weren't so bad thank goodness. I went back to my area and prepared for the second rush hour as it was nearly 4 and stocked up some of the shelves and cleaned up a little. Again it was the cold and flu supplements that were being targeted not much of anything else was moving. Most of my new stock there was gone and it would be 3 to 4 days before the franchise would replace it. I got my clipboard and started writing up a list of all the supplements that I knew I could get from API the pharmacy supplier of drugs as I knew they always delivered first thing every morning. After finishing the list and adding other products that I wanted I went up to the Chief Pharmacist and explained the situation, he agreed and ordered them while we were talking. I asked him if he had ever seen anything like this before and he said no, we had a little run during the SARS outbreak and not much happened during the Pig Flu a few years back except the Intern got it. The day was nearly done so I took my evening dose of supplements and packed up my gear and did my usual mad dash to the Railway Station. Getting off the train I went to the Coles car park where I normally parked the van and decided to go into Coles and stock up my Vitamin C and Tea Tree Oil. Their shelves in the Cold and Flu area had taken a beating to but I found what I wanted and got two bottles of 300 tablets of 500mg Vitamin C and two large bottles of Tea Tree Oil.

Day 4

No mention of anything on the early TV news, they have to say something soon. Caught the train to work and noticed it was a bit emptier than usual, but they all seemed healthy enough. Checked out all the discount book stores between the station and work as I normally do once a week as I get a lot of good medical books at a very cheap price. I found some small pocket books on Homoeopathy and Herbal Medicine for $2 each so I brought 20 of them thinking I'll put them away for the future and sell them when I do the markets again. Was very pleased with myself when I arrived at work and put my feet up for half an hour thinking I could easily sell them for $5 each and they would go well with all my animal books which I used to sell at the markets, especially when I was traveling and prospecting. The books had financed my prospecting and traveling for nearly a decade now. Did my usual walk around the shop when I started and noticed there were two boxes of stock in my aisle from API mostly of Ease A Cold and similar formulas and lots of Vitamin C. Looking at the boxes reminded me to go to my draw and dose myself up with my usual supplements and while I was there I filled up my pocket with Eucalyptus cough sweets. I decided to pull forward and neaten up the shelves in my aisle before putting the new stock away as I would have to make special places for them and move the other stock around. As I was half way through pulling the stock forward a customer sort me out. I recognized him as a customer who was staying in the 30 story Hotel above us as he had been in a few times before. He looked really sick and said he wasn't feeling very well, Looking at him I said come with me so we can sit down. I took him into the Pharmacy waiting area where the chairs were and made him sit down and said what happening. He told me he felt feverish and his chest was congested and now it was really hurting when he breathed in. I asked him how his condition had started and he said what I was expecting, with a sore throat and then a cough which went down to the chest. I told him that he really should see a doctor but he said no, Australian doctors are too expensive, I am going home soon, the reason I said you should see a doctor is because of the pain when you breathe in, that can be a sign of a secondary infection starting. Wait here and I'll get the Pharmacist and we will see what he has got to say but before I do give me your name and mobile so I can check on you tomorrow, here write it on the clipboard. While you are doing that I will get the Pharmacist. I told the Pharmacist the symptoms and what I said and left them to talk. I finished neatening my shelves and started on the new stock, the Ease A Cold was easy but I had to make room for the others. One of them a new formula made me laugh, the herbs used in it were Echinacea, Olive Leaf, Elder Berry and Andrographis, in other words the best cold and flu ingredients from the Mediterranean, Europe, America and Asia. Obviously they didn't have to think to hard when they made that formula but still it would be effective. Sometimes when new products come out and I read the formula I can figure out just where the Naturopath who wrote it has been to on their latest holiday. A bit quieter today even the first rush hour wasn't so bad so I had plenty of time to think mainly about the new flu, it was a nasty piece of work as it came on slow which was unusual for flu but when it reached the chest then the virus seemed to replicate extremely fast and make the patient's condition worse very fast. Though when you think of it a warm wet humid chest is an ideal breading incubator for any germ. Maybe that's why it was upsetting the Asthmatics, maybe with them or some of them being immune compromised through their steroid treatments it could miss a step and go straight to the lungs. I can see this flu's going to be a problem as no one's going to figure out what's going on till it's too late. For something like this you have to really hit it hard at the beginning to be successful because it's too late when it reaches the chest. I'll give Erick a ring; he's fairly clued up and always ahead of the rest. Erick is a fellow Homoeopath who also works in the city as well as being an Herbalist and Iridologist like me, but he's more into the manufacturing side and has the equipment that allows him to make most of his own medicines but he also has the best gossip. I rang him and told him my thoughts and what had happened. He seemed to be of the same opinion as me, I asked him about the Asthmatics and he told me most of the hospitals were full of them and it would probably be today or tomorrow that they would get the test results back and then they would know what they are really dealing with. I said the Asthmatics would take the focus off everyone else and they would only get a warped view of what was going on, this is unusual because it takes so long to become nasty and that guy I was dealing with from the hotel he was really sick and to make it worse he's basically a super spreader wandering around infecting everyone. We both agreed that things were beginning to look a bit disturbing and that the media weren't getting involved because asthma attacks were fairly boring but we could both see the potential for this to spread and get out of hand. You know what makes this worse I said, nah what, Tamiflu really only works if you use it in the first 48 hours of the infection, with this they won't know what they have till it's too late. Oh well you know what we've got to do, yeah we've got to make a disease nosode of it. Yes I replied, I'll come round Saturday morning and help you, I'll give you a ring before I come round. I went back to sitting down and sorting out where I was going to put the new stock which was really just an excuse to sit down and think. I decided that I had better get my own stocks of medicine up just in case, it's been a long time since I have had all the flu remedies. I went back to the phone and rang Newton's Pharmacy in Sydney and placed a personal order to be sent by 24 hour express post to my PO Box so I could pick it up on Saturday. The order was for bulk herbs all at 1 kg which latter I would process into herbal tinctures. I ordered Cats Claw, Olive Leaf, Yarrow, Elder Flowers, Echinacea x 2, Boneset, Licorice x 2, Andrographis x 3, Willow Bark, Elecampane, Horehound, x 2, Mullein and Pleurisy Root x 2. I went back to finish the shelves feeling a little happier now that I was doing something and would have the disease nosode by Saturday. Just before the second rush hour another really sick tourist from the hotel came up to me asking for help. I took him to the pharmacy area again and sat him down and asked the usual questions, he also had the new symptom of breathing in hurts and he said it hurts the walls of my chest. Again he did not want to see the doctor but this is fairly common with tourists. In all my years here I had only seen one tourist go the doctor and she was an Italian with a sore left hand in which I could not find a pulse and it was fairly obvious in the end that she had a clot blocking blood supply. In that case the pharmacist who was watching me dragged us both off to the doctors. As I had done to the other hotel guest I got him to write down his name and number and told him I would call him in the afternoon to see how he was and then handed him over to the pharmacist. I went out the back and washed my hands and then headed to my draw of supplements for another pocket full of Eucalyptus sweets putting two in my mouth as I headed back to my row. Our second rush hour was quieter than usual, it had been a fairly quiet day compared to normal Thursdays as most people in the city get their scripts on payday. Now that I had a bit of time I thought I would go and talk to Cam one of the girls who helps run the shop and works in dispensary now and again. Cam was a pretty Eurasian of about 23 and one of the few people I could confide in and trust. I told her my thoughts and what I had been talking to Erick about. I also told her of the two sick hotel guests. She said she had heard about a lot of people getting sick and some of her friends were to. I told her I was beginning to get a bad feeling and that I thought things might get out of control if they carry on at this rate and nobody really knows what the hell is going on. I am going to put you on the same regime of supplements as me, it should act as a preventative after all I haven't got it yet and they've been breathing all over me for weeks. I took her to my draw and showed her what to take and doubled the dose for her first time. I told her I would have the disease nosode by Saturday and that's as close as you can get to a vaccination at this stage. It was time to pack up and go home. I spoke to the Pharmacist on the way out saying we don't need a big order but you might as well do it because their stock must be getting low by now and better us to get it then someone else. I made my mad dash to the Railway Station thinking I should go to Coles on the way home and get more supplements but also get some candles and LED torches to add to my collection.

Day 5

Again there was nothing on the morning TV news; this was getting to be annoying. The train to work was not as full as usual but still, they all looked healthy. Friday was the day I always checked out my favorite toy shop in the city as it was loaded with military models, figurines of stars and models and even a big Dalek. I checked out all my favorites then headed off to work. After putting my feet up for half an hour I started work by heading to my supplement draw for my usual and then tracked Cam down to make sure she had taken hers. Started my usual lap around the shop, went outside to check the bins and came back via my aisle where I found 2 boxes of stock from API. Started pulling forward the stock on the shelves starting from the front of the shop working to the back and then started on the new stock. It looked as though the pharmacist had made the right decision because the shelves were emptier then when I left last night. There is a big population living in the city now compared to what there was a decade ago as there are now lots of high rises with permanent residents and with the shop being open from 7am to 8pm the residents make good use of it. Had about the normal amount of people for our first rush hour, more than yesterday and they all seemed to be coming down with what I now presume is our mystery flu that no one seems to know about, which reminded me about the hotel guests I said I would ring, but that can wait till after the rush hour. Most of the people I was seeing were showing the whole range of symptoms ranging from sore throat to chest congestion and a sharp pain in the chest upon breathing in. I was beginning to think that the breathing in chest pains were the result of inflammation rather than a secondary infection because some of the people getting it were young and healthy and had never had respiratory problems before while secondary infections are more common in the elderly or those with a preexisting respiratory problems. Maybe we should be prescribing that new Lemsip because as a tea they would absorb the whole dose fairly fast and it's meant to be for fever, pain and inflammation. Maybe I should think of Aspirin as well, started early so its anti-inflammatory action is already working before it's needed, then again I should really think of the anti-virals first because it's better to take out the cause then the end result. As the rush hour was dying down I decided to ring the Hotel guests upstairs and see how they were doing. Neither of them answered so I waited 10 minutes and tried again. After no reply the second time I decided to give it half an hour before the next try. On the third attempt at not getting through I went to the pharmacist and told him what had happened and said as I am off to the toilet which is near the hotel reception I will stop in and tell them about it. I told the hotel reception the story and said the guests had been strongly advised to see the doctor twice but had refused and I said that they had been told that we would check on them in the afternoon. The chief of security was sent for and told the story; he then found the room numbers matching the names on my clip board and went into the back office to get out the master keys. Coming out he said follow me and we headed to the elevator. It was not long before we were at the first guest's room where he knocked on the door, there was no reply, he knocked again and called the gusts name and said this is security we need to talk to you. There was still no reply. He knocked louder and called his name and said this is security, I am opening your door with the master key this is security. The door opened into the lounge and we walked through to the bedroom where we found him in bed. He was having difficulty breathing and his lips were blue, he did not look well at all. I said to the security chief respiratory distress, his lips are blue and we need oxygen fast and an ambulance. He notified reception and another security man was on his way up with an oxygen bottle. I suggest we get on either side and lift him into a sitting position as it sounds like he is drowning in his own fluids. Just as we got him into the sitting position the security man with the oxygen bottle arrived and began to administer the oxygen while we supported the patient. After the oxygen was set up I said we better check the other guest. He said come on and told the other security man to notify reception and stay with the patient till the ambulance arrived. He went through the same routine again because there was no answer, as the apartment was the same layout as the other we headed straight to the bedroom and found the bed unmade with no one in it. As we left the room we saw a body on the floor of the kitchen, he walked over and bent down and felt the pulse at the neck looked up at me and said he's dead. I said to him that I think you are sitting on a time bomb here; those two would of infected lots of people. I have to get back to the chemist, wash your hands well and don't touch your face till your hands are washed. I have to go down and tell the pharmacist what's happened. Come down and see us when you've got this sorted out and I'll give you some anti-viral face masks for you and the rest of your team as it would be better wearing them next time you have to do this. I went back and told the chief pharmacist what had happened and he said oh shit. We are in big trouble the hotels probably a time bomb waiting to go off over our heads. I need some Tamiflu I've been handling someone about to die and one who has (a little lie can go a long way) and Tamiflu only works in the first 48 hours, with my damaged lungs I don't stand much of a chance. He opened the draw next to him and gave me a pack. Thank you. The chief of the Hotel Security is coming in to see us soon; I promised him and his men some of our antiviral masks that we've got under the counter in case of an epidemic. I'll go dig them out for you. I got the mask and the kit that went with them for I was the one who buried them, mainly because I was not very impressed with it as the kit said wear the masks and hand them out in a pandemic and keep washing your hands. I took them over to the pharmacist after putting a big hand full into my draw and said you might as well put in a big order for Tamiflu, maybe one for each of the staff and I would also hassle State Emergency and be the first to place an order on their emergency stocks, that might force the fools into getting their act together and maybe start doing something. I went back to my area and concentrated on calming myself down as the adrenaline was still surging through the body. Cam came up and said what the hell's wrong with you, your pacing up and down. I told her the story of what had just happened, her reply was oh dear were in deep shit. I told her that I would come over later on Saturday morning straight after Erick and I had made the Disease Nosode and give her three bottles, one for her and one each for her divorced parents. Telling Cam reminded me to tell the chief pharmacist as he had just done the decent thing for me so now it was my turn to return the favor.

I told the pharmacist that Erick and I were making a Homoeopathic Disease Nosode and at mid-day on Saturday I would bring him in 17 bottles which would cover all the staff and I also told him what Erick said about the asthmatics in the Hospitals. Our second rush hour was about to begin so I went back to my aisle taking my first Tamiflu as I went. This was the busiest rush hour I had ever had everyone seemed to have been holding off about doing something about their colds and flu's till the weekend. By the time it was over the usual stocks were empty again. I was feeling very exhausted by now, it had been a long week and with the plan beginning to form in my mind it would also be a long weekend. I told the Pharmacist that we had better do another API order for me as the shelves were empty again. Then I went to my draw and took my usual supplements before going home. While I was there I took the Tamiflu out and pulled a sheet out and cut in half and put the rest into my pocket. I slowly packed everything up and got ready to go but before I left I went over to Cam and gave her half a sheet of Tamiflu and told her not to tell anyone. I told her she had to use them in the first 48 hours of symptoms beginning otherwise they wouldn't work. Did my mad dash for the train and while on the train I decided to hit Coles again for more supplements, candles and maybe a few more LED lights. I didn't really need food as I always squirreled away a few cans of food and bits and pieces every week so as to build up a large supply for my next prospecting trip, but I think I will get myself a few beers as I need to unwind and a few beers will help me sort out my new ideas and see them from a different perspective because I don't think I can stay in the city for much longer.

Day 6

I slept in till about 9am as I needed a rest then got my act together and gave Erick a call and told him I was on my way and asked if needed me to bring anything. He was short of 60 15ml bottles and about 3 liters of pure alcohol. I had lots of bottles as I had recently brought a pack of 500 so I put about 100 in a bag. As my 25 liter bottle of alcohol was fairly new I could spare 3 liters easily. All Homoeopaths usually have alcohol licenses as most Homoeopathic Potencies are made from near pure alcohol and some of our tinctures such as Calendula are made from a solution of 90% alcohol. I packed what I needed and got into the van and headed off to Erick's. When I arrived Erick was at the back in his work room and was just finishing making the Nosode. I came in and put the bottles and alcohol on the workshop table and sat down and made myself comfortable. So where did you get the Nosode from I asked. He replied the Nosodes made from 3 peoples mucous all with serious congestion of the lungs who were about to go to hospital. They were potentized to 15C separately and then mixed together and potentized to 30C. There's a 100ml bottle for you over there of a 16C mix for you. We worked together and filled and labeled all the 15ml bottles. The label read Influenza Nosode 30C with the next line having the date with strain next to it. Now that the work was finished we sat down and relaxed and Erick mixed the Nosode with water in two glasses gave one to me and said cheers. We talked as we sipped with Erick saying we Homoeopaths have been doing this now for hundreds of years, it was probably Napoleon who made our Nosodes famous when he was marching his legions through Europe spreading typhoid in his wake. Our Nosodes saved a lot of towns back then and since then. He raised his glass and said here's to us let's hope we get through this one. So what are you going to do? After you he said. So I told him that I was going to head out to a Lake in the middle of a National Park in the middle of nowhere. You can always survive by a Lake as there are fish and all the wild life go there for the water. I don't want to be in the city when it collapses and all the fruit loops take over. I am leaving on Monday evening after work. We are going on Monday too Erick said. We are off to the wife's parents as they have a big place in the country so I'll take my gear and set up there and start planting some herbs. Have you got any seeds to spare I asked just give me your old and out of date ones. He went out and got me a bag of about 20 to 30 seed packets and said have these I don't know if they will work. I packed up my gear and said my goodbyes to Erick and his wife and wished them all the best. Next stop was Cams; I had three bottles of Nosodes for her. As soon as I got there I prepared a Nosode for her 8 drops into a small wine glass size of water. You haven't just brushed your teeth or had a cup of coffee I asked, why she said, because they both can upset Homoeopathic potencies, she shook her head and took the glass. I told her to sip it slowly and not to eat or drink anything for an hour or more and to give the same instructions to her parents when she gave them their Nosodes. While she was taking her medicine I told her I was leaving on Monday evening after we hopefully get our pack of Tamiflu each. What she said after all these years you're just going to bugger off like that! I'm not staying in the city after Monday as everything's going to start falling to pieces, anyway you saw what happened to me last time I got the flu, when I got over it I was still having trouble breathing for a week after, if I get this one I am history. Where are you going Cam asked? South across the border for a while then a couple of hundred Ks inland to a large National Park with a lake in the center of it. What are you going to do camp next to the lake or something? No, I know an old man down there who lives next to the Lake. Does he know you're coming? No he doesn't have a phone and he is also a wanderer, actually he's an old alcoholic, did I ever tell you the story about John. No. I met him about six years ago in the high country in the dividing range in winter. The rest stops there have a kind of half enclosed bus shelter with a big fire place because it's bloody cold. Anyway he let me share the fire with him and his dog and gave me a few beers that he brewed himself. He took me around to the back of his old Holden and opened the boot. Inside were two big 25 liter brewing bottles bubbling away and all the rest of the gear he needed for bottling. He was brewing the beer as he traveled. He was making the beer with water from fresh water springs that he used to travel to. He gave new meaning to drinking and driving. I went to the next town early the next morning and after I had done what I needed to do settled down for the night in their really big rest area and then John turns up. John lives next to the Lake I was telling you about and when he gets bored he packs what he needs into the car and goes walk about. So John invited me back to the Lake with him for a few days which I did taking a dozen bottles of Coopers Red with me. I stayed with him again about 3 years ago when I was returning to Queensland. If I stay in the city I will either die or get knocked off by someone who wants the Tamiflu or the Nosodes. Take me Cam said I don't want to stay here by myself. I was hoping you were going to say that. Have you got a long flat suitcase, yes, let's see, Yep that will do as it will fit nicely behind the driver's seat. Now start packing with all your warm clothes and good shoes and boots. Don't worry about food as I have 4 large boxes already that I was going to use for my next prospecting trip. Start packing now so I can take it when I leave and fit it in when I load the rest of the van in the tomorrow. We will go after work on Monday. Stay at home over the weekend so you don't get yourself diseased. Sort out your parents with the Nosodes and tell them what is probably going to happen. I left Cam and headed back into the city to the pharmacy and parked outside in the loading zone. I went in and gave the boss 20 bottles of Nosodes and told him what the score was and how I was leaving on Monday evening with my new pack of Tamiflu hint hint. I told him to look at it as though I was taking a few months holiday and if everything turned out alright I would be back. He knew the risk I was taking working here with my damaged lungs and I needed a break anyway. He appreciated the situation and I said see you on Monday. By the way Erick's running away to the country with his family on Monday to. I went to my PO Box on the way home to pick up my parcel of herbs from Newton's Pharmacy and grabbed the newspaper to see if anything was in it. Also went to the supermarket to stock up on candles, LED torches and rechargeable batteries suitable for my solar recharger. Went home and started packing as I had 16 foam boxes to fill that were going to make up the flat base on the van floor for my double mattress to fit on.

Day 7

Up early as it was going to be a long day. After breakfast I checked out the van for water, oil, brake fluid and even gearbox oil and then drove to the service station and filled up with petrol, LPG and slightly over inflated the tires so as to deal with the added weight. Went home and fitted my small single draw filing cabinet with 2 small draws at the top into the van by bolting the side of it to the fire wall of the engine at the back of the driver's seat using a block of wood as a spacer so as to let the draws open and close when they weren't locked. Next I put the camping fridge which looks like a mini version of a normal fridge on top of the filing cabinet and strapped them together with a ratchet strap. After doing the hardest part I put Cams case between the gap of the seat and the cabinet where it was a snug fit and out of the way and then went in for a rest. The next job was to lay the 16 boxes on the floor in order; I always have the food boxes at the front by the fridge and then started loading the filing cabinet with food, sauces and pots at the bottom muesli bars and snacks at the top. There were three boxes of food and one of water and one of gas cans for the stove along with batteries, torches, candles and other spares. The next row of five boxes with three behind them were all my medical supplies and equipment along with my main medical references. I had 2 boxes for clothes and boots. The last 3 boxes at the back were filled with tools, oils, jacks and spare parts. After all of that it was time for another long rest but before that I got the portable stove and put it behind the fridge. The next job was the one that I was not looking forward to and that was getting the double bed into the van. After much thinking I decided to reverse the van up to the door as close as possible and slide the mattress outside and into the van. The difficult part was having to curve the mattress so as to reduce its width to get it through the van door. As it was the beginning of winter and we were going to a cold place I made the bed a special way that I had figured out while prospecting in some very cold places in Victoria, after the sheets I used an army blanket followed by a long quilt you could tuck in with another army blanket on top. I have found that sandwiching the quilt keeps the heat in. The top blanket was a quilt in a cover sitting loose so you could pull it up and wrap it around your neck if you had to. Last came the pillows and a couple of small cushions and that was another job out of the way. With the mattress pushed back to the rear door on top of the boxes you get an area like a couch at the front on which I always put a piece of thick ply and a few thin cushions so as not to damage the boxes. Next was to prepare a bathroom bag. Before calling it a day I started taking all the information I needed off my computer and into the laptop and memory sticks. After finishing with the laptop I took it to the van a hid it under the mattress. Finally it was time to sit down and put the feet up and watch the TV news. They had a story about the Asthmatics taking up all the hospitals life support and lung machines, they went on to say that there was a new strain of flu that seemed to be targeting asthmatics and that all asthmatics should be careful. I wondered how much they really knew and hoped that they had not been side tracked about the asthma because the asthma victims were just the beginning; the dead man at the hotel was young and fit and did not have asthma.

Day 8

Watched the early news but they didn't have any more to say, they just repeated what was said yesterday. Left for work in the van at 9am so most of the rush hour traffic was gone and headed to the city. It was going to cost a small fortune for all day parking in the city but this was my last day and you have to do what you have to do as all my instincts were screaming for me to get out of the city before things got out of hand. Being all packed up and ready to go kind of gave me a new found confidence and purpose. It would be good to get out of the city and into the peace and quiet again. Arrived in the city and parked in the new underground car park close to the central railway station and walked from there. The streets seemed to be a little less busy then usual and there seemed to be less people to. Got to work my normal half an hour early and sat down and put my feet up in the lunch room. Looked into the time expired box to see if there were any more Eucalyptus cough sweets or anything else interesting but found nothing. Started work in the usual way by walking around the shop and seeing what's different, checked the outside bins and then headed over to my section. In my aisle the cold and flu shelves were nearly empty and there was no stock from API to replace them. Went to the back to see the pharmacist and find what had happened to the stock as it was fairly good last time I saw it on Saturday. He said there had been a big run on them on Sunday afternoon. I told him I would write out an order for him and that we might as well get it from API on top of our normal franchise stock because it's going to sell anyway. After sorting the order out I went to see Cam to see if she was alright and had sorted out her parents. So you all ready. Yeah what about you? All sorted the vans fitted out and ready and is in the underground car park by the station. Your parents get the Nosodes. Yeah dad picked them up and took it to mum. You don't look all that happy what's wrong. Two of the staff are sick and I'm virtually running the place by myself but the boss says he's got two coming in at lunch time. I went back to neatening up the shelves and had a much needed sit down. Our lunch rush hour was very slow, I only had to help a few people which made me wonder if they already knew our stock was low. I decide to ring the other stores to see if I could do a stock transfer to get the levels back up but found that they all had the same problem. The casuals had taken the weight off Cam so she was much happier; I told her that all our other chemists had the same problems of sick staff and most of the cold and flu remedies gone. I told her it's time for our midday supplements and took her to my draw. As we were taking the supplements the young pharmacist came over and gave us each a packet of Tamiflu and said put it away and don't let anyone see it. I said to him and what are you going to do, he just looked at me and smiled. I said you bastard you've been on them all week, he just walked away. Cam looked at me and said should we and I said no, lets save it till we need it I've taken four but that was after dealing with those sick guys upstairs, best to leave them till we need them. A lot of the other staff must have got Tamiflu to as everyone seemed happier than they were before. The day dragged on slowly, there was defiantly less customers then normal and when I went outside and looked at the streets they seemed emptier than normal. The day slowly drifted on to the second rush hour which again did not live up to its name, people were coming over to my area and looking at the shelves and then leaving the shop. I went over to my draw and started sorting out what I was going to take with me and then started sorting out my briefcase making sure I had all the references and gear I would need. Finally at 6pm the work day came to an end. I gathered up all my gear and wished all the others the best of luck and said I hope to see you all again soon. Cam was in the lunch room getting her things together so I waited and we left together. We walked to the car park not saying much both lost in our own thoughts. When we arrived at the van I opened the sliding door and put my briefcase at the back of the fridge with Cams bag and the supplements on top. So does the van meet with your approval? Yep sure does. We started out of the city which was fairly easy with rush hour being nearly over and headed to the motorway. It was a good run to the Gold Coast without much delay so we kept on going. We went on for an hour crossing the border and stopped for fuel and dinner. We might as well take our time and have a decent feed and rest I said. After dinner we relaxed for a while then headed off again. We turned right and started heading west inland, we had a few hundred Ks to go but I knew of a truck stop rest area with a toilet about a hundred ks away which would be a good place for us the spend the night. After a long 80 minutes of driving I finally found the rest area, with a sigh of relief I turned in. It was deserted except for a lone tri axle fully loaded and tarped with its legs down sitting in a corner, I headed to it and pulled up on the other side of it letting it shelter and hide me from the road. It was close to 11pm now and I was feeling very tired. I got out of the van and said to Cam I got to use the loo, she said me to so we headed over to the toilet in the middle of the rest area. On the way back to the van I noticed it had got very cold, it seems that every time you headed west over the dividing range in winter the temperature dropped by about 5 degrees. When we got back into the van I told Cam just to take off her jumper and we will go under the covers with our clothes on just in case we have to make a quick getaway. I don't really like being in rest areas overnight all by myself, there is always safety in numbers and with heaps of gray nomads on the roads these days you can usually find the numbers. After finally settling down and getting warm I said to Cam thank god the days finally over, it was taking so long to end at work and thank god we got some more Tamiflu. Yeah that was really good of him. Do you think it's going to get really bad? I think it will and my instincts tells me it will and I have learned to follow them as they've saved me too many times now to ignore. The scary part is that its attacking the young, those guests in the hotel were young and fit with no previous health problems. The hospital probably thinks they had asthma. Flu usually takes out the old and the sick, when it takes out the young that's when you really start paying attention and as the young make up most of the population that's a bad sign.

Day 9

Woke up to a cold morning but the sky was blue and the sun was only just above the horizon. I said to Cam we might as well sleep in, I always feel safer in these rest areas when the sun is up. So we snoozed for a few more hours till the sun warmed the van. When we were warm we got up and headed off to the toilets, on the way we noticed a Police car hiding behind some trees at the end of the rest area no doubt hiding from his victims. Had a breakfast of muesli bars which I had filled the top draw of the filing cabinet and got ready to go. You can drive for a while Cam, time you got used to the van, its fairly user friendly but on gas it's got about a quarter less power so change gear at about 2500 to 3000 revs because you're not going to get any more power out of it. We got in the van and started on our way, as we were getting close to the exit I noticed something strange about the Police car and told Cam to stop close to the car but on an angle so my door opens close to the cop's door. The cop looked as though he was sleeping with his head in his hands on the steering wheel but I had a feeling he was dead. I got out of the van and knocked on the window, are you alright, but there was no movement or reply, so I looked at him through the front windscreen and he didn't look to healthy. Is he alright Cam asked, I think he's dead. I went back to the van, opened the glove box and took out a face mask and a pair of latex gloves and went back over to the Police car and opened the door and pushed the body back from the steering wheel onto the seat and tried to find a pulse in the neck but it was obvious that he was dead but to be sure I ripped the rear view mirror off its stalk held his head straight and put the mirror in front of his mouth and nose. I held it there for about 20 seconds and then pulled it away. There was no water vapor on the glass, he was dead. Looking down at his waist I was thinking you don't need your weapons belt anymore but I do. I lifted the lever to recline the seat and undid the pistol belt. Jesus Mark what the hell are you doing. We need his gun more than he does now. I raised the seat up again and put the cop back into the position I found him in then lifted the gun belt away from his back and opened the side door of the van and lifted the bed mattress up and laid the gun belt flat on the boxes and dropped the mattress down again, I closed the door then locked and closed the door of the Police car and got back in the van and told Cam to drive away normally. I took off the mask and gloves and waited till we were a few Ks down the road and threw them out of the window and opened a packet of wet ones and washed my hands and used a separate one to wash my face, then threw them out of the window. I went through my pockets and pulled out four Eucalyptus cough drops and gave two to Cam and had two myself. It looks like things are getting worse I said to Cam. How long till we get there she asked. A couple of hours, you can drive for about another hour till we come to the main turn off then I'll take it from there because after that there are a few turnoffs we have to take and I'll have to rely on memory. At the turnoff I took over the driving and told Cam that we were looking for a gravel turnoff on the right about 20 minutes away. We found the turn off all right and then it was a short 10k drive to the turn off to the Lake. At the Lakes turnoff there was a big wooden sign saying National Park etc so we turned down the road and I stopped and parked in a clearing close to the sign. What are we stopping for asked Cam? I got to go to the loo and then I am going to take that sign down. Why she asked? So unwanted visitors will have a hard time trying to find us, the reason I picked this place is that not many people know about it. Let's keep it that way, when things get worse there will be a lot of weirdo's wandering round with guns like me. She replied sarcastically ha ha very funny. Years of prospecting had taught me well how to deal with National Park signs and gates. The old T bar wheel brace was the answer for it fits all the bolts on signs and gates and as I had only 4 bolts to deal with it would not take long. After the signs were down I carried them a fair distance into the bush so they would be hard to find. Now that the signs were dealt with we went on our way, we had only 30ks to go before the Lake. Finally we arrived, Johns place was easy to find because it's about the only street there is and his house was the last one. I swung into the driveway and drove round to the back of the house like I normally did when the driveway was clear. I went to the back door and knocked and patted his little dog sitting on the step while Cam hung back and waited. There was no answer so I went to the front door and knocked, again there was no answer, the little dog that had followed me started to whimper which gave me a very uncomfortable feeling. I went round to the back again with the dog following me and whimpering more and tried the door which was unlocked so I opened it and went inside. The dog raced in front of me and went to John's bedroom door and started whimpering and scratching the door. I opened the door and entered the room and saw John was in bed and as I went closer I could see that he didn't look good at all. I shook his shoulder and called his name but he did not respond, I could see that he was breathing but it was shallow and I could hear his lungs gurgling, I opened the curtains to let light into the room and decided to open the windows to let some fresh air into the room. The extra light let me see just how bad he was. The face was pale and damp and the lips were blue. Cam poked her head through the door and asked if he was alright. I said no, he's about had it.

I told Cam we are in big trouble we've got to decontaminate the house, basically wipe and clean everything he may have touched or coughed on with disinfectant but first we have to find him some oxygen or he's going to die. There's no phone here and we need oxygen right now so we are going to have to go next door. But first lets clean our hands and face, try not to touch your face as that's how you infect yourself. I went next door and knocked on the door then stood back a fair distance as I didn't want to disease them. A pretty long haired blond lady opened the door with a young girl peeping out around the side of her and looked at us questioningly and said can I help you. I said that I was a friend of Johns and that he was really sick and going blue in the face and that I needed oxygen and asked if she could ring an ambulance for us. Come in she said but I said no, I don't want to give you what he's got as it's really bad. All right I'll ring. I said we will wait out here. She came back about 5 minutes later and said they can't do anything, the systems overloaded and they can't cope. There's a garage down the road so he should have a gas axe could you give him a ring and tell him the score and see if he can take the oxygen bottle off and bring it over here as we need it fairly fast. It wasn't long before she was back and said he's on his way. What's your name I asked, she said Angela. Thank you Angela I am Mark and this is Cam. As we were going back I said lets go to the van and get the masks and gloves, better safe than sorry and I'll get some for the bloke coming. A few minutes later a white Ute pulled into the drive. I told Cam to put her gear on and open the front door for us and went out and greeted him, put my hand out and said Marks the name, he said Allen. Cam had the door open and I helped Allen with the trolley and oxygen bottle, it was a very large bottle.

Cam held the door open, before we go in Allen put these gloves and facemask on, he gave me a strange look and I said believe me this is bad I have already had one dead one and it's not even lunch yet. When we go in we will try to sit him up, one on each side, lift him into a sitting position then well figure what to do with the oxygen. We left the oxygen at the bedroom door and went on each side of the bed and put a hand under each armpit and dragged him forward and up. He looked terrible and was struggling to breathe, I asked Allen to set up the oxygen bottle while I tried to wake John up. I held his head up straight and shook his shoulder. John wake up you've got to wake up. Allen was about ready so I said go for it maybe it will wake him up, but try to get the oxygen going as slow as you can. After a few minutes of me holding his head up and Allen giving oxygen I tried to wake him again. In the silence following I noticed I couldn't hear any gurgling so I felt for the pulse at the neck and couldn't find it, then I tried the wrist and there was no pulse. I walked around the room looking for a small mirror and there was none to be seen. I think he's dead, I was looking for a mirror to make sure, and then Cam came in with a small shaving mirror saying found it in the bathroom. I took the mirror and put it in front of his nose and it didn't vapor up. He's dead, damn it, I should of opened a bottle of beer and waved it in front of his nose, that would of brought him round. Thanks Allen but I think it was too little too late. What are we going to do now Allen asked? I don't think anyone is going to help us, to many people are dropping dead at the moment, so we will have to bury him in the back yard. I'll get you to help me take him to the back and then ill bury him. I took the blankets off John and rolled him up in the top and bottom sheets. I asked Cam to see if she could find some big rubbish bags and checked Johns pulse and did the mirror test again just to be sure he was dead. Cam returned with some big wheelie bin liners and then we rolled him up in a blanket and I then put one liner on the bottom and another on the top of John. I asked Allen to help me put the body on my shoulder and went out into the back yard and headed to the back left corner of the section by the bush and decided to bury him there. I went back to the house with Allen and asked him if he could help me take out Johns mattress outside, which we did and laid it on the boot of John's car in the sun. I was hoping the direct sunlight would decontaminate the mattress. I helped Allen put the oxygen bottle back into the Ute and asked him to come back with us to Angela's. Cam knocked on Angela's door then came back down so as to keep her distance. I told Angela that we were too late and that John had died so she had better cancel the Ambulance and while she was there to ask them what the hell's going on. Tell them I am going to bury him in the back yard. But while I have got you and Allen here together let me tell what I think is going on. Before I could say anything I noticed Cam was beginning to shiver, I moved forward behind her and held her tight. Poor Cam I said it's not even 12 o'clock and you've seen 2 deaths already, but I know how you feel, remember what I was like on Friday when I came back from the Hotel upstairs after they died. Yeah she laughed you were pacing up and down your aisle. OK this is what I think is going on. There is a new strain of flu turning epidemic and most likely pandemic. This flu is strange because it starts slow with a sore throat, cough, and then it goes to the chest where it goes berserk. It also attacked most of the asthmatics who went downhill very fast and filled up all the hospitals life support machines. Through this happening they were distracted from the real issue. Because of the amount of time that it takes to do viral tests they are probably just getting the answers now, but I think it's too late and I think it is just starting to get out of hand now. That's why Cam and I left the City. Now for some good news, I and another Homoeopath made the Disease Nosode from this flu on Saturday which Cam and I have already taken, this is the closest to a Vaccination as you can get and they are not going to have a vaccine for a while as they don't know what the disease is yet. I'll give both of you the Nosode soon and show you how to decontaminate yourselves. If you treat this flu from the very beginning you've got a chance, if you leave it till your lungs become congested your history. I have a van full of medicine with a lot of it I am going to have to make up myself in the next few days so there's a good chance we are going to be alright. I'll just go to the van and get the Nosodes, Angela you might as well make that call and see what's going on. I'll be back in a minute. From the van I got 2 bottles of Nosodes, wet ones, Tea Tree oil, some plastic cups and a water bottle. I gave a bottle of Nosode to Allen and said don't take it now because we will decontaminate other selves in a minute and I want to tell you and Angela about it at the same time. Angela came back out and we all asked what they said. He said pretty much the same as you, lots of people are getting sick and the hospital is full and they can't cope. When I said you were burying him in the back yard he said do what you must no one will be able to come out for a few days but I have recorded everything. Well we are 70 to 80ks away from everything I said. Ok here is a Nosode for each of you, what you do is get 20mls of water, add 6 drops of Nosode to it and slowly sip it swirling it around your mouth. Take it 2 hours after you have eaten then repeat before going to sleep and that's it. Now I want to show you how to decontaminate yourselves, you're alright Angela but the rest of us have been in contact with John. First clean your hands with the wet ones then your face concentrating round the mouth and nose. The main way we infect ourselves is by putting our hand in contact with our mouth or nose which may put the virus in contact with the mucous membranes, so when you are around infected people or areas try never to touch your face. When you do your face make sure you do the first part of your nose put the wet ones tissue around your finger and put your finger in your nose and twirl it around a few times and hopefully this will kill the virus. Now for the Tea Tree Oil. When you first get a cold it starts in the nasopharynx area, it usually goes dry and irritated and you usually get your first pain from this area. That area is usually where the virus first starts to replicate. Put 3 to 6 drops into a small wine glass of water, 6 drops is starting to get a bit hot. Now gargle it and try to get a few drops into the nasopharynx area without choking yourself to much. This is the best way to kill an infection before it begins. From now on always do this when you come into contact with an infected person or infected area and always never touch your face because if you transfer the virus from a surface area to a mucous membrane you've got it.

Afterwards I told them that they both should go shopping now in case everything falls to pieces, stock up as much as you can get, don't forget candles and torches because the power may go out latter on and get heaps of Tea Tree Oil, Vitamin C, Echinacea Garlic Zinc and C together in a formula and get lots of Garlic Oil Capsules. I told Allen to take his Nosode latter on in about an hour's time as strong things like Tea Tree Oil can ruin Nosodes. We will leave you both to it. Come and tell us what you saw in town I would be very interested. We said our goodbyes and set off to start digging the grave for John. John had a garden shed at the back so we headed there and inside found a shovel, spade and rake. I said to Cam we might as well get this over and done with then we will open all the doors and windows in the house and begin to decontaminate it, then we will have a hot shower and change our clothes. I think it would be better to sleep in the van tonight and give the house overnight to decontaminate. Just as we were about to start digging I said let's get something to eat first. After lunch we started the grave, luckily for us the ground was soft and it was fairly easy going. It took nearly an hour to finish the grave and we had a few sore muscles. Once John was in the grave it took only about 10 minutes to finish and then we put all the largest rocks we could find on top to hopefully stop any animal from trying to dig him up.

Let's decontaminate the house Cam said and get it over with. We got into our gloves and masks and went into the house. Starting with John's bedroom we opened all the windows wide and pulled back the curtains. Then we went into the lounge and wedged the door open and opened all the windows and curtains there. Next we went into the second bedroom at the back of the house and saw it was half filled with beer. Beer was John's main hobby; he used to know where all the fresh water springs were and make different beers from them. I said to Cam it looks like we are going to have a few drinks tonight, you don't need to drink much of Johns beer, he makes it really strong. Other than the beer the room only had an old single steel frame bed and lots of newspapers and magazines. The kitchen was a mess, he hadn't done the dishes for a while and there was rubbish everywhere. I opened the fridge and it was mainly leftovers and bottles. I opened the freezer and it was nearly overflowing with meat and frozen food packets. There was another freezer on the opposite side of the kitchen that one was a top opening freezer and I found that it was also full. I said to Cam that we should start eating out of the freezer because if the power goes off we will lose everything. Under the kitchen sink I found what I was looking for which was disinfectant, spray bottles, sponges and most of the equipment we needed. We opened all the windows and moved on to the bathroom, toilet and laundry. Starting with John's room every handle was sprayed with disinfectant, doors, draws, windows, wardrobe and every area at hand height around the doors, nothing was left to chance. Blankets were gathered up and taken to the clothes line, hung up and sprayed with disinfectant and left for the sun to do its share. We finished by doing the tops of the bedside draws, chest of draws and windowsills. As I was finishing I sprayed a gentle mist over the carpet. Next the lounge was given the same treatment. I asked Cam if she wanted to do the kitchen next or the bathroom, toilet and laundry. She took one look at the kitchen and said you can do the kitchen and promptly left. I did the usual, handles, door area and surfaces and then made a start on the dishes. I washed half of them and then started drying with a clean tea towel and was about to put some away in the pantry when I realized his hands could of touched the top surfaces of all the other plates so I decided to take them all out of the pantry and wash the lot. I even emptied the salt and pepper and washed them to. With the plates all out I disinfected the pantry. It was getting late into the afternoon before we were finished but I was feeling a bit happier and safer now that we had finished. I decided I would get the fire place ready for a fire tonight as it looked as though it was going to be a cold one. As I was getting the fireplace ready I heard our neighbor's car pulling up. Angela and Jodie had returned from their shopping. We went out to see Angela and asked her what it was like out there. Fairly good she said a few places were closed but the supermarket was crowded and some of the shelves where getting empty but I got everything I needed and I filled up the car too. Don't forget to do the Tea Tree oil and take the Nosode before you go to bed I said to them before we left.

The End Of The Beginning
Day 10

We slept till the sun made the van to hot and got up at about 9 am feeling better from our long deep sleep from the exhaustion and stress of the last few days. We had a breakfast with bread from the freezer and whatever we could find in the fridge along with some coffee and talked about what we had to do today. First on the agenda was to get Angela to introduce us to the neighbor on the other side of her so we could get to know them and give them a Nosode as we wouldn't want them to become sick. The idea now was to get to know everyone and give them a Nosode. After breakfast we went off to Angela's and knocked on the door, she opened it and invited us in. Who lives next door I asked. An old man called David, he's very quiet and does a lot of fishing you hardly see him at all. I'll get you to introduce us to him as we need to see if he is alright and to give him a Nosode. His fishing could be handy in the future if food gets low and thank God you've got chooks. Angela said lets go next door and find David. She knocked on the door and after a while David opened. Are you alright David, after watching the news last night and not seeing you for a week I thought I better check? Yes I'm fine there's nothing wrong with me. I want you to meet Cam and Mark they are friends of John. He came down and shook our hands. Angela told David about John and how we tried to save him with Allen's oxygen which didn't work and how we buried him yesterday. She also told him that the ambulance couldn't come because they were too busy. She told him about me and the disease Nosode that I wanted him to take.

David said I didn't realize things were that bad. It's getting bad David I said and I think it's going to get worse fairly fast. With what Angela Told me yesterday about the last time John went out I worked out that the disease has a 5 to 6 maybe 7 day incubation period which means that there are a lot of people with the disease that don't even know they are infected so we could be at a point that we can't really stop the spread. I am sure that Hong Kong is very sacred because when the disease settles in the chest it becomes very similar to Severe Acute Respiratory Syndrome more commonly known as SARS. So they must be getting a bit confused especially when they only get to see people in the last stages. Anyway the important thing is do you need to do any shopping, have you got candles, torches and lots of fuel. Yes I can see what you are getting at said David. You should go with Angela and really stock up I said as I don't think money going to mean much in the future. It would be a really good idea to stock up on seeds I said to Angela. Cam and I can look after Jodie, there's no need to take her, best to keep her away from people for a while, she can help us make medicines. Don't forget to get lots of fuel and 2 stroke mix for your boat David as we could all be living off fish soon. I got the Nosode for David as they were getting ready to go and told him to take a dose now and one before bed.

Jodie, Cam and I headed to the van; the first job was to put the mattress on John's bed. Just as I was pulling the blanket off the bed I remembered that the Policeman's gun was under the mattress and that I had better not let Jodie see it. I got Cam to carry the blankets and loaded Jodie up with the pillows; while they were gone I put the pistol belt into the box with my clothes in and hid it under the clothes. When they came out again I had the mattress out and ready to go. Cam and I took the mattress in with Jodie trailing behind. I left Cam and Jodie to make the bed and started taking the medical boxes from the van into the kitchen putting them on the floor and just under the kitchen table. Cam came in and said that's the bed done. Let's go back to the van and see what's left I said. Tools, clothes and food were all that was left along with the 25 liter bottle of pure alcohol. We will leave the rest for latter I said. Back in the kitchen Cam started sorting out the pantry to make room for all the supplements in tablet form along with the Tea Tree Oil and Nosodes while I started getting prepared to make Tinctures. The main problem was going to be finding enough big jars for making the Tinctures. I had about 15 packed into which I had loaded the bags of herbs so as to save space. I decided to make what I had and go searching for jars latter. I started with Licorice and Echinacea, to make it easier for me instead of using 45% alcohol which I should of I used I used 50% so all I had to do was make a half and half solution of alcohol and water. I told Jodie the alcohol in the solution extracts all the oils out of the herb while the water takes out of the plant all that is water soluble so between the both of them we extract nearly everything out of the herb. Making herbal tinctures is fairly easy, it's just adding the water and alcohol solution to the herb usually at about 5 to 1, seal the jar, shake and put on the window sill in the sun. Every morning you shake the jar for a few minutes and carry on doing this for about 2 weeks. When they are ready you double filter the liquid and then bottle it as an herbal tincture. The main reference for making tinctures is The British Herbal Pharmacopeia as this tells you the proportions of herb to liquid and the strength of the alcohol for each herb. By the time Jodie and I filled all the jars it was lunch time. I said lets watch the news before we have lunch. The news was not good, it was mainly about the disease which they said had been found to be a Bird Flu Human cross which they said makes it very contagious as most people will not have any immunities to it. They went on to say that because so many asthmatics had been affected early on it made the Doctors slow to realize what was really happening. They said the UN was already working on a vaccine and that there was going to be an announcement by the Government this evening at 7pm. I turned off the TV and said oh well at least they know what it is now but they have left it far too late. We went back into the kitchen and finished making the tinctures and then I left Cam and Jodie to tidy up and organize a place for everything. It was fun working with Jodie; she's very bright and intelligent for an 8 year old and was very interested in making the medicine and learning what each one can do. It was such a nice change to work with a pleasant happy young girl who was nearly the mirror image of her mum with Cam and I thinking of calling her mini Angela.

While Jodie and Cam finished off in the kitchen I decided to explore the rest of the house starting with the big double linen cupboard in the hall. Inside on the floor was all of John's beer making equipment. The next shelf was filled with large home brew cans of many different types and brands. The rest of the shelves were filled with blankets, sheets, overalls, sleeping bags and clothes. As I was closing the door I noticed that the top blankets in the corner were out of shape as though concealing something, so I got on my tip toes and moved the blankets away from the corner of the wall and saw the butt of a rifle. I got a chair from the spare bedroom and stood on it so as to get a better look at what was up there and found an old Bruno 22 rifle with telescopic sights and 4 boxes of 200 rounds ammunition. I was happy with my discovery as I used to have the same rifle myself and knew them to be a very accurate and reliable rifle. I pushed the blankets back and decided I would tell Cam latter when Jodie went home. I went on and explored the rest of the house and found lots of useful things but the best finds were in the garage which was full with all types of tools hoarded away over the years along with a good supply of timber.

I heard a car pulling up next door and saw that it was Angela and David returning from town. Jodie and Cam had heard as well and came out of the house and we all together went over to greet them with Jodie running to her mum and hugging her. So what was town like I asked Angela? It was chaos, everyone was there and there were cues everywhere. A lot of the shelves were empty in the supermarkets and there was a long cue at the service station. We got a lot of stuff, I took your advice and brought up big, between Dave and me the car is full. I told them that the Government was making a special announcement tonight a 7pm. And then we left them to their work and went to our new home and made some coffee and put our feet up for a while. I told Cam of the rifle I had found along with the ammunition and said I would put the policeman's gun up there with it. I said that we should start taking the Tamiflu till we have finished 1 pack each and save the last one as a reserve. None of us were showing any symptoms but with the incubation period being so long we might start getting them soon and as Tamiflu only works best in the first 48 hours I thought it was best to run the course of medicine now and not take any chances especially since we were living in the house of one of the diseases victims.

After our break we continued cleaning the house and organizing it the way we wanted while taking note of what we had inherited. We threw away very little for now our futures were uncertain and you never know what you may need in the future. In the back of our minds all that afternoon was what they were going to say on the 7pm news. We made a large dinner that night as there were still lots and lots of food in the freezer and I was scared that the power might go off sometime soon in the future and did not want to waste any of the food. Finally 7pm came around and we sat down to watch the news. This is the 7 o'clock news. We start this bulletin with a special announcement from the Prime Minster. Due to the rapid spread of this new strain of Influenza Australia will from 8.30 this evening close its boarders and as from now quarantine all new arrivals. The Government has activated its emergency Pandemic Procedures and all points of entry into Australia are now under quarantine and will remain so till further notice. The government has decided to follow this action more as a preventative measure. Under the Emergency Procedures and working for disease prevention the Government has decided to release the emergency stocks of Tamiflu which are now being moved to the hospitals and supplied to Emergency Service Personal. After this supplies will go to the Pharmacies which will allow your local GP to prescribe. Be assured we have a vast stock and don't foresee any shortages. There has not been reported any mass outbreaks but I have been informed that most city hospitals are full with people who already had preexisting respiratory problems as this flu seems to target them rather than healthy people. Please stay calm and continue as normal and we will give you more information as it comes to hand. The news carried on saying lots of other countries were also closing their boarders and how Doctors from all over the world were working together in real time on the internet for a vaccine and cure. I turned the TV off as they were beginning to repeat themselves. Well it looks like the beginning of the end has begun; it's time for a beer.

After a while of sitting quietly I said I think they have got it wrong. I think this disease has an incubation period of 5 to 7 days but for those who already have respiratory problems I think it's a 1 to 3 day incubation period and then the virus misses out a few steps that healthy people have to go through and goes straight to the chest and goes nuts and multiplies flat out leading to a massive inflammatory response that's more responsible for killing the patient then the virus. I think healthy people have to go through the sore throat and other symptoms just to make the conditions right in the lungs for the virus to go berserk then kill them. If I am right that means those in the hospital are the first wave and the second wave is soon to follow. The whole confusing thing about this disease is the really long incubation period, no one would expect that. Oh well thank God were out of the city said Cam, I would hate to be in the Chemist now and the shop would be filled with diseased people from the Doctors next door. Well time for bed let's see what the world brings us tomorrow.

Day 11

Slept in and relaxed. Decided to have a lazy day as all we need do now is lay back and relax. Got up had breakfast then watched the news on TV, not much new just a world closing down and shutting its boarders. Now it's just a matter of wait and see. Glad I don't have to go out in the world today, no doubt there will be big rushes on fuel and food after the PMs Announcement last night. Jodie and Angela came round about 10am and introduced us to the Reverend Lovejoy an old retired hippy who lives in the last house on the lake front. He's the only religious practitioner in the area and looks after a flock of about 30 people covering about a 50 kilometer radius, mostly farmers and loners. I asked him about John and was told that he wasn't really interested in religion and that they had just a nodding relationship. He told me he had a service in the hall twice a month on Sundays as his flock wasn't really a religious lot but usually made an effort for the children and to see what everyone else was up to. It's kind of the only social event in the area. We had coffee and Cam cut up and buttered some of my old fruitcake which she had been making fun of for years. The Reverend was a likable guy who didn't take himself too seriously, so I told him our story and what we had seen. I told him about the Nosodes and the very long incubation period of the disease with the exception of those who already had respiratory problems such as asthmatics and how this would confuse the Doctors. I told him that you had a chance of stopping the disease before it got to the chest or a least making it less severe but after the disease settled in the chest there was not much hope as the inflammatory action of the immune system would take you out before the disease. The only way to go with this is prevention and to attack it hard with preventive measures and not to stop. As soon as someone comes down with the disease isolate them and try to keep them away from the healthy, especially in the last stages of the disease when the virus is replicating fast. The Rev excused himself and said I had better go and check on my flock, I was thinking of doing it anyway after last night's news but now you've made me more anxious. I can give you 20 small bottles of Nosodes to take round; for families just give them 2 bottles and that should hopefully cover the 30. Theres more if you need them. I'll get a few things put together for you, while I am doing that Cam will explain to you about the Nosodes and how to take them. Come on Jodie you can help me. Jodie get 20 bottles of Nosodes out of the pantry and put them into that small foam box and while you are doing that I will make 20 bottles of Tea Tree Oil from the big bottle of oil. Thank goodness we have hundreds of those small 15ml bottles. You finished? Get that big jar of Garlic Oil Caps and 20 more bottles and fill them. When Jodie and I had finished we went out to the Rev and gave him 2 foam boxes filled with what he needed. I got a black felt pen and marked the first box Nosodes, These are in a foam box because they are heat sensitive I told the Rev that they couldn't go over 40 degrees. The next box has Tea Tree and Garlic Oil. I'll get you a pen so you can write this down. At the first indication of infection use Tea Tree Oil. Get a small wine glass full of water, add to it 2 or 3 drops of oil. Gargle with this liquid and try to splash some into the back of the nasopharynx area. The oil is a very potent germicide and if you can get some in the nasopharynx area which is the main incubator for colds and flus you could win the fight at the beginning. Now for the Garlic oil, it's antiviral, antibacterial, ant fungal and heaps more and as it is in oil form it moves from the gut to the bloodstream very fast. You've heard of garlic breath, well it comes about because of the oil in the blood. When blood comes into the lungs to pick up oxygen and release carbon dioxide it also releases some of the Garlic. So now you can see how I am targeting a strong antiviral right to the areas where it is needed the most. How are you going Rev, you've just been given heaps of info in a short time can you remember it all. Yes I took a few notes but it kind of makes sense the way you explained it. So the Nosodes are to protect them, Tea Tree Oil is the first line of defense and the Garlic Oil is the second. How are you going Doctor Jodie, she replied with a sweet smile. I've been thinking about what you said about keeping the sick away from the healthy said the Reverend, what about using the Hall for the sick, I'll leave you the key. Angela told me about the ambulance not coming for John so it will no doubt be worse now. If you have a look under the stage in the hall you will find it full of camp beds and other equipment as the scouts come down here three times a year so it might be ideal for the sick. We will go down and have a look I replied. Reverend Lovejoy made his goodbyes and said he must be on his way. We went out of the house to see him off and then decided to all go down to the Hall and have a look after lunch. Before you go Jodie you can help me shake all the tinctures we made yesterday so you can see what happens. Jodie and I went to the kitchen where I started on the first jar of tincture. See how pale the liquid is inside; now watch what happens when you shake it 20 times. After this the liquid inside became noticeably darker. See how its darker I said, she nodded, the alcohol in the mixture extracts all the oils from the herb while the water in our half and half solution extracts all in the herb that is water soluble. So between the two we extract virtually all the medical properties out of the herb. For the next couple of weeks we will do this every day and it will keep on becoming stronger. After lunch we all got together and walked down to the Hall. The Hall was on the front corner of the park by the lake with a little lane running next to it going to a car park and then straight down to a boat ramp and the lake.

I opened the door of the hall and we stepped inside. Have you been in here before I asked Angela? Yes Jodie and I come here every fortnight it's about the only social function we have here. It's a big sized hall I said, whats at the back of the stage area. There is a kitchen and a big spare room. Let's go and have a look. The kitchen was a decent size along with the spare room which had a few empty wardrobes and sets of draws. We went back into the hall and over to the stage which was raised about 4 feet and had 3 sets of big cupboard style doors, one at each end and one in the middle. We opened the center doors and found they were filed with fold out camp beds and large plastic sealed boxes which when we opened them contained 3 single air mattresses. We took out 6 beds and 6 mattresses. We looked in the end door and found that it was filled with large tents and then went to the last door and found it full of barbecue and kitchen stuff. I'm going to go home I said and get the face masks, gloves and medicines, keep hunting around under the stage, I am hoping that there is going to be a big first aid kit and maybe some food. At home I gathered the masks, gloves and another set of prepared Nosodes, Tea Tree Oil, Garlic Oil Caps, Vitamin C and a large bottle of floor cleaning disinfectant and 2 empty spray bottles. When I arrived back at the hall they had 6 beds set up along with tables and chairs. Jodie had found a really big first aid kit and upon a quick inspection I was pleased to find that it had everything you needed including splints. As there were 2 boxes of gloves in the kit I took one of them and added them to the others. A little voice from under the stage said I think I have found some food, so we all went over and saw Jodie pushing some boxes forward towards the door. They were big boxes and fairly heavy, when I opened them we saw that they were big tins of corn, peas and baked beans the size usually used by the military or institutions. Jodie rounded up about four boxes and then went back to her exploring. That's a really good haul I said,

I'll take them to the kitchen. By late afternoon we had set up the hall to our satisfaction, we had 6 beds set up and Jodie had found army blankets under the stage for them and had enjoyed her afternoon of crawling under the stage. All that was missing for the beds were sheets so I presume the scouts bring their own. We had the table and chairs set up in a comfortable manner for Angela had suggested that we set it up as a meeting room which we all agreed was a good idea. Let's go have a break, we're finished here for now I said, so we locked the hall and set off for home. On the way home I told Angela that I would start taking down the fence in the back yard so she could make one large garden which would be enclosed and still safe for the chooks. She said she had a good design in mind and would draw it out for me. It would also be a good idea to expand the chickens I said. Johns got a lot of wood stored away so we should build a bigger and better home for the chooks so I'll get you design that to.

When we got home Cam and I had a snooze for a while then made dinner continuing our effort to empty the freezer. Just as we finished dinner there was a knock at the door, it was the Reverend, he said he had a car coming to the hall with very sick people in it. They are a family, I have their two young girls in the car and their son is driving them to the hall. Ok we will be right over; before you go I'll give you some sheets for the beds. After he had left I told Cam that we should gargle some Tea Tree Oil mix now so as to create a kind of barrier and we might as well do the Garlic Oil to, you can't be too careful. Then I went down to the linen cupboard where I had seen Johns large collection of overalls and grabbed a couple pairs, luckily they were about our size. Here, strip off and put these on, that way we won't contaminate our own clothes and we can throw these into a tub of disinfectant when we get back. We marched off down to the hall carrying our gloves and masks in our hands. The Rev was waiting outside the hall with the girls beside him looking worried, he should have been here by now and there they are now. The car pulled up with what must be the young son driving who quickly got out and opened the rear door by his father and started to help him out. The Rev quickly went over and helped him and they took him into the hall to one of the sheeted beds. The father didn't have much strength left and the others were virtually taking all the weight. There were no pillows so I quickly folded up an army blanket and used it as a pillow. The patient was very red in the face and agitated and restless constantly moving his legs and arms while looking around the hall trying to catch his breath. I squeezed his wrist and he looked at me, I said try to relax yourself and concentrate on your breathing. Try breathing very slowly but deeply while trying to relax. I felt his pulse while he was tying this and it was hard and rapid. Just concentrate on relaxing as we want to get your pulse and blood pressure down. I headed to the next bed where his wife now was and said to the son and Rev let pick up the bed and turn it round so they can see each other and communicate. Having done that I found that his wife was the same as him and gave her the same instructions. Rev I need you to go to Allen's and get the oxygen but keep Allen away as the less people we contaminate the better and you had better keep your distance from him as you are probably a walking biohazard by now too. I looked at their son and held out my hand and said Marks the name, Bruce he said shaking my hand. Now tell me their story. It started 5 to 6 days ago, they just kept on getting worse, I kept trying to ring an ambulance but they just had a recorded message saying this service is not currently available please consult your local GP. What were the first symptoms when it first started? It started with a sore throat and then turned into a cough, and then it just kept getting worse with aches and pains and a headache. Then they got a fever with chills and shakes which kept going on for days. Now that seems to have stopped and they are weak and having trouble breathing. Have they been eating? No not for days only drinking and now they are not drinking much. I went back to his father and said I am just going to feel your glands in your neck; they were very swollen and tender. I went to his wife and did the same and said you must try to do what your husband is, try to breath slowly and deeply, I felt her pulse and it was the same as her husbands and I said to her to try to relax as we need to slow your heart a bit and get your blood pressure down. The Rev should be here soon with the oxygen which should make your breathing a bit easier. While we are waiting I will take your temperature. They were both nearly 103 degrees which is why they were probably restless. You're not getting chills anymore I asked. They both shook their heads. The Rev arrived with our Jerry rigged oxygen and Bruce helped him with it up the stairs. Put the bottle on the floor between them in the middle, while they were doing that I got a couple of chairs which I put at the head of them both so I could sit down and give them oxygen. Cam came over and told me what the girls had said which was fairly much the same as Bruce. OK I said what we need to do now is to decontaminate Rev, Bruce and the girls. Wash hands and face, get the wet ones and get them to wrap it around a finger and swab out each nostril then get them all in masks and gloves and try to stop them touching their faces with their hands. Rev did you have the Nosode. Yes he replied. Next everyone has a Nosode and Rev and us will join them. In an hour's time we will all do the Tea Tree Oil and Garlic. I'll leave it to you Cam to explain everything to them. After that get them to decontaminate their car as it will keep them occupied for a while and it will show them how to decontaminate their house when they get home. After that we had better find some food for them. Aye Aye Captain Cam replied and said to the others lets go sit down and get comfortable. I started giving oxygen at 2 minutes each then built it up to 5 minutes each, I talked to them and told them that the best thing they could do was sleep. They seemed to be more relaxed now with the oxygen but still a bit agitated. Going back and forth to them I noticed that their pupils were really big and that their movements were still jerky and spasmodic like. There is something wrong with the nervous system. Sitting down I had time to think, this disease is very similar to the last stages of SARS, it's just a massive inflammatory response with the immune system going berserk, there was something nagging me at the back of my mind I was trying to remember what I had learned about over reactions of the immune system and then I remembered. Symptoms caused by the flood of immune chemicals can be fever, headache, body aches and usually when this happens it is where the virus first entered the body that becomes the most inflamed, in this case it's the neck. The next part I remembered was that the rupture of the countless dying cells spilling there toxic wastes in the blood stream overloads the lymphatic system and swells the areas glands. The patients were dying before my eyes and there was nothing I could do. Herbs would be to slow and I doubted that the digestive system would be functioning enough to absorb the dose anyway. Even if I was a Doctor and had access to all the anti-inflammatory drugs I doubt that they would survive. I remembered that the Chinese had some good results with SARS by using an injectable form of Licorice that they had made. Licorice has strong anti-inflammatory actions and is also antiviral. Come to think of it Licorice is good for stress and supports the adrenal glands and also has a demulcent soothing action. That just leaves Homoeopathy and the one remedy that really screams out for this condition is Belladonna. Actually the more I think about it Belladonna is about the only remedy I can give because it covers the eyes with the large pupils, the red face, the swelling and congestion of the neck, the nervous system symptoms and spasms and the burning hot feeling of the skin. I was just about to get up when Bruce came over and asked how are they? It's not good but I have got them relaxed and comfortable and I've just thought of something else I can do so you can take over here while I get it. Come sit down where I am, take the oxygen hose and put it close to the nose, I am giving them each 5 minutes at a time now, I went over to my kit and found the bottle of Belladonna 200C in Homoeopathic Potency and added 4 drops to 10mls of water twice in to small plastic cups and gently gave them both their doses. I threw the cups in the rubbish thoughtfully set up by Cam and grabbed a chair and went over to Bruce. Move your chair back and I'll sit here and we can pass the hose back and forth. What's that medicine meant to do Bruce asked? It covers all the present symptoms and I am hoping its going to stop all their twitching and restlessness and any pain they may have but it's too late to cure them, it's basically their own immune system that's doing all the damage now. Think back to when the symptoms started and tell me who you think might have given it to them. I don't know they hadn't been anywhere; we kind of had a big project on. We were replacing all the old pig fencing which was a mess and putting up the right pig wire. Is that the mesh type of fencing I asked? Yes he said we get it in rolls. We had been doing it for a week and neither of them had gone out. So you were replacing all the posts then as well. Yes we were replacing the whole lot we even got heaps of those new fancy wind up strainers. So they hadn't had any contact with anyone for about 5 days? I think it was about 6 or 7 days since they last went to town. Well in that case they have definitely got the pandemic flu; you just confirmed it with the 6 to 7 days because that's the incubation period. So they aren't going to get better? No I replied I think they only have a few hours left. I carried on talking so as to allow Bruce to get himself together. I went on saying that as we are talking about 50% of the planet is getting sick and most of them are not going to get better. You've been watching the news so you have a fair idea of what's been happening; now I'll tell the real story of what probably happened. There are two types of this flu but they are really the same. The second type of flu which your parents have has a 6 to 7 day incubation period which is a hell of a long time as most diseases are about 2 to 4 days. This long incubation period before symptoms begin to show is going to confuse the hell out of Doctors and scientists as they are not trained to expect the unexpected and none of them presently alive has ever had anything to do with a pandemic. flu outbreak. The first type of flu has a 2 day incubation period but this one only attacks those with existing respiratory problems such as asthma, bronchitis or anyone with a bad chest especially those that have been using steroid based medicines for a long time and are immune-compromised anyway. What happened at the beginning was all the asthmatics got hit first, I remember them all coming into the chemist in a bad way seeking help. We had to sit a lot of them down as they were breathless and panicky. After that they all started filling up the hospitals taking over the life support machines and probably worst of all they took up most of the attention of the Doctors and media while the flu with the long incubation period slowly went about its work unnoticed till now, and now it's far too late. Some of us saw this happening and knew it was a time bomb waiting to go off so we made the disease Nosode and left the city to its fate, I came here with Cam and Eric went to a country town with his extended family. So we are on our own now said Bruce. That's what it looks like and that's what Cam and I have been preparing for, the only problem though is that we have got to survive first. I checked the patients again and noticed that they were calmer and seemed more relaxed but I had a feeling that they were slowly losing consciousness. I lifted the eyelids and looked at their eyes and I saw death, the eyes had lost their shine, it took me a long time to learn that lesson when I was younger on a farm, when the lights go out it means they have given up or can't go on, it's now beyond what anyone can do. Bruce must have seen my face and asked what's wrong. It's getting close to the end now, the bodies beginning to shut down, I'll go get the girls as this may be your last chance to talk to them and say your goodbyes. I'll leave you in peace until you call me. I went over to the girls who looked nervously up at me and said go sit with your parents for a while and help your brother. I sat down with Cam and the Rev; I was feeling really tired and sad. Cam asked what was that medicine you gave them, you didn't knock them off did you. Actually now that I think of it I may have inadvertently have. I gave them a Homoeopathic remedy in a high 200C Potency mainly to stop the twitching and relax them and ease any pain but now that you mention it I've just remembered the last part about using 200C. What's that Cam asked? They say that if you use it close to death that it gives a peaceful and easy death. So you did knock them off Cam replied shaking her head. Where are we going to bury them Cam asked the Rev. I was thinking of at the back of the hall as there are no picnic tables there. I was thinking the same thing I said. We talked quietly for about an hour until we heard what must have been the last breath of the father. I'll get the mirror I said. Armed with my mirror my tool of last resorts I walked over to their father and felt for a pulse and couldn't find it, then felt the neck for a pulse and there was none, then placed the mirror over the nose and mouth for what seemed a long minute, then checked it and found no vapor. I showed Bruce the mirror and shook my head. I checked their mothers pulse and was surprised not to find one, so I checked her neck and used the mirror. Again there was no vapor; she had died quietly without anyone noticing. Mums gone to I said, there was a stunned silence and Cam and the Rev began to walk over. I thought I better say something then my mind flicked over to his father's signet ring which I had been admiring before and an idea came to mind. I went to the ring and took it off and said this rings yours now Bruce and took his hand and put the ring on his finger. The farms yours now make it work and grow. I went over to their mum and noticed that she had a wedding and engagement ring so I took the wedding ring off and gave it to the oldest girl Amanda who was about 11 this rings yours and the house is yours now turn it into a home again. I took the engagement ring off and gave it to the youngest girl Jessie who was about 8 and said this is an engagement ring it signifies hope for a happy future take it with our wishes that you will have a happy future and for remembrance of your mum. The Rev said amen. I'll leave you to say your goodbyes the Rev and I have some work to do. Cam came with us to the door and said you're going to do some digging? Yeah were going home to get some tools then we will start digging. We returned with a shovel and spade and begun digging. Luckily the soil was soft at the back of the hall and with the outside light on and a full moon we had plenty of light for the task. It was my turn in the grave and I stopped and had a rest. Looking up out of the grave I could see the Rev resting his chin on the shovel handle with a full moon at the back of his head like a halo. I said to him never in my wildest dreams did I ever think I would be digging a grave at midnight under a full moon with a Reverend. The Rev laughed and said yes it's strange where we end up isn't it. At last it was finished and I thought now comes the really nasty part. The Rev, Cam, Bruce and I carried them out each using a corner of the sheet and gently placed them inside the grave which was a lot easier said than done. We placed the top sheets over them and then filled in the grave. When we had finished the Rev told Cam and me to go home. He said he would have a service with the others tomorrow. Don't forget the Tea Tree oil and Garlic I said and take the Nosode again first thing in the morning. I went up to Bruce and shook his hand and said I'm sorry we didn't meet under better circumstances. Cam and I will see you in a few days as I've got to make up some more medicine in case you start to show symptoms, anyway I am looking forward to seeing your farm as I haven't been on one for a long time. Bruce said thanks for everything then Cam went up and kissed him on the cheek and said I am sorry and then we finally went home. When we got home Cam stripped off her overalls and said I'm in the shower first. I filled the laundry tub with water and disinfectant and put the overalls in and then put away the shovel and spade. After a while I heard I'm finished so I stripped off the overalls and had a shower and decontaminated myself making sure to gargle the Tea Tree Oil water mix and clean out the nose. I found Cam in the kitchen thinking while staring out into space looking very sad. I went over and gave her a hug, but it was a strange hug, it was more like two desperate people clinging to each other as tight as they can. I said I think we will have a beer before going to bed as I don't want to think to long before I go to sleep, John's beer is really good for knocking you out.

Day 12

We slept in till about 10 as we were both exhausted and emotionally drained. After a long breakfast we decided to start work by pulling down the wooden fence in the back yard between us and Angela. I said to Cam that we better make sure our yard is chook escape proof before we take down the fence. It looked good, the only place they would be able to get out would be down the sides of the house and it would be very easy to make a wooden fence between the house and the remaining fence. Johns shed I knew had a big roll of chicken wire stored in the back along with a very large collection of 4 by 2 building studs. It was a pleasant day and the work was easy and gave Cam the chance to learn basic carpentry and get used to using hammers, saws and clamps. Soon the frames were finished and it was time for the wire. Fortunately John had all we needed so armed with a good cutter and small staples that we had found in a jar it was all over very fast and the sides of the house were made chook proof.. After that we went next door to get Angela to inspect our work and see if it was chook proof. Angela along with Jodie following came to inspect our work. She asked what happened last night I heard the reverend come and get you and heard you come back late. Cam said Frank and Margaret Tanner died last night and we buried them at the back of the hall at about midnight. Oh dear said Angela this is beginning to get really scary especially with all the bad news on TV. How are the kids, are they alright? They seem to be though they will be in shock for a while I said. I'm going to spend this afternoon making up some medicines just in case anyone starts showing any symptoms. Your only chance is to stop this thing is in the beginning and even then you're going to have to hit it hard because you've got to reduce it before it gets to the lungs, that way you might have a chance. So what do you think of the fence, chook proof or what? It's good they shouldn't be able to get out. That's good now we will start taking down the main fence, we can use the wood to make a new chook house which I will get you to draw up a design on paper. I found a breaker bar and another hammer in the shed and we started work on taking the fence down by removing the planks first and the main beams last. By 1pm we had finished and had all the planks and beams all de-nailed and stacked out of the way. Time for lunch I said and I think we might share a bottle of beer as all this work has made me thirsty. After lunch we turned on the TV and watched the news on the news channel. I was wandering what was happening after missing the news last night. The Government had closed down the schools which they said were a temporary measure to stop the spread of the flu and later on we heard that 25% of the work force was sick and had failed to turn up to work other than that everything else was just a rehash of what had already happened though I laughed at the last part when they said that the Government had now issued all of its stock of Tamiflu. Cam looked at me strangely and said what's so funny about that? I told her that about a month ago I was talking to a drug rep at work and he was saying that the Governments stock of Tamiflu was just about to go out of date so it looks like they got rid of it fast. We had better start making some medicine in case anyone starts getting symptoms, especially us. It looks like the Revs going to be the main man as he knows where everybody and everything is, so we have to make it easy for him because he will have lots to explain so we better make this mug proof. After a long discussion we came up with a plan. First we would introduce them to the disease and the symptoms, next the preventative medicines which we would take out of our stocks. After that would be the first medicines to use when the symptoms began which we had yet to work out. First was to introduce them to the disease, especially to the different incubation periods and we did this as follows.

Pandemic Flu Symptoms Onset

A/. This flu has a 2 day incubation period in those with respiratory conditions such as Asthma, Bronchitis and any other chronic condition of the respiratory system.

B/. For all other people in good health the incubation period is about 6 to 7 days.

Leading Symptoms In Order

1/. Day one - Scratchy throat, can get severe making it hurt to swallow, swollen neck glands, sore throat getting worse.

2/. Days 2 to 4 - Cough begins following sore throat and becomes persistent without any phlegm, can get severe. Headaches begin and can get severe with watery red eyes. There may be muscle aches and pains especially in the back but can be in the whole body. There may be fever with chills; temperature can be as high as 102 degrees.

3/. Days 4 to 5 - The disease goes to the chest causing massive inflammation along with a massive immune response which usually leads to death. When the virus starts it attack on the lungs the virus replicates extremely fast usually way beyond what the immune system can deal with and at this stage the spread on infection is the greatest so patient must be isolated and decontamination procedures must be followed. A mask should be worn at all times.

4/. Day's 6 to 7 - Pleuritic chest pains, sharp pains breathing in, extremely ill, administer oxygen.

5/. Day 8 - Prostration, overwhelming malaise, fatigue, exhaustion, coughing lasts as infection breaks. Now is the time to concentrate on building the patient up again.

The next info sheet we made follows

Disease Presentation
Information Sheet

As this pandemic is now in a very advanced stage its better now to stay at home and wait it out. As the disease has a 7 day incubation period in healthy people it is best to start preventive measures immediately. You have been issued with by the Reverend Lovejoy Preservation Society Tea Tree Oil, Garlic Oil Caps 3000 mg, Echinacea Garlic C and Zinc Tablets and a Pandemic Flu Disease Nosode. The last is the most important as it is the closest you can get to a vaccine at this time.

Use As Follows

1/. Tea Tree Oil - To half a small wine glass of water add at least 3 drops of oil. Gargle with this morning and evening. You must try to get a few drops of this gargle into the nasopharynx area (up in the back of the nose area) as this is where the germs begin to multiply for the start of their conquest. Use immediately after you have come into contact with a diseased person.

2/. Garlic Oil 3000mg - For the current emergency take 3 capsules 3 times daily. Garlic is an antiviral. Garlic leaves the body via the lungs and throat, hence garlic breath. By using Garlic we are placing an antiviral in exactly the area we want it to work on so look at it as targeting an antiviral. If symptoms appear double the dose. If they continue triple the dose.

3/. Echinacea, Garlic, Zinc and C - Echinacea stimulates the bone marrow to make more white blood cells which in turn go out and kill the viruses. Zinc is one of the main minerals used for supporting the immune system. Take 1 tablet 4 times daily.

4/. Vitamin C - Is the main antioxidant to the lungs and boosts the immune system. Take 1000mg night and morning. This is on top of what you are taking in the Echinacea Tablet above. If symptoms begin double the dose. If symptoms continue triple the dose.

Ok let's have some dinner, afterwards ill figure out that formula and you can type up the info sheets on the laptop. We ate well for dinner again and still hadn't really made much of a dent in the freezer. We cleaned up fast so we could catch the beginning of the main news. Just as we got comfortable the news started. The news of the day was that Perth had blockaded itself from the rest of Australia. They had blocked off the 2 main highways one to the east to Adelaide and the other to the north to Darwin and had successfully cut themselves off from the rest of the nation and the Prime Minster was not impressed at all. Overseas news told us that most nations had now closed off their boarders except for the English who said it was a little too late to bother about it and most of the arrivals were English anyway trying to get home. The other main overseas story was that there were mass riots throughout most of the Middle East. We turned off the TV and got to work, Cam with the laptop typing up the info sheets and I started with the formula I had been thinking all day about covering the onset of the flu and the sore throat going to severe and hard to swallow. I knew I had to hit it really hard at this point and try to break it or reduce it as much as possible or the battle was lost at the beginning. I decided on the following formula and strengths.

First Flu Remedy
Information Sheet

Licorice @ 25% of formula
Astragalus @ 30%
Baptisia @ 30%
Poke Root @15%

To make this formula more effective I have decided to make it as syrup so it would coat and line the targeted area and stay in contact with it for as long as possible. Licorice would aid this as it coats and soothes inflamed areas with its demulcent and anti-inflammatory actions. This way the combined antiviral actions have more time to do their work on the targeted area which is the throat.

Formula is in 50% syrup.

Licorice - Improves macrophage activity (white blood cells) and increases production of interferon.

Astragalus - Stimulates production of interferon which helps to stop viruses from replicating, immune booster.

Baptisia - Anti viral, used for tonsillitis, laryngitis, inflamed lymph glands, reduces fever, stimulates immune system.

Poke Root - Anti viral, cleans lymph glands, tonsillitis, diphtheria, this is a very strong herb not used much anymore and I'm using it in a very strong dose because of the emergency

Dosage

The adult dose for this will be 10mls 4 times daily. Each individual dose is to be taken in 2 parts. For example, take 5mls then wait 10 minutes and then take the last 5mls of the dose. This way we will have the greatest possible time of the dose in contact with the targeted area eg the throat.

Just as I finished there was a knock at the door. I answered and saw it was the Rev and invited him in. Come in, sit down, put your feet up, how's Bruce and the girls. They are OK but a bit lost and confused, it's not the best way to start life but Bruce is fairly mature and knows the score and has a lot to keep him occupied with running the farm. We said we would go see him tomorrow; I am actually looking forward to seeing his farm. That's good I won't bother seeing them tomorrow then, they need all the friends they can get at the moment. I told the Rev what we had been up to and of the 3 info sheets we had made for him and that Cam was just typing up the last one now. Cam gave him the laptop so he could read them for his self. We tried to make them mug proof I said. He laughed when he came to The Reverend Preservation Society. I went into the kitchen and got 3 bottles of beer and glasses and mentally thanked John for his dreamless sleeping tonic. The Rev finished reading the info sheet and said that's really good it's a pity the Government didn't do something like this. We will put it on a memory stick so you can transfer it to your own computer and print it as you need. In the morning I will make up the medicine and give you 10 lots of everything. I'll try to have it all done and drop it off to you by 10am then we will go and see Bruce. We talked for a while then decided to call it a day.

Day 13

Up early with an early breakfast and then started to make the new formula. I used my big 1 liter medicine bottles because I needed a lot and it's easier to make liter quantities when you are using a percentage system. So 25% of licorice was 250mls, 30% of Astragalus was 300mls, 30% of Baptisia was 300mls and 15% of Poke Root was 150mls. Soon the bottle was filled and the formula made. Then I shook the bottle. I was going to use golden syrup (treacle) as the syrup because I noticed that John had heaps of it especially in the cupboard with his brewing gear. I was beginning to wonder if this was his secret ingredient in his beer. I got another liter bottle and half filled it with golden syrup and filled the rest of the bottle with the herbal formula and then shook it well. Next I got 5 x 200ml bottles and filled them up with the mixture. I repeated the process twice so in the end I had 15 small bottles of medicine. I got Cam to write out the labels as she had nice neat writing compared to mine. While she was doing that I got 15 of each out of the pantry of Nosodes, Tea Tree Oil, Echinacea Garlic and Zinc and Vitamin C putting them in separate bags. John had stored away a small collection of small foam lidded boxes which I placed the medicine in keeping the Nosodes away from the others. Next we had some coffee and cake to full our tummies and then headed out to the Revs place. We gave the Rev the boxes and he placed them on his office chair. Angela, David and Allen haven't got theirs yet I said to the Rev, but I will take Bruce's lot to them and we will grab a couple of copies of the info sheets from you to. As the Rev was getting the info sheets I asked him how many people he would be seeing today, his reply was 3 to 4 I hope if they are still there. Some seem to have gone, maybe to sick relatives. Well we will leave you to it and head up to Bruce's. Bruce's place was meant to be just under 10 kilometers up the road, on the right and then up a long driveway going uphill with bush on either side. We found it easily and drove up the driveway and got to the top of the hill and stopped for it was an impressive view. It was like looking down on a big rectangle that had been cut out of the bush starting where we were at the top of the hill going down into a valley and then up again to the top of the hill.

The orchid parts were on the hills running down to the valley and in the valley was a stream which was damed twice, first at the beginning of the cleared property and the second was at the end of the property then the stream ran back into the bush. Cams word said it all wow. I continued to the house which was down the hill a bit on the left and tooted the horn a few times to let them know we had arrived. There were two equipment sheds next to the house and a large workshop next to them. We parked in front of the garage under the house and got out of the van. Amanda and Jessie came down stairs to greet us. What a lovely place you've got here I said while Cam went up and hugged and kissed the girls. Bruce is down doing the pig fence said Amanda; we will walk down and find him. We walked down the valley and over a bridge built for the tractor. To the left as we started to walk up hill was a Goose house with the birds outside giving us the evil eye as we walked past. I like Geese they always look so regal I said. Above us on the hill was a large pig paddock centered on the property with orchids on each side. I said to the girls that the pigs and Geese must be happy with all that fruit to eat and they smiled at me. Bruce was in the far top corner of the paddock and saw us and came walking over. G,day Bruce I said shaking his hand, what a lovely place you've got here. Yep I like it he replied. Cam went over to him and kissed him on the cheek. You're fencing just the pig paddock or the whole lot. Just the pig paddock for now, I kind of got to rethink things again now. Yeah I know what you mean, things aren't getting better, I think everything's going to fall to pieces in 3 or 4 days and I think we will lose the power to. Maybe you should start eating your freezer, we are. I was thinking about that last night, things don't look good. Come on girls you can show me the house said Cam and we will leave the boys to talk. I said to Bruce lets go to the top of the pig paddock and sit down so I can see the view. We walked to the top and sat down and I admired the view. You know when I drove down the driveway I expected a dog to run out and start barking. Sorry about that said Bruce he died about a month ago. You're not having much luck are you? Well what can you do? Unfortunately I think it's only going to get worse I replied. I don't think I am going to get the flu because I have been around it too long and as I have damaged lungs I would only have the 2 day incubation period instead of the 7. I believe our prevention measures will work because they saved me years ago when I had my accident and damaged my lungs, if I had caught a cold or the flu then I wouldn't be alive now. I was too scared to cough for 2 years because I didn't want to drown in my own blood again. What I have really been worried about all along is that there might be a mass exodus from the cities to the country areas and having heaps of armed weirdo's wandering around, that's why I pulled down the sign for the lake on my way here. How many people do you think are going to die asked Bruce? The worse scenario is about 50% of the population but I think this one will take lots more maybe 80% and add more for rioting, violence, greed and natural causes. But the real problem is that flu comes every year, so this year's flu is going to be next years mutated flu and we will still not have any immunities against it as we don't adapt that fast but we should be able to survive the year after. Though there is a bright side sometimes when nature knows it's had it and can't win it will kill off the victims fast to slow the spread and protect the species, I think that may be happening now and it could save us from next year's flu. That's not what I was hoping to look forward to said Bruce. Now you're beginning to see why I took the sign down and chose a lake to hideout in. Lakes always have fish and crayfish and all the local wild life will come to them for water and it's the biggest dam you can get for growing your crops so one way or another you're going to survive and that's what it is all about. You've thought about this a lot said Bruce. I'm a survivor I said I've always survived against the odds and I think you are to. But I'm only a young boy Bruce replied. Not anymore I answered. All right then what the hell do we do now. Well the first thing you can do is start eating the food in the freezer as the power is going to go out soon. Second is to camouflage your driveway maybe get the posthole digger and put a hole in the middle of the driveway and sick a dead tree in it, sweep away all the tire marks and scatter maybe some more dead trees in the gaps so no one will know you are there while they are going past and watch out making smoke in daylight. Next thing is that you and your farm can probably keep the Revs flock alive, so think and plan for that and don't hesitate to ask Cam and I for a hand especially when you've got a project planned. So basically Bruce said we have to become self-sufficient. Yes until we know civilization has become civilized again. Another thing I've been thinking of is that there is a truck stop at the end of our road and about 20ks either side there are 2 more. When I was in Melbourne years ago I used to load trucks for the supermarkets and other big retail out lets and I know that lots of them use that highway. There's a good chance we will find a food truck in one of them and 20 tons of canned food would come in handy, also we want the CB radios from the trucks so we can see what other survivors are up to and we want the diesel for you tractor. Another thing for you to think about is that refined fuel only lasts a year so after that we will have to make bio-diesel. I reckon that we should try for the trucks the day after the power goes out, it's going to be messy because there will be bodies in the sleeper so get yourself prepared for it. We have only really got each other now so we have to look after ourselves, so have a good think about things and see what you come up with. We have all got a lot to think about because in a few weeks it's going to be a different world. So how are the girls taking their new situation? They haven't really being saying much; in fact none of us have been saying much but just doing what we have to do. I think that's about all you can do, I know I won't be happy for about a week or ten days until I know we have a future and I get so angry at this all happening when I'm getting old and not at my best, but as you say what can you do. Let's go back to the house and see what the girls are up to. As we were walking back to the house Bruce said you're in a van aren't you, I can't sell the fruit anymore so I was thinking of giving it to the Rev so he could hand it out in his travels, could you deliver them to the Rev. That's no problem I said, better the fuel going to a good cause, I will bring the van down to the shed. We loaded the van up with about 40 boxes of fruit. You want the boxes back; yeah we may not be able to get anymore. We went to the house to see what the girls were up to. Cam had already shown the girls the info sheets and medicine so I quickly ran through it with Bruce and noticed it was nearly midday. Turn on the news Bruce it just about to start, let's see what's happening. The news reader said we start with a special announcement from the Government by the head of The Emergency Services. Because of the hospital situation throughout the nation and the swift rise in the number of patients with flu we have decided to call a state of emergency. All hospital car parks are now to be turned into field hospitals. All mobile Blood Donation Buses and Trailers are being requisitioned along with similar vehicles. These will be placed in front of the field hospitals and used for screening and evaluating patients as they come in. All people with cars in hospital car parks please remove them now. The military has been activated to set up, run and supply these hospitals. As we speak military helicopters have started transporting drug and medical supplies and have taken over control of supply. The Government still has vast supplies of Tamiflu which is now on route to all hospitals. The Government intends to give all citizens Tamiflu all you have to do is produce your Medicare Card.at the nearest hospital. Further information will be given this evening. Due to the State of Emergency the Government has decided to call up all military Reservists. Further information will be given throughout the day. Thank You. The news then turned to local state news with reports that refrigerated Semi Trailers had been seen leaving hospitals supposedly full of bodies and that there were mass graves being dug in public restricted areas so people could not see what was happening. I said to Bruce I think we've seen enough. It looks like things are beginning to fall to pieces and will rapidly get worse. Though with the Governments opening field hospitals and giving out Tamiflu to the public makes it better and safer for us as it may stop the exodus away from the cities and the flood of refugees to the country. Bruce said should we go to the hospital and get Tamiflu. I think if you were going to get the flu you would of all got it by now I replied, but if you start getting symptoms then yes go and get it fast but if you have no symptoms and you go you are putting yourself at risk and if the disease has mutated slightly you may be open for infection. I will talk to the Rev, maybe we can all give our Medicare Cards to one person and send them out and then quarantine them for 7 days when they get back. I was talking to a drug company rep a few months ago and he was telling me that most of the Tamiflu that the Government have is nearly out of date so it would be best to wait a little while till they get rid of the old stock because we really need some that we can put away till next year when the seasonal flu comes back slightly changed. In a week or 10 days we could just go in and get it ourselves and no one would be around anyway. You sound as if you don't have much confidence in Tamiflu Bruce said. I don't know, it seems to be most effective in the first 2 days of infection where it's meant to reduce the symptoms and slow down the spread rate but I think if it was really effective things would not be as bad as they are now. They might have left it too late. Anyway we had better be off as I have to figure out another formula for the next stage of the disease but I will find the Rev and see what he says as he may know someone going to town, so go find you're Medicare Cards. On the drive home I asked Cam how the girls were getting on. They seem to be doing well, Amanda's bossy and has taken over the house and she and Jessie decontaminated the house themselves and did a good job from the sound of it. I think they have kept themselves so busy that they haven't had time to think about what has happened to them, though I was watching her while she was watching the news and she seemed to know what was going on. Yes it's all getting worse, maybe she's got the right idea, just keep yourself going and busy instead of flipping over into headless chook mode and start running around in circles. How do you think Jessie is going? She's quiet but I think she is all right. She's one of those who needs lots of affection and hugs but I think when she's sick of Amanda she can go off and find Bruce. We stopped at the Revs place but he was not there so we left a note about the Tamiflu saying maybe it would be better if one person went or maybe if we wait a week. Then we headed home. At home we decided to sort out the fruit first as we had decided it would be best to put 3 different fruits into each box so everyone could have a variety box. It took about 90 minutes to turn them into variety boxes then we reloaded the van and took the first box over to Angela's. Angela and Jodie seemed well so we headed next door again to David's. David answered the door and we gave him a big box of fruit. How's it going there I asked, been fishing lately. No I haven't been doing anything really David replied just watching TV and seeing what's happening. It's getting really scary out there isn't it? Yes I agreed but there not much that we can do about it, we've done what we can but I will be glad when it's over so I can just lie down and relax again. Anyway we had better go we've got to give a box to Allen. We headed back to the van and drove to Allen's and knocked on the door. After a while Allan answered and we gave him the box of fruit telling him it was from Bruce as he couldn't get to market anymore. Allen told us he had decided to go into town. I've been thinking of getting more supplies for a while now and after watching TV and hearing about them giving Tamiflu to everyone I've finally decided to go. We were just talking about that before I said. We left a note about it on the Revs door. What did you say asked Allen? We said it might be a good idea to get someone to go into town with all our Medicare Cards and get the Tamiflu for everyone, that way we don't have lots of people risking infection. Do you think they will let us do it that way Allen asked? I don't know but it would be worth a try, we could all give you a note giving you permission and the Rev could give you a covering letter. Well I suppose there's no harm in trying. I've got to make some more medicine after this but Cam could come back and give you our cards and a note and get Angelas and David's to. It could be better to wait till tomorrow before you go as we don't know if the military helicopters have got there yet. As I was telling Bruce I was talking to a drug rep the other day and he was telling me that the Governments stock of Tamiflu are nearly out of date so that could be the real reason they are being so generous so the latter you get there the more the chance of getting some of the new batch as we really want them to help save us from the next seasons strain of flu which will still be probably lethal. So you reckon next year's strain is going to be a killer. Yes, usually by the third year your immune system has figured it out. Before you drive to town take a dose of the Nosode and make up some Tea Tree Oil gargle that you can take before you get out of the car when you get to town. Wear a mask in town and try not to touch your face. When you get back into the car throw away the mask and do the Tea Tree oil again then the Garlic Oil. Don't take any chances Allen. No I won't thanks Mark. I'll leave you to sort it out with the Rev then; we are going over there now to drop off the rest of the fruit. See ya latter. We carried on to the Revs place. Well that solves that problem with the Tamiflu said Cam, the Rev and Allen can look after it. Yes its good, I don't really want to go back to town with it full of people, we've taken to many chances already, I will be happy when it's all over I said. We reversed the van to the Revs door and as he was not home we unloaded the boxes and piled them up on the shady side of the stairs and then added to the note on the door. On the way home I asked

Cam if she could sort out the Medicare Cards so I could start putting together the new medicine. I had been thinking about a formula all day and now was fairly sure of what herbs I would use. Cam followed me into the kitchen and we sat at the table. I got the pad and paper and wrote a note giving Allen permission to get my Tamiflu, signed it and taped the card to the paper. That's the way to do it I think, do yours the same way. When Cam had finished hers she said I will take the pad and tape and get Angela's and David's and take them to Allen's. Instead of making the formula straight away I decided to write out the info sheet first.

Information Sheet For The Second Flu Formula

This covers the end of the second day to the fourth when the fever, muscle aches and pains begin and the disease slowly begins its path to the chest. This is the last phase of the disease where our attacks can be effective as the disease is preparing the chest for its last main and fatal assault. All efforts are now to minimize the strength of the disease so as to not be lethal. Consider everything mentioned in the previous Information Sheets especially the Garlic Oil which we will now use as a constant background remedy. Also raise the Vitamin C dose too about 4 x 1000mg or to bowel tolerance in fit and strong people as this works in the lungs as a natural antihistamine as well as an anti-oxidant.

The Formula
Licorice @ 15%
Astragalus @15%
Boneset @ 35%
Elder @ 35%
Licorice - Anti viral, demulcent (coats and soothes), anti-inflammatory.
Astragalus – Anti-viral, makes interferon, immune booster.
Boneset - Immune booster, possible anti-viral, flu specific.
Elder - Traditional specific for the flu, covers most symptoms
Dose - 4 to 5 times daily at 5mls

Cam had just returned and said you make the formula and I will type up the info sheet. I decided to make about 12 bottles and would give 10 of them to the Rev along with the info sheets. In 45 minutes the work was done and the info sheet ready for the Rev. Time for dinner, I'm starving I said. We had a large evening meal and cleared up. Want to see the news Cam asked. No I think it will just be a repeat of what we saw before, they haven't had much time to set up yet so we might as well leave it till tomorrow. Let's go for a walk down to the lake and walk off dinner. We left the house and walked up to the main road. The Rangers house was on the right on the corner. It was more a big yard with sheds for the tractor, slashes and other equipment along with the house. We had never met him and according to Angela he had been away for well over a week now so I doubted he would ever come back. Instead of going to the end of the road we followed the back fence line of the Rangers yard which had a driveway like track that lead to the big picnic table field in front of the lake. At the end of the fence we turned right and followed the bush line to the end of the field and to the lakes edge. We followed the lake to the hall walking through the empty park with all its picnic tables and a bandstand in the center. It was a nice colorful sunset so we carried on past the hall with the freshly dug grave out the back over to the boat ramp and through the car park and back up to the main road. We turned left at the main road and started walking back home past the Revs house which still had the note on the door and then past the little shop. Next was Allen's house followed by the little two pump service station with a garage. Next followed the seven holiday houses all empty and directly opposite them on the corner was the Rangers yard and our road back home. Cam said she had found some games in the main bedroom wardrobe and said what about a game of monopoly. So we played monopoly and had our usual beer and ended another long worrying day.

Day 14

Woke up to a nice sunny morning and slowly got our acts together. Cam said I am so tired of waking up each morning and checking to see if I am sick. I will be so glad when this is all over its like being locked up on death row. Couldn't have put it better I said, just the constant worry gets you down, then there's the worry of if we survive how are we going to survive. Got up and had breakfast and watched the early news. A Government statement said most hospitals have now been reorganized and the supply chain has been taken over by the military with military aviation supplying crucial drugs when needed. The Rail System was going to cease from 3pm this afternoon as there wasn't enough staff to keep the operation safe but all lines were being cleared so military personal could run special trains when and if needed until the emergency is over. Trade and especially the Transport System were breaking down with a 50 to 60% sick rate among workers nationally. It looked as if things are beginning to grind to a halt. I said to Cam we are going to lose our power soon. Overseas was just as bleak, no one was winning against the disease and even a few ships had been beached because the crews were sick. There seemed to be problems with a vaccine and even if they could figure that out would there be anyone left to make it. The news ended with people should stop bringing bodies to hospitals but should bury them in their back yards, you can go to the hospital and they would give you a body bag with instructions and a form to fill out. What a mess Cam said. I think it's worse than that a 50 to 60% sick rate is massive. I remember reading a paper on the Spanish Flu and they were saying that the death rates were so high because the disease was 50 times more prolific then ordinary flu and had a massive rate of viral replication. This flu that we are dealing with has already gone way past that and what makes it worse is that next year's flu is going to be the same. Angela and Jodie came over and showed us the design she wanted for the chook house and another one for a veggie garden. She said the medical herbs would have to be scattered all around as they all needed different climates and conditions to survive and some would even have to be inside. The chook house was going to have ten nesting boxes twice as many as before. We will use the wood from the fence first I said, well we might as well get started. John had a large pile of old paving slabs which we decided to use as a floor because of their size 2 foot by 2 foot. We ended up by putting 3 down by six going across centering them on the old fence boundary, this size allowed us to get away without having to cut down the wood from the fence. We lifted up the corner paving and put posts in the corners then chiseled the corner off the paving so they sat flush against the posts when we put them down. With the floor and corner posts done it was time for lunch. We made an attack on the heaps of frozen pies in the freezer in our effort to empty it as fast as we could and with the help of the microwave they were soon ready. We decided to have a cold beer with it as we were hot and sweaty from our work. After a long lunch break we started by putting the center posts in and just as we finished Allen arrived and started to walk over to us. I've got them he said. I'll get the others I told

Allen. I left Allen with Cam and went over to Angela's and told her Allen's back, then to David's and we all headed over to Allen. What happened I asked tell us what it's like out there? Was there anyone on the road? No there was hardly anyone on the road. Were there any trucks in the truck stop? Yeah about 2 or 3. Anyway in the whole 90ks to town I doubt if ten cars went by the other way, there was not much traffic at all. I went to the hospital first, there wasn't as many people there as I thought there would be. The Army was there and seemed to have organized it well they had a big sign up saying Tamiflu with an arrow. I went there and told the soldier the score and he got his officer and I told him again. He said that's alright and it was a good idea and went through each letter got the Tamiflu while the soldier punched the Medicare Cards and stamped issued on the letters along with the quantity. I asked them how things were going and they said not well. I told them what had happened to us and they said we were fairly lucky. He said at the hospital all the old folks in the home at the back went first and the hospital took over the area but things seem to be slowing down now especially today. The Armies taken over the school down the road from the hospital and uses the football fields for the helicopters and from there trucks everything to the hospital. On the way home I noticed a backhoe digging at the end of one of the school fields so they are probably burying people there to. Other than that most of the town was closed and looks a bit like a Sunday afternoon. I went over to my garage supplies and he was there so I managed to get what I wanted including oxygen, and he was telling me that it's fairly bad with most people being sick and some shops mostly food ones are just opening for a few hours in the afternoon. He said you have to listen to the local radio now to see what's open when. It doesn't sound good at all I said, it's like the towns slowly going to sleep. Anyway here is all your pills Allen said handing back the Medicare Cards and giving us each a pack of Tamiflu. Angela got 2 packs because of Jodie. Shall we start taking them now Angela asked? Everybody have a look at the expiry date I said. It turned out that all the packs had only two months left on them. I think we should all go through at least 3 quarters of the pack and save the last quarter for an emergency, Tamiflu only works best at the beginning of the disease and we have nothing to lose any more so we might as well start taking them now. You want to tell the Rev what we are doing Allen. Yeah I'll do that see ya all later. Don't forget to decontaminate yourself properly I said.

Don't worry about that I am not going to get the flu. Let's have a coffee break I said to Cam. We went in and had a break. Cam asked how big the Town is. About 10 to 15000 people I said, it on crossroads and is one of the main truck routes, you go straight up for north Queensland mostly to access the inland towns or turn right to head to the coastal highway going North, it's the main truck route if you're coming from Western or Southern Australia or Melbourne. So it's very unusual that he only saw about 10 cars go by the other way usually in that small run you would expect to see at least 20 trucks go by not mentioning the hundreds of cars. He also said he saw a few trucks in the truck stops which is good for in about a week I want to check them out because I want a food truck. You think one might be there Cam asked. Yes there's a good chance, I used to load them years ago when I was working on the rail side. Bruce and I were talking about it the other day; we also need the CB radio so we can see who's out there, along with the batteries and diesel fuel in the trucks. You were planning on taking me asked Cam. Of course I said, I really only want to do this once, I want 2 trucks one with 20 tons of food and the other with whatever and we have a good chance of getting them, after that we go into hiding and see what happens. Let's do some more on the chook house said Cam. We went out and put the 2 center posts in and to finish the day's work I put three beams across the roof short ways so as to hold the posts at the required measurement for when we timbered the sides tomorrow. Time for dinner said Cam. We were finally making a dent in the freezer. After dinner as the sun was going down the Rev paid us a visit. You look tired I said, come in, sit down and put your feet up. Have you eaten yet, no I haven't got home yet. I will put a couple of pies in the oven for you; I am trying to get rid of the damn things. I came back from the kitchen with a beer for each of us and a glass for the Rev then he told us his news. He had been round to everyone and handed out the Tamiflu, 2 families had left with only one leaving a message saying they had gone to sick relatives and he didn't know what had happened to the other. He had seven packs of Tamiflu left and they were all short dated. How's Bruce and the girls I asked. They are all fine and keeping themselves busy. Did Allen tell you about town I asked? Yes doesn't look good though the Army seems to be doing a good job. One of the loners who lives fairly close to the highway has come down with the flu; he wouldn't let me come near him as he didn't want to infect me. He didn't take the Nosode I gave him or any of the medicines I gave him days ago, said he doesn't believe in Natural Medicine. I get that all the time I said especially from men, they usually leave things far too late so there's not much you can do for them. I kind of believe now after all these years of being a Naturopath that some people just aren't meant to get better and I think that a lot of people about my age with cancer are just looking for a good excuse to leave the planet and get away from a marriage they don't like or other personnel problems. He's got all the info sheets and medicines he needs the Rev said and now he has Tamiflu. It's like the old saying I said you can take a horse to water but you can't make him drink. The oven bell went so I went and got a tray with the pies, sauce and knife and fork for the Rev. There you go enjoy an unhealthy meal while you can I said. Anyway the Rev said I will go and check up on him tomorrow and see what's happening. The Rev demolished the second pie and finished his beer, thanked us and said his goodbyes saying he was exhausted and going to have an early night and would see us later. Cam said I'm buggered we might as well call it a night to.

Day 15

Another nice sunny morning. Cam and I got up early as we were anxious to see the early news. Our daily routine with pills and gargles were becoming a habit and while you were doing it you would always be checking yourself for the telltale symptoms. Wiped out some more pies from the freezer for breakfast. Getting so sick of pies but I suppose that in six months' time we would be longing for them again. Made coffee and settled down in front of the TV for the news. The lead story was about a vaccine for the flu, it was proving to be far harder than they had expected and with the staff shortages it looked as though it would never get there in time. In Africa some countries had gone off the air and broadcasts had ceased. Lots of cities in the Middle East were on fire with no one attempting to put them out and the same thing was happening to a few cities in the USA made worse by wind storms and a shortage of firemen. There were food riots in South America while not much news was coming out of China and Russia. Lots of ships were beaching themselves as harbors were full and in lots of cases blocked by floating vessels not under control. At home it was becoming noticeable that a lot of the TV personalities where missing and shows were being canceled. TV journalists were beginning to disappear to. There was a lot of speculation about the countries death toll which was generally thought to be in the millions now with no end in sight or cure either. The disease had already surpassed the Spanish flu and there was still no end in sight except for the worst. Apparently they were not impressed with Tamiflu either saying it was too little too late and very over rated. We turned the news off when they began repeating themselves. Oh well at least they are talking about the death toll now and have finally pulled their heads out of the sand I said to Cam probably because their mates are disappearing one by one. Let's finish the Chook house Cam said. We both went outside and looked at what we had already done. OK we need a roof a side wall, chicken mesh for the front and a door on the other side. But we better do the nesting boxes first. I'll start on the nesting boxes and leave you to find the chicken mesh, iron for the roof and everything else. I started on the nesting boxes, we wanted ten of them. I had found a long wide plank that would give me all the partitions I needed so I set to work cutting them all out. Soon it was done and I was very pleased with my new saw that I had brought recently that was razor sharp. I decided to use fencing planks for the roof and floor of the nesting boxes so as to not waste any wood but as they were 6 foot lengths I would have to make two boxes of five. Cam called from the shed to come take a look at this. I went over to see what she had found and heard her say look what I found under the corrugated iron. It was an old coal fired cast iron stove about five foot by 2 foot with a couple of broken legs. It had two small round elements and a big square one on top with an oven on one side and a coal door on the other. It looked as though John had worked on it as there was a new pipe coming out of the top back. On the floor behind it was the rest of the chimney. I said to Cam it looks as though he made it so the chimney comes out of the side of the house and then goes up in the air instead of going through the ceiling. It's a good find Cam and it's a good time to find it as the power will go soon. That's going to be our next project after the chook house. I finished the nesting boxes while Cam put up the chicken mesh. I raised the nesting boxes about a foot off the ground by putting legs on them and then screwed them to the back wall. After that I cut the planks at the back of the boxes and put hinges and bolts on them so as to make it easy to remove the eggs. Then we started on the side wall and made half of the side wall on the other side a door which could drop down like a ramp. Then came the roof bearers and the corrugated iron for the roof. After that we got Angela who was working in the garden and showed her the finished house. That's good she said and the door at the back of the nesting boxes will make it easier to get the eggs. What are we going to do with the old chook house I asked? I will strip out the water and feeders for this one and from the old one we might make a mobile chook house and use it later as a chicken tractor system; anyway I will take over from here and get the chooks moved in. Time for lunch Cam said I'm getting hungry. While we had lunch in the kitchen we tried to figure out where we would put the coal stove and in the end decided that the best spot was where the fridge was sitting now which was in the center of the wall against the back end of the side of the house. We thought that here it would have a lot of room around it and heat up the whole room while at the same time being safer. This would make the kitchen the main room in the house especially in winter. After lunch we went into the shed to check out our new coal powered oven. It's going to weigh a ton so we had better strip it as much as possible before we move it. I'll start striping it and you can set a wire brush on the parts and get rid of the rust. I removed the elements two round ones and a big square one and noticed that they had a big indentation in them for some sort of tool to remove them when they are hot. I showed Cam and told her we had better find something to fit it. Next I managed to get the oven door off and then the door to the fire compartment and gave them both to Cam. John must have cleaned all the inside and it looked to be in very good condition. I got Cam to help me roll the oven on its front and put some wooden bearers on the floor so it would not lay flat for it was still very heavy and then started work on removing the legs. In a few hours we had the oven finished and ready to go. We will leave it here till we are ready for it; I don't think it will be long now. We went next door into the garden to see what Angela and Jodie were up to and found them turning the earth over and breaking it up on a large plot that Angela had laid out, so we got our shovels and started helping them. Half way through I said Cam and I can finish this you might as well start laying out another area. Close to dinner time we finished and put our tools away and sat outside on the steps watching the chooks check out their new home. After dinner we sat down and watched the news which was mostly a repeat of the morning's news except for a mention that food supplies were holding out and some farmers were still even delivering to the Vegetable Markets though there was a problem with milk. I said to Cam maybe the foods holding out because there are fewer people to feed because far more are dead then what they think. There had not been the exodus to the country from the city like what I was expecting it was as if everything was just very slowly grinding to a halt. There was no more rush hour traffic news telling you of crashes and backed up traffic because there just wasn't that much traffic anymore or as many people on the streets. Later in the evening the Rev popped in for a visit. You don't look very happy I said something bad happen? You know that loner that I told you who had got sick, I nodded, well I went to see him this afternoon and there was a note on his door, he didn't want to wait for the flu to take him so he dug a hole at the back of the house got in and shot himself. Come sit down mate and I will get you a beer. I came back with a beer for each of us and sat down. You know I said I think I am getting hardened to all of this and it's getting hard to feel anything at all anymore. I think I know how he feels and I am not all that patient either. I am beginning to feel a little like that myself said the Rev. I found that I wasn't all that surprised and just did what I had to do without thinking too much about it. The worst part I said is that it's all out of your hands and there's not anything that you can really do about it, you've just got to wait it out and try to make the best out of what's left. Cam opened a large bag of chips and we all helped ourselves. You see anyone else today Rev? I saw Bruce and the girls this morning, they are alright and have hidden the driveway like you said so I doubt if anyone could find them now, I went straight past in the car. They seem to be alright and are keeping themselves busy. Do you think the Ranger will be coming back I asked, he's overdue isn't he. I don't think he will be back. Have you got his phone number so you can contact him? Yes, at home I have, I will do it tomorrow, why, what are you thinking the Rev asked. When the power goes I am going to check out what he has in the sheds, I'm hoping for a generator. I am also going inside the house to see what's in the freezer and Rangers also usually have a weapon for putting down animals so I want that and the ammunition, better us to have it than anyone else. Also the fence that goes all round that property makes it good for a protected garden as kangaroos can't get over it and mess up the garden, and I was hoping that I could extend the fence into the park. The wild life and Kangaroos are going to be our worst enemy in the future especially to gardens; I remember all the problems I used to have on the farm. If we get really hungry we will have to shoot some roos to survive though we got fish and crayfish in the Lake and we could always get some pigs and geese off Bruce to breed. Also another thing we have been talking about with Bruce is going to the truck stops soon and bringing in a food truck or whatever and parking them at the back of the Rangers place along the back fence, 20 tons of food would make me very happy and feel a lot more secure. The truck would also give us lots of diesel, batteries for power and CB radios to see whose left out there when everything has ground to a halt. I see you've been doing a lot of thinking the Rev said. Sure have, tomorrow I start setting up the solar panels and batteries and this morning Cam found a coal fired stove so we have to get that installed to. Well at least it will keep you busy and a truck load of food would go down nicely just as nicely as your beer has done, I will pop in and see you soon, it's been a busy day and I think I will have another early night. We walked outside with the Rev to see him off, don't forget to ring the Ranger I said. No I won't, I will see you all latter, goodnight. We might as well crash too Cam said its getting really cold.

Day 16

Woke up to a cold cloudy morning, the type of morning that you just don't want to get up, so we didn't and had a nice long sleep in. Today might be a good day for a fire said Cam. That's a good idea, we should also start gathering wood for the fire and our new stove and start storing it as it's just going to get colder especially since we are near the Lake, soon it will start getting foggy as well. We better get up and watch the news and see what's happened. We had a quick breakfast then made some coffee and settled ourselves before the TV and put it on the news channel. The main local news was that a couple of the commercial TV channels had gone off the air due to staffing problems the speculation was that all their main personalities had gone sick so they had temporarily closed down. There was not much coming out of China or India in the way of official news but on the internet they said there were lots of bodies in the main rivers and the hospitals and medical systems were pushed way beyond their capacity and that people were fleeing some of the cities. Al Jazeera one of the main overseas news companies had stopped broadcasting, whether they had closed down themselves or been closed down by the Government no one knew. Riots and food riots seemed to be happening everywhere and it looked as though the infrastructures of the world were finally collapsing. At home all the hospitals especially those in the cities were overflowing even with their new extensions into the car parks but they all seemed to be functioning alright and the Army was still getting supplies through and they must be helping with the staff as well. I wondered what they were doing to prevent sickness. The Army had also taken over the Railway and was arranging for special food trains to the cities and asking anyone with rail experience who wanted to help to ring a National Number. As the news began repeating itself we turned the TV off. Well it looks as though the military is holding the country together; the rest of the world is a bit of a mess though. I'm glad we are here in the middle of nowhere said Cam. Have a look at these I found them yesterday in the spare room. Cam passed me over a couple of ring binder folders, I think these are Johns notes on brewing beer, I am going to take over and start doing it myself she said. He's got a lot of gear and stock and it's a pity to let it go to waste so I might as well put it to good use. The hardest and most important part of brewing beer I said is the cleaning and sterilizing of all the bottles, but his beer I reckon is some of the best in the world so if you can duplicate his recipes you are going to get some nice beer. You might as well take over the spare room and turn it into a brewery. I'm going to concentrate on batteries and solar panels today and get ready for when the power goes out. We both set off to do our work, I decided to get Johns car out of the way first. I went to the garage at the front of the house where the car was in the garage with the mattress still lying on the boot which I was getting sick of seeing but didn't really want to touch. It took a while to start the car which finally burst into life on the fifth try and slowly settled on a smooth idle so I relaxed for a while and allowed the motor to warm up. With the motor warm I reversed the car out of the garage and down to the end of the street where it was out of the way. Leaving the motor running so as to charge the battery I walked back to the house and to the shed where I got the trolley and put a hose and fuel can on it and headed back to the car. I turned off the car and opened the bonnet and removed the battery. There was only a quarter of a tank of fuel in the car which I siphoned into the 20 liter can nearly filling it to the top. I took the fuel and battery back to the house and poured the fuel into the van. While I was with the van I took out the vans camping battery which had its own special container with plugs and took it into the house and started charging it with my battery charger. I took Johns battery to the shed and started charging it on his charger. I went through all of my electrical gear and removed all of the batteries and torches along with my two ten watt solar panels with charging computers built into them. The panels had served me well over the years and with all my torches and lights being LEDs my power consumption was always very low. I started removing the special interior lights that I had put in the van, they were two units each having 34 LEDs in them and gave bright light to small areas, I was thinking of putting one in the kitchen and the other in the lounge over the couch. Next I sorted out the batteries into rechargeable and throw away. I charged all the rechargeable using the power charger and my two solar charges, I was thinking that I should use the rechargeable all the time and only use the throw aways when I must. I decided to put a torch in every room and the shed next to the light switches. After searching for hooks I finally found a box of curtain hooks so I went around each room and put a hook and hung a torch below the light switch. I put my 12 LEDs torches in the big rooms and the little torches in the small rooms. I told Cam what I was doing as I put the torch in the spare room. Cam was getting her first batch of twenty bottles ready and organizing the room so she could do two brews at the same time in the big twenty liter brewers. I mounted the solar panels on the porch roof as it was fairly flat and the sun would go across it from morning to evening. I put a wooden box in the inner area of the porch where I could place the batteries when they were being charged. Next I started on the 34 LEDs lights, the first light I mounted in the kitchen under the cupboards above the bench by the sink as this would light a small work area very brightly making it easy to work on something difficult at night. I was beginning to have second thoughts about putting the second light over the lounge. After a lot of thought I decided that if the coal oven was going to be in the kitchen then the second light should be there to as the kitchen would become the main room of the house due to the need to keep the oven going. I went to the spare room where Cam was working on her brewing and told her of my decision and asked her what she thought. Cam thought it was a good idea but said if the kitchen was to become the main room of the house then it should have the lounge in it so as to make it more comfortable as it would fit nicely along the wall and then put the light over the kitchen table. When the power goes out there will be no need to keep the fridge, electric oven and freezer there so we can clear them out and have more room to move. I agreed with Cam that the best place for the light was over the kitchen table as that would become the main meeting place of the house especially when we had visitors. Time for lunch I said let's get rid of a few more pies from the freezer. After lunch I quickly finished the wiring and the light over the table. The next job was the coal oven. I remembered seeing a large sheet of asbestos in the shed which was almost three and a half times the size of the oven and decided to put this on the floor so as to fireproof it against the oven. I cleared a space in the kitchen and then went and asked Cam to help me carry it in. After the sheet was in place I told Cam that this would fireproof the floor in case we dropped burning ashes on it from the oven and that I would use the asbestos planks in the shed on the wall to fire proof that against the back of the stove. I said that I would leave a gap of about 3 and half feet between the wall and the back of the stove just in case and that we could use that as a drying area especially for clothes. I glued the asbestos to the floor and then brought in four concrete blocks which would replace the missing legs on the oven and placed them into position away from the wall. I was not looking forward to the next part which was bringing the oven over. I found the trolley and checked the tires on it and decided they needed more air so I over inflated them due to the weight of the oven. I got the trolley in place and made sure the oven was fully stripped bare. I managed to get the oven to stand on its side and get the trolley under it and then managed to get the trolley and the oven to the back door of the house in one piece, then went and found Cam to give me a hand. I got Cam to control the trolley while I used a large piece of wood as a lever under the trolley so as to get it up the stairs. With the worst part over it was fairly easy to get it into the kitchen and place it into position by the concrete blocks. After a lot of effort it was over and the oven was in place. Now came the wood working bit of fitting the chimney. John had designed the pipe to come out of the oven at a 45 degree angle going through the wall and then straightening out about three feet away from the outside wall going up and about six inches away from the guttering with a bracket that could bolt on just below the guttering. There was another large bracket with a clamp for the pipe and two large arms that could be bolted to the house. The sun was beginning to set as we finished and we were both tired and hungry but happy with the work we had done. Dinner was concentrated on trying to empty the freezer which was finally getting down, we had steak with chips and mixed veges along with gravy. After the dishes were done we settled in front of the TV and watched the news which was virtually a repeat of the mornings. There was a knock on the door and it was who I expected, the Rev. Come in and make yourself comfortable. So what's new I asked. Nothing really everything's the same since I last saw you and everyone seems to be keeping well. Did you manage to get hold of the

Ranger I asked? No, he's not answering his phone or emails so it doesn't look good. I will get you to pass on a message to Bruce, tell him we will go truck hunting the day after the power goes off. What do you think your chances are the Rev asked? I think we have a good chance as there are two main truck stops one each side of us and if we can find a food truck then we are set up for years. When the power goes off we are going to go into the Rangers place to get his food in the freezer and all the other food we find we will put that in the Hall with the food we found under the stage. What I really want from the Ranger place is his rifle and the keys for everything. After that we can make a start on putting a garden there as it is a big fenced off area which will keep all the kangaroos out. In the future the roos and what we can get from the lake will be our only source of easily available protein. Well I think it's time for our daily ration of beer, Cams started brewing as John had so much stock it would of been a waste not to. That's good to hear said the Rev at least it will keep you occupied for a while. We spent the evening drinking and chatting which was far more pleasant than watching the mess on TV and after a few hours called it a night.

Day 17

Woke up to a cold but bright sunny morning, got up and had breakfast and then headed to the TV to see what was left of the world. I turned on the TV and flicked though the channels and found most of them missing, that's strange I thought and went through all the channels again but slowly so as to take note of what was missing. The only channels left were the Government ones. I said to Cam all the private channels are gone and then went to the main Government channel just as the news was beginning. The news said that a lot of the private channels had gone off air and said that in some cases this was from power outages especially in Victoria and South Australia and that this could get worse due to the shortage of essential services personal, they were asking people with past experience in this field who could volunteer to ring the number on the screen. Overseas news was bad as lots more countries had dropped out as their infrastructure and Government had collapsed, it seemed as though most of the world along with our country was sick, but the news finished on a bright note with the military still working well with lots of volunteers and were still getting most of the essential supplies through. We turned off the TV and didn't say anything for a while as we were lost within our own thoughts. We better sort out the oven with wood and stuff, I think I have lots of fire starter cubes in the van and we have lots of paper but I haven't seen much kindling. Cam said there's a big basket in the spare room that we can fill up with wood I'll take it outside. We went outside and found Angela and Jodie working in the garden. Angela was marking out two big plots that would need to be prepared and have the soil turned over. Well it looks as though we have our mornings work all set out for us I said to Cam. You sure have said Angela with a big smile, I have most of the garden sorted out now, and it's just the small parts left to do. Jodie came over and I smiled at her and put my arm around her and crushed her against me. I told Angela about our talk last night with the Rev about the Rangers place and told her that when the power goes off we would go there and empty out the freezer and put the canned food in the hall with the other food we found under the stage. But what we really need are his keys for the sheds, gates and tractors etc and his land because we can make a big fenced off garden there and he has a lot of water tanks for irrigation as well. So when you are finished with this garden you will have to start over there and get some chooks ready for there too. That will be a lot of work said Angela, its fairly large but the fence would be good for the chooks, but still it would be good and keep me busy because when I am not working all I do is worry. How are you going for when the power goes off I asked. I've been worrying about that too she said. Come see what we have done. I showed her that every light switch had a torch under it, then took her to see the kitchen and showed her our new oven. On the way out I showed her where the car batteries would be charged and where the solar panels were. You have been busy haven't you said Angela. Have you got enough torches I asked her? Yes we got heaps last time we went to town but I like your hooks idea, I think I will do that too. I suppose we had better start on the garden. I went to the shed and got a couple of pairs of shovels and gloves and we set to work. By lunch time we had finished and were feeling very tired, our level of poor fitness was really beginning to show. We lunched from the freezer and decided to spoil ourselves and had a bottle of beer each as we were hot and sweaty. After a big lunch and the beer we decided it would be nice to have a snooze so we had a siesta for a couple of hours. After getting up for the second time I said to Cam that we had better do what we were going to do the first time we got up. What was that asked Cam. Get some wood for the stove. We soon had the basket filled with wood and also found a lot of small kindling from

John's wood supply and I gathered together all my matches, lighters and fire starters so we could have everything in the one place for the time being. It was about three in the afternoon so we still had a few hours of sun so I said to Cam let's climb the hill at the back of the house and see the view; it might make a good lookout. Might as well said Cam. As we walked out of the house Cam saw Jodie in the garden and asked her if she knew the way to the top of the hill. Jodie said yes so we asked Angela if she could take us to the top of the hill. We followed Jodie who led us down the road passed David's house to a track which was not all that well used and hard to see. The track seemed to lead directly up the hill then when it reached the steepest part began to zig zag to the top. It didn't take long to get to the top as the track must have been about a kilometer long and taken us to a height of seventy meters. The view at the top was good, looking towards the west you could see our house and the lake, north was all bush, south you could see the park and the hall along with the road, and looking east you could see the main road coming into the lake. It would make a good observation post because it showed you the whole area and would be good for fire watching. Any other tracks leading up here I asked Jodie. There's another one by the sailboat club said Jodie. Let's go down that way so I can see both tracks I said. You had a good view nearly all the way going down and the track was fairly easy going and came out on the east side of the boat club. We will have to take a look in the boat club when the fuel runs out I said to Cam. We walked down to the lake and came back via the rear of the Rangers place following the fence line. At home we put our feet up for a while and then attacked the freezer for dinner having nearly the same meal as we had the other night. When dinner was over it was time for the TV news which again was just a repeat of the morning news and all the private channels were still not working. We carried on watching for a few hours as a couple of good programs came on and then called it a night.

Day 18

Woke up to another nice sunny day. Breakfasted from the freezer which was now only a quarter fill and had coffee. After breakfast we went to watch the news. I picked up the remote and turned the TV on and nothing happened. I think the powers gone. We just had the kettle on half an hour ago said Cam. I turned on a light and nothing happened. Let's go see Angela and see if she's got any power. We knocked on the door and she opened it and said no power? The same with us I said. Could you try your car radio and see if you can pick up any of the local radio stations I asked. We all headed to her car and watched while she turned the radio on and there was nothing there. Well that stations gone let's see if the others are there. All the stations had gone off the air. Well it looks like we are on our own. There's no point in going into town as we would be just in endangering ourselves for nothing. David next door to Angela came over to us and said you've got no power to? I said no and all the radio stations are gone as well. How much food do you have in your freezer Angela? About a quarter full said Angela. Same as us said Cam. What about you David. About the same. I think it's time to see what's in the Rangers place as I don't think we are going to see him again, we will take what's in the freezer and put all the cans and none perishable stuff in the Hall with the other food we found. What I really want is the keys to the sheds as I am hoping that there will be a generator in there and we could keep a freezer running and load it up, a sort of communal freezer. Johns got a massive bolt cutter for cutting reinforcing rod which should get the gate open I will go and get it now then we will all go. In a few moments I was back and all five of us started walking to the Rangers place. The chain on the gate was small so I used the cutter to slice through that and opened the gate. We walked up to the house, the front door was of solid wood so I went to the back to see what the other door was like and found that it was the standard old door of three glass panes so before anyone could change their minds I smashed the center pane and opened the door. I said to the others that I would open the front door for them so they would not have to walk over the glass. I opened the door and let everyone in. You want to sort out the kitchen Cam and I will try to find the key box. I found the office and there was a key box on the wall and also found what I hoped was a rifle cabinet. The key box was locked so I checked the office draws and found some keys but none fitted. I put the keys in my pocket and went out of the office to the back of the counter where I found a tool box from which I took a hammer and a strong screwdriver. The key box was easy to open; I just banged the side in with the hammer and flicked it open with the screwdriver. The box was filled with keys all labeled. I took out the one that said cabinet and tried it in what I thought was the gun cabinet and it opened. There were two rifles there one an old 303 which had been sports modified and now had telescopic sights and the other was a Sterling .22 bolt action and it looked as though there were sights for that at the bottom of the cabinet. I closed and locked the cabinet pocketing the key and took the keys marked shed out of the key box and went to the kitchen to find the others. How's it going I asked Cam. The freezer was full and he's got heaps of food in the pantry. I found the shed keys I said; I had to break open the key box. If the freezer here is full then we are going to have to find a generator to run two freezes, the one here and we will have to add to it a communal freezer where we all put what's left of our own in. Let go take a look at the shed and see what we have got. It was a very large shed that had three roller doors side by side and enough room for two more but this instead had a window and a door. I decided to open the roller doors so as to let in as much light as possible. With all the doors open we could see well in the shed, behind the first door was a tractor with a slasher and at the rear of it on the floor was a big water tank with a pump and hoses which fitted the tractor and ran off the power take off. This was obviously set up for dealing with fires. Next was the Rangers Ute which was a four wheel drive diesel which was well stocked with tools and equipment. Next was a four wheeled trailer with a big plastic 100 liter caged tank with a petrol powered pump at the back of the trailer. He's really geared up for firefighting I said. I went into the workshop part and found what I needed, there was a generator on the floor with two twenty liter cans of fuel next to it along with two big out door extension leads and a couple of power boards. Help me move the generator in front of the fire trailer I said to Cam, there's enough wire here to make it to the house and the generator is still in shelter. We might as well have a barbeque tonight as it will help us empty the freezers and God knows when we will be able to have another one. That's a good idea said David. I have a good barbeque that I haven't used for a while and I need to get it going again. We might as well have it here as the generator should be able to power a few lights as well. If everyone takes out of their freezer meat, sausages, bread etc and start thawing them out now they should be ready for tonight. I will try and bring the Rangers fridge out here and plug it in and we could keep the leftovers in that for tomorrow. Sounds like a plan said Cam, we will have to tell Allen and the Rev. Angela said she would go see the Rev and Allen. I will stay here and get things organized and clean up the glass and fix the door. I said to Cam that I would start by cleaning up the glass and measuring up the door for a board then I was thinking of getting our trolley and taking our freezer out of the kitchen and bringing it here. Might as well said Cam, I'll go home now and meet you there, by the way did you find a rifle. Yes there are two of them in a cabinet I've got the keys for it in my pocket. See you at home. It didn't take long to clean up the glass and I found a tape measure in the toolbox under the counter so I soon had my measurements. I decided to cut two boards as that way it would be a fast fix and it would sandwich the broken glass in the door making it safer. I went home and found Cam all ready to go with the trolley already under the freezer. It took only a few minutes to cut the ply boards down to size and then we were ready to go. The freezer was light and went down the steps easily then we wheeled it to the Rangers and left it outside the back door till we figured out how we were going to do this. We walked into the kitchen and looked around and decided to take the table and chairs outside as they would be useful for the barbeque tonight and that will give us room for the freezer but first let's get those boards on the door. When I was finished the door there was just the table to take outside. Let's get our freezer into the kitchen. We put our freezer between the Rangers fridge and freezer and plugged them all into a five point adaptor and ran the extension lead back to the generator. I checked the generator over then filled it with fuel. The generator looked new and burst into life on the first start. I waited for the motor to settle down and then plugged the extension lead in and turned on the power. The generator seemed to accept the load alright so I left it to do its job. Cam yelled from the kitchen that they were all going. I went over to Cam and said let's take some stuff out for tonight's barbeque. Has the Ranger any beer in the fridge. Yep about twelve VB stubbies. That's good we will add about five bottles out of our stash to that and it should be about right. We went through the freezers and pulled out steaks, sausages, bacon and bread and put them in the fridge to thaw out, we can use the eggs here to and I'll put in the onions from the pantry so everything is in one place. Let's find some boxes and get the canned food out of here and into the hall. When we had finished I said we might as well use the Rangers Ute to take them to the hall and went to the key box and got the keys marked Ute. The Ute was new and started first time and drove easily to the back door, we left the motor running as we loaded it up with about three boxes of nonperishable food then drove to the door of the hall. I still had the hall key on my key ring and soon we had the boxes in the kitchen where we loaded them away with the other food. Just as we were finishing the Rev popped his head around the corner and said hello making Cam jump. You scared me Cam said. How's it going the Rev asked? Good so far I've got two freezers and a fridge running off the generator but we really want to finish the food fast so as to not waste much fuel, but then again fuel only lasts for about a year anyway. You got any food in your freezer Cam asked. Not really it's nearly empty. Did you find your guns the Rev asked? I found two rifles one a 303 and the other a 22 but I haven't found the ammunition yet as I haven't had a chance to look but by law you are not allowed to keep the ammunition with the rifles so the ammos going to locked up some separately. Do you know if Allen's got a rifle I asked the Rev. I don't think so but I will ask him, why? Because I was thinking of giving the 22 to him and the 303 to you. Why the 303 to me. Because it's a high powered weapon and their won't be much ammunition for it because it's very expensive, twenty years ago I was paying a dollar for each bullet for one of those The rifle is very accurate and has a range greater than most modern weapons which gives you a tactical advantage and is powerful enough to go through a cows skull which is what we shall probably use it for in the future. So it's a rifle that will be used sparingly but needs to be well looked after. It's better and safer for all of us if the rifles are spread out and don't forget there are going to be a lot of hungry dogs wondering around in packs out there soon after their masters are all dead. Ok point made I will look after it for you and talk to Allen. I'll bring you over the cabinet so you can keep it locked up. Tomorrow Cam, Bruce and I are going truck hunting. Yes I remember you telling me about it well keep safe and good luck said the Rev. I intend to I said, will you be coming tonight. Yes I will be there said the Rev see you then. Cam drove the Rangers Ute back so as to get used to it. When we got there I said to Cam see if you can find that ammunition, this is the key to the cabinet and it has other keys on it which I think is for the ammunition so see if you can find what the keys fit. I am going to check the freezers and carry on setting up for tonight. While you are searching keep an eye out for anything useful and any first aid stuff you find put it on top of the counter as I was thinking of turning this place into a first aid post. I left Cam to it and went back to check the generator. Everything thing was going fine and we had the table and four chairs outside so all we needed now was a light and a few more chairs. I found two work lights each having a long lead and hung them on the porch and got them ready to go when we needed them. Angela and Jodie arrived carrying bags for the freezer so I showed them the set up and said anything you want to have for tonight just put in the fridge. As Angela left David arrived in his car with his food and barbecue. I showed him the setup and then helped him with the barbeque. As David left I went inside to find Cam. How did you go? Found them all, they are inside the cabinet now. There are about a hundred 303 rounds and four packs of two hundred .22 rounds. I put a packet of .22 rounds in my pocket and closed and locked the cabinet. We might as well drop the cabinet off at the Revs. We loaded up the Ute and Cam drove to the Revs who opened the door as we arrived. The Rev helped me with the cabinet while Cam did the doors and we placed it in his office. I gave him the keys and told him what was in it. I said you can give the other rifle to Allen. I told the Rev that the Ranger had an extensive first aid kit which we have got set up on the counter. I said we were going to leave the place open and the gate unlocked and that it would be a good first aid post for anyone who needs it. Good idea said the Rev what are you going to do for the rest of the day, not much, have lunch and then in the afternoon prepare tools and disinfectant spray for the truck hunt tomorrow. OK we are off as I am getting hungry, see ya tonight. We had lunch and then a rest for a while and talked about what we were going to do tomorrow. I said to Cam that she was going to be security. She would drive the van and stand guard over us while me and Bruce checked out the trucks, we would start from one end of the Truck Stop and work our way to the other first checking them out for people and then selecting which ones to further investigate. Food trailers were the priority but we would take whatever was useful as they would come with batteries and diesel fuel which we could use anyway. While we are there I want to take a look at the solar panel that works the lights and phone and see if we can get that along with the battery. Its time you learnt how to handle and use the pistol I said to Cam. I went to get the pistol and said we will go in the kitchen and use the table. I brought out the belt with the pistol and everything else attached that we took off the policeman in what now seemed like another lifetime ago. I took the pistol out of the holster and removed the magazine and opened the breach to see if there was round in the barrel which there wasn't. With the safety on I tried to pull the trigger just to check it worked then took it off and pulled the trigger so as to get a feel of the trigger tension. I gave the pistol to Cam and said this is yours, it's a fifteen shot semiautomatic which means all you have to do is pull the trigger fifteen times to empty the magazine. If you are ever in trouble or know you have to use it for real put the magazine in load a round in the barrel, put the safety on then take out the magazine and replace the missing round then replace the magazine and you have a sixteen shot semiautomatic pistol and it will really upset someone who has been counting off your shots and now thinks you are helpless. I taught her how to check the pistol and load and reload the magazines and soon she was familiar with the pistol and we knew all the magazines were fully loaded. Next I showed her to shoot using two hands with the magazine out of the pistol. I told her pistols are not all that accurate and most of the time you will miss so if you ever have to use one in anger always use both hands to keep it as steady as possible and always fire three shots at a time at the target. If you use one hand the recoil will shake your hand all over the place, aim low in the center of the target and let the recoil take the bullets up. Cam spent the rest of the afternoon shooting imaginary targets while I got my tools and equipment together and loaded the van and prepared it for tomorrow.

At 4.30 we headed over to the Rangers place and found David already there and getting set up for his cooking. Do you think I should start now David asked? You might as well I said it will start getting dark at 5.30 so get the worst part over now while you still have light. A little latter Angela and Jodie arrived and we sat down and started talking. At 5pm the Rev turned up with Allen so I went to the fridge and gave them along with David a bottle of home brew then got another couple for Cam and I. Do you want a VB I asked Angela it's not as strong as the home brew. Yes thank you she replied. There's some lemonade for Jodie. I returned with the drinks and sat down with all the others. I said welcome to the end of the world party which was greeted by a long and thoughtful silence. Angela said do you think there are many people left. There's always survivors I said but I think they will be in isolated pockets like us, the only way to survive a virus as strong as this is by isolation and even then the virus will have mutated again by next year's flu season and will carry on doing so, I think it would take about 3 years till a virus this strong has mutated into something our immune system can handle. This kind of makes a trap for other survivors who after a year will want to start coming together and make a bigger community which then could be wiped out by the next season's flu because it's still too complex for our immune system to deal with. Flu has always been a case of the Grim Reapers lotto as the numbers have to come up sometime, we have just been lucky that it's taken so long. Allen said but we still need to see if we can get outside news. I've been thinking of that too, Johns got an old monitor radio which has got short wave and long wave on it so we should be able to get all of Australia and some overseas countries to and tomorrow I hope to get some CB radios from the trucks we get. If we make a radio log and record the time and station and date etc. and note what we received we would soon have a fair idea of what's out there though we shouldn't broadcast till we are all agreed as we don't want to make ourselves a target for some one. This could be a good job for you I said to Jodie, have a think about it. Allen said he was going to fix up the paddock at the beginning of town and get some livestock and try and find some horses with the Revs help as he knew where most of the livestock was in the area. I'm going to ask Bruce for a breeding pair of pigs and put them next to the garage and experiment with methane gas. I am also going to turn one of the holiday homes into a barn and put some stalls in for horses, I was brought up on a cattle farm so I know how to handle animals and how to butcher them to. Angela said her piece next. I am going to keep going with the garden and in a few days will start on the Rangers place as I am just starting to get my ideas together. Marks given me a Permaculture Designers manual which teaches you how to set up ecosystems that support themselves with very little work needing to be done after the initial set up, so at the moment I am learning that and Mark and Cam have said they will help me. So when you see Bruce ask him if I can have a breeding pair of Geese for the Rangers place she said looking at Allen.

David decided it was his turn to say his bit and said from tomorrow he would start fishing, he would launch his boat tomorrow and leave it permanently in the in the lake and moor it at the end of the park by the Rangers place where it would be easy for him to walk to. He said he would leave set lines and crayfish pots out overnight and bring them up in the morning. Next the Rev had his say. This has come altogether nicely, it's good that we all have things to do and keep us busy so we don't dwell on all that is lost, we only have each other now and as from tomorrow it's going to be a very different life then what we were used to as we all adapt to life without any power supply. Well it's time to eat said the Rev and I think I will have another beer. It was a good night maybe the last fairly normal night we would have in our new world and we had all come together with a purpose. We called it a night at about 9.30 and shut the generator down as the cold night air should keep the fridge and freezers safe.

Day 19

Cam and I were up early as we knew we had a long and busy day ahead of us and just wanted to get it over with. We went over to the Rangers place and turned the generator on and made our breakfast from the fridge. I had a nice steak and bacon sandwich with a glass of lemonade. After breakfast we headed home and got ready to go and took all our preventive medicines. To them I added a strong Ginseng tablet which would keep us alert and give us energy if needed; I also find Ginseng improves my thinking especially under stress. I gave one to Cam who was another Ginseng fan after I introduced it to her years ago. Cam grabbed the gun belt and was about to put it on when I told her not to wear it as people would see she was armed straight away. I said when you get there carry it like this and took the pistol making sure the safety was on and pulled the back of my shirt out and slid the pistol down my spine and under the belt. This way no one can see you're armed and it is fast and easy to draw and if someone is watching you just pretend you are scratching your butt and draw. It's a good place to hide knifes too. I gave the pistol to her and told her to practice it a few times. When she was happy with the new technique we headed to the van. Cam drove to Bruce's and we parked just after his camouflaged driveway and walked up to the house. We saw Bruce in the shed next to the houses so we headed over to him. I shook his hand and said how's it going. Good said Bruce we are all fine. Got any power I asked. No it went out yesterday. So you ready for some truck hunting? Yeah I've been wandering when you would turn up. On the way back we should pick up the girls and take them back to the lake, I've opened up the Rangers house which can be your home away from home. We will see what happens Bruce said I will be a lot happier when we are finished. I know the feeling I said. We went in and saw the girls, they looked fine and I gave Jessie a hug and said hello to Amanda as I was little weary of her and had left it to Cam to figure her out. We told the girls what we were going to do and I told them that we would be back before 5pm regardless if we got anything or not so they were not to worry till then. If everything goes alright we will pick you up on the way back and take you to the lake with us and stay there over night. We left and told the girls we would see them soon. While Cam drove to the main road I told Bruce about the barbeque last night and what everyone was doing. I told him Allen would be asking for a breeding pair of pigs and Angela would ask the same for the geese. I told him that Allen was going to take over the paddock and holiday homes and turn one into a pig sty and the other into a barn or stable with horse pens and how he and the Rev were going to find cattle and horses or any livestock they could. Allen was also saying that he was brought up on a Cattle farm and he knew how to butcher. Cam had reached the main highway so I told her to turn right which would take us in the opposite direction of town and into a fairly isolated area mainly of bush and hills. We had all been quiet on the highway looking for other cars or any other sign of life but the road was deserted. The sign for the truck stop finally appeared saying 500 meters on the left. Ok Cam lets slow down and go in very quietly. Soon we were at the entrance and Cam turned in and slowed down to a crawl, we could see five trucks, three before the rest area and toilets and two more after them, but what we all noticed first was a body on the road by the third truck which also had the sleeper door open, it looked as though they had fallen out of the door. I told Cam to hide the van behind the first truck so no one could see it from the road. Cam parked at the back of the truck using the trailers tri-axle to hide the van from the road. This is what we are going to do. I go to the first truck go up the steps knock on the widow and say is there anyone there and look through the window to check, when I am sure no one's inside I check to see if the keys are there. Bruce you do the same for the second truck, then we will both do the third truck, then me the fourth and you the fifth. Cam you follow at the rear keeping a distance and looking on both sides of the trucks as you go. OK let's do it. Bruce went first heading to the second truck while I went to the first. The first two trucks had tarp covered trailers and we went up to them and banged the sides asking if anyone was there and looked through the driver's window. No one was in my truck and it looked locked and I couldn't see any keys. I stepped down and looked at Bruce who shook his head and I did the same to him. Bruce walked slowly to the third truck allowing me to catch up. The third truck was a pantec trailer fully enclosed with two big doors at the back so there was a good chance that this one may be a food truck. The body on the ground looked as though it had been there a few days as the crows had been having a feast and now the body was covered with ants that were getting their share. I will do this truck I said but first I will put my mask and gloves on. When I was ready I climbed up and knocked and said is there anybody there and upon no reply looked through the window. No one was inside and the driver's door was locked but the keys were in the ignition. I stepped down and told Bruce and said lets finish this. The next two trucks were both pantec trailers. I did the routine on mine and found it locked and empty. I went over to Bruce who was still banging and saying wake up. When I got there he said there is someone in the sleeper but I think they are dead and the keys are in the ignition. I went to the other side of the truck and looked through the window and could see the back of what looked like someone sleeping, I banged hard on the sleeper but the body did not move. I went back to Bruce and said I think he is dead. Let's check out the toilets and rest area now. Both the toilets and rest area were clear, we were alone except for the dead. Alright let's check the loads starting back at the van. We started undoing the tarp of the first truck and lifted it up to see the load. It was a very mixed load with paint, fencing wire, wood, boxes of hardware and maybe some outside sheds, this must be a delivery to a hardware place said Bruce, I agreed and said this could be handy and started tying down the tarp again. We went over to the next truck and started undoing the tarp. This one was filled with bags of cement and paving grout all on pallets. We retied the tarp and headed to the pantec. I took the wire cutters out of my pocket and cut the security seals on the door then opened the doors. We could see cartons of canned food on shrink wrapped pallets. You want to get in there and have a closer look I asked Bruce. Bruce climbed up, its food all the way and it looks as though they have partitioned the load twice with boards to protect it. Excellent I said and it's the one with the keys in. We shut the doors and headed to the rest of the trucks with Cam keeping her distance and watching our backs. We opened the doors of the fourth truck which was another pantec and looked inside. We could see pallets of shrink wrapped cartons of all different sizes. Bruce went inside and looked around and said it's a mixture of clothes, books, shoes and allsorts probably a Kmart or Woolworths load. We shut the doors and went to the last truck which was another pantec and opened the doors. This turned out to be a load of car and machine parts which were not much use for us. I said it's the food truck and hardware truck for us. I agree said Bruce. We went over to Cam and told her what we had decided. We will do the hard one first I said. We went back to the van and I got the tools I needed and told Bruce to take the wheel brace and smash the passenger's window and get in and unlock the driver's door. I waited by the driver's door till he unlocked it and then I opened the door. I asked Bruce to go to the van and get the disinfectant spray and spray everything you think was touched by the driver while I try to get this started. I had a very small cold chisel used for cutting metal which had a hexagonal end on it; I placed the blade part on where the key would go and used the hammer to smash it in. Next I put a socket on the hexagonal end of the chisel and attached a T bar to the socket with an extendable pipe on the end so as to give more leverage. I slowly added weight to the T bar and heard the crunching sound as the locking mechanism broke and carried on gently till the ignition lights and the low air alarm came one. I got into the driver's seat and checked the gear stick for neutral and checked all the other gauges noting that the fuel tank was three quarters full and the engine kill lever was in. I moved the T bar further taking the accelerator pedal to quarter and the motor burst into life. I let the motor run on a low rev watching the air gauge move slowly up until the alarm stopped and then gave it a few minutes more. Bruce gave me a big smile and the thumbs up. I told Bruce that I was going to drive up next to the food truck and that I would meet him there. I released the brakes and reversed back a bit so I could clear the truck in front and slowly drove up and parked parallel to the food truck. I left the motor running and walked around to the cab of the other truck and found that Bruce was already in the driver's seat with the door open and decontaminating it with the disinfectant spray. Open the door on the other side I said and went round to the other door and got in. I checked the gear stick and found it was in neutral. You might as well start it I said. The motor burst into life straight away along with the air pressure alarm. I told Bruce to run it on a low rev till the alarm stopped. This is a fairly new truck I told Bruce so it should be easy to drive, we are just going to take it slowly, remember to swing out and use the entire road for sharp corners. What's the fuel I asked, half a tank he replied. OK release the brakes and drive forward a bit then stop. Right we will head back now. Follow me and Cam will take the rear, I will get Cam to pick up the girls, we are going to park the trucks at the back of the Ranges place along the back fence line, I will go first and drive down till the end of the fence line you can park behind me. I jumped out and told Cam what we were doing and went back to my truck. I drove out slowly and took my time and did everything in slow motion especially the doubling of the clutch as it had been nearly thirty years since I had driven a truck of this size. The modern trucks were a lot easier to drive then the old ones as the gear selectors were far more positive than some of the old worn out things that I had to drive when I was younger. I took it slowly and drove just under 80ks and it took us about twenty minutes to reach the turn off to the lake. Bruce didn't seem to be having any problems and I could see Cam following behind. I turned off the highway and kept the speed to 50 to 60ks and we slowly made our way home. I slowed down at Bruce's place and gave a long blast on the horn and heard Bruce do the same. In another ten minutes we were home and now came the tricky part which was to turn the truck so as to get it to follow the fence line which was a very sharp turn, I slowed down to a crawl and went over to the other side of the road and way over the verge and waited till the triaxle was close to the corner and swung the truck in and slowly coming round without hitting the fence. I gave a long victory blast on the horn and drove to the end of the fence stopped and killed the motor and breathed a big sigh of relief as it was all over and nothing had gone wrong. It looked as though the Rev had been praying extra hard. Bruce shut down and jumped out of the truck and smiled at me, I went over and shook his hand and said thank God that's over, I feel safe and secure now with 20 tons of food. We went to the back of the truck and saw Angela and Jodie walking over and opened the back doors of the truck. I looked at Jodie and said just the person we need, can you get into the truck Jodie and tell us what each pallet has got on it? The truck had a very mixed load and a lot of the pallets were mixed cartons so you would not really know till you had the pallet out but it seemed as though 80% of the truck was food. Cam arrived when Jodie was about half way through, I said hello to Amanda and Jessie and gave Cam a big hug. Soon after Allen and the Rev turned up. Where's David, he's gone fishing Angela Replied. We stood there listening as Jodie went from pallet to pallet, sometimes getting her to dig a little deeper in the pallet. By the time Jodie was finished we were all very happy. What's on the next truck Allen asked. I smiled at him and said you are going to be very happy we were thinking about you when we got this truck. Bruce if you climb on top of the tarp we will undo the side ropes and pass them up so you can pull up the sides that way it will be easy to tarp again. We soon had the sides up so we could get a good look at the load. It was a mixed load, at the front were two packs of structural pine batons for building houses, these together took up about four pallet spaces on the floor, on the back were four pallets of fencing wire barbed and normal, the normal wire had fence pickets standing up in the middle of it and there seemed to be a lot of fence pickets of different sizes spread out through the load anywhere they could fit. The twelve pallets in the center were a mixture of paint and boxes of different types of hardware. Allen was very happy with what he saw and kept on saying excellent. I said to them all that it feels like Christmas, let's have another barbeque tonight and celebrate. Everyone agreed and we were all very happy. A huge weight had been lifted from our shoulders and now we had hope for the future where before there was doubt and worry. I said to everyone that you will have to excuse us for a while as we are going to decontaminate ourselves and then head over to the Rangers fridge for lunch. After we had decontaminated our self's we headed to the Rangers fridge as there was still enough to feed us. After we had eaten I showed Bruce and the girls the Rangers house especially where the main and spare bedrooms were and told them to make themselves at home as this would be where they would be sleeping tonight. I had better get some food out of the freezers for tonight I said heading out side. Look what I found said Cam who had opened one of the hall cupboards. She pointed to the floor and we saw two cartons of beer, most of the other shelves were filled with towels sheets and blankets. I'll take one of those for tonight I said; I'll put them in the fridge now. After we had the evening meal sorted out I said we might as well start emptying out the food truck while we have extra hands. Could you bring the van over to the truck Cam and put our trolley in the back too, we will load the van with what food Bruce and the girls want. I will get the Rangers Ute, I was thinking of putting all the food along one side of the hall as that way it would be easier to pick and choose what you want and you can see what you have got at glance. Cam came over and dragged me aside and said that's not a good idea. Bruce and the girls probably don't like the hall after their parents died there. Oh crap I forgot, it seems so long ago now. Well not for them Cam said. I think we can handle it Bruce said, I will go talk with the girls they can stay here if they want. Cam and I went to get the cars while Bruce talked to the girls. I reversed the Ute back between the trailers open doors so we could get out most of the first two pallets into the Ute by standing in the back. Bruce and I got the first two pallets out while the girls grabbed what they wanted and put it in the van. The girls didn't want to go to the hall so while we were gone I got them to try and find some chips and nuts for tonight. We drove to the Hall and I reversed the Ute right up to the Hall steps. You want to pay your respects to your parents while I open the hall up and get set up I asked. Bruce nodded and went round to the back of the Hall. By the time I was ready Bruce was back. I will stay up here for half the load then we will swap. I had the trolley so I loaded it right up before I wheeled the cartons over to the back corner of the Hall and kept repeating the procedure till the Ute was half empty then I showed Bruce what I was doing and swapped jobs. In half and hour we were done. We drove back to the trailer and I saw that Cam had taken the pallets out so I reversed in again. You girls can have a go now while Bruce and I have a rest. It looked as though it was going to be tins in cartons all the way till the first partition. By just after four in the afternoon we had about a third of the load out and were fairly tired so we called it a day. Cam had filled the front passengers floor and seat with cartons of what she wanted so we drove home and emptied her load into the kitchen. Before I had left I told Bruce and the girls to go to the Rangers place and make themselves at home and maybe have a rest for a while, that's going to be your home away from home I said so set it up how you want it. After the van was empty we had a rest for a while too. What a good day we have had Cam said we should be able to survive well for a while. Yes I am feeling pleased myself and fairly happy about our future now but still it was strange not seeing any cars on the road or any sign of life, that highway was always busy, it's the main inland highway it just seemed a little unreal, but I am pleased with you, I felt very safe and secure with you guarding me in the rest area you did a good job. I think you would have made a good soldier and no doubt we will have to do things like this in the future. We staid quiet for a while lost in our own thoughts. Just before five we got up and headed over to the Rangers. Bruce and the girls were outside with David who was just about to start cooking. David greeted us and said I see you have had a good day. Yes we did well how did yours go? I caught three fish with the rod which I am just battering now but I have two set lines down and four crayfish pots so we will have to wait till tomorrow to see what happens. Did you see any life out there David asked? No, Cam and I were just talking about that there was nothing at all even the body we found on the road of the truck stop had been there for at least a couple of days it was and felt very strange especially with it being such a busy highway. Angela and Jodie arrived next, Angela had thoughtfully brought along three outdoor chairs for our guests. Jodie quickly went to the other girls and they all started talking, it was good to see her in the company of her own age. David soon had the fish ready to eat and we still had plenty of bread and someone had even found some tartare sauce. It was the nicest and freshest fish I had eaten for years so I took my time and savored the taste. The Rev and Allen came over just as I was finishing the fish. You missed out on the fish I said it was really nice. David had the barbeque on now and was loading it up with food. I went over to the freezers and checked out how much food we had left and said to everyone that it looks as though we have one more night of feasting like this and then we are back to our new reality, so let's enjoy it while we can. I went to the fridge and saw we had about twelve stubbies and twelve bottles of beer and someone had put cans of soft drinks in the fridge to for the girls. Soon all had drinks and were happily talking. Allen told me he was really happy with the hardware truck and it was just what he needed. I told him that I thought there were a couple of farm gates in the center between the pallets. When I am finished with the food truck I was thinking of parking the other truck outside your place so we could both go through the load together and then load what you don't need into the hall. That would be good Allen replied it would make easier work for me. I asked him if he had any ideas what we could do with the pantec when we had finished unloading it. Why don't you drive it alongside the hall, that would make it easier for you to unload and we can use it as a future storage space and you could use the empty pallets as a stair case for going into it. That's a good idea, well that's my work cut out for tomorrow. I told Allen that Bruce was taking the prime mover on the hardware truck home as it has got about three quarters of a tank of fuel in it while the others just got under half a tank. Also he can use the batteries for lighting and I was thinking he could use the CB to communicate with us like what we were talking about with the radio and Jodie. Bruce was listening to what we were saying so I told him how we were thinking of getting Jodie to monitor the radio and CB, he and Jodie could agree on a time and band for transmitting, but its best to stay quiet on the airwaves in case someone is listening because they can easily get our position. It's a bit paranoid I know but its best to see who's out there first, but it would be good for emergencies anyway after Jodie's been listening for a while we will know what's out there. Jodie came over to me and touched my arm and said you're talking about me? So I quickly explained what was said and told her that it was a very important job and if we were in the military she would be known as the Intelligence Officer because she would be the one gathering outside information and putting it all together so as to tell us what's happening in the outside world. This is where your log is an important tool for we will have the time, date, frequency and what the transmission was, with this log we can work out patterns as when to expect transmissions etc so the log is a very important tool.

On top of that I am going to teach you medicine, all those tinctures we started making have to be finished in about four days' time so we have that to do as well. Are you happy with that I asked her? Yes she said I like medicine and I am happy with you she said giving me a kiss on the cheek and going back to the girls. Well it looks like you have made a friend there said the Rev. Cam punched me in the shoulder and said I'll have to watch you. David had our feast prepared and all were hungry and ready for it after smelling the aroma for so long. I thought I might as well make a pig of myself, we only had one more day of this and then we would have to accept our new reality. After we had eaten I went to the fridge and got another beer for us and soft drinks for the girls. Most of the evening was spent discussing our plans and ideas with an interesting one being David's idea of smoking fish which Allen said could be easily adapted to pigs. Bruce was happy with the idea of supplying a breeding pair of pigs and geese and had actually been thinking of the idea himself so he had already selected the animals he just didn't know who to give them too. Allen and Angela were happy with the animals he described to them and he also suggested that we should take all his young fruit trees.

I told Bruce that Angela was learning Permaculture so that would be very handy for her as she could add them to her design. You are going to have to come up with a plan for the whole Lake side park I said to Angela. She poked her tongue out at me which made Cam and me laugh. At about 9.30 we called it a night. I left it to Bruce to turn off the generator and gave him a torch and said I will see you in the morning. Lying in bed Cam said these last two nights have been very productive in organizing ourselves and getting things done. Yeah it's amazing what beer can do, the social lubricant, we are only just really getting to know each other and trust each other, we were lucky that we fell in with such a good bunch of people, but you are right maybe you should suggest to the Rev we do this monthly and have a party and get slightly bent and discuss everything, as the chief brewer you have a big responsibility now. I suffered my second punch in the shoulder for the night and finally gave up and surrendered to sleep.

Day 20

Slept in till about 8am and spent half an hour thinking about getting up. Cam and I finally went to the Rangers place for breakfast at 9am. There were lots of leftovers so we ate well and were joined as we were finishing by Bruce and the girls. So what are your plans for the day I asked Bruce? We've got to go home this morning to make sure the animals are alright. You might as well come back after that and stay the night again as there's enough food left for one more night like last night, the same goes for the beer. After that it's all over we're back to being primitives with no power, how's this for a plan. We will get both trucks going and drive the hardware truck and park it at the garage for Allen and me to unload and I will park the food truck parallel to the hall. Then we unhook your truck and bring the van over and load the sleeper up with food, then you can go home and do what you have to do and come back, by that time we should have more food unloaded and have a fair idea of what's left in the food truck and then you can load up with more and different food tomorrow after a long sleep in. Sounds like a good plan to me said Bruce, you happy with that, girls? They both nodded their heads enthusiastically. When we all had finished eating we headed over to the trucks, you drive the hardware truck I said to Bruce so you can start getting used to it and park it in the garage but leave the motor running so we can unhook it. I watched him start it using my new starter mechanism which he soon mastered and the truck burst into life. Just go straight ahead and drive through the park and I will follow you. The girls jumped in with him for the ride. I went to the food truck and went in along with Cam and followed Bruce through the park and back on the road, he turned in the garage and straightened up while I went passed and turned right and drove down the side of the hall leaving the rear of the trailer level to the front of the hall. I shut down and walked over the road to Bruce and the girls. Jump on to the back of the truck Bruce I said and take the air hoses off, they just twist off and then take the plug out for the lights. OK now jump off, we have to wind down the legs now, I'll show you first. There's two gears in the winder, I straitened the handle then turned it and found that it was in the fast gear, this is the fast gear and its used to get the legs down fast, then I stopped and pulled the handle out toward me and it went into the next gear which is the slow gear, use this when you start lifting the weight of the trailer. I got out of the way so Bruce could do it. He pushed the handle in and started winding the legs down, when the legs touched the ground he took it as far as he could in that gear and then changed into slow. I said look at the turn table and keep going till you see a bit of light. When he stopped I said now you pull the lever out of the turn table. Now jump in the truck and take it out nice and slowly. Soon he was out. Now take the truck for a drive, you're going to find you're really bouncy with all the weight off. It looks as though this truck is designed to carry steel or a low loader for bulldozers so the suspension is highly sprung so if you hit a big pothole at 60ks you might jump off the road. I have in the past so be careful, now go for a drive to get used to it and find a pot hole. Take Cam so she can get the van and bring it back so we can load your food.

I opened up the hall and took the trolley over to the truck and opened the doors and put the trolley inside then got in myself. I started taking the cartons off the pallets and used the trolley to wheel them to the door. Bruce and Cam came back and started emptying the van into the trucks sleeper. When Cam had finished she drove over and reversed to the back of the food truck. Bruce came over and gave us a hand. When the van was fill Bruce said we will go home now, see ya when we get back. See ya then. It was a busy morning and by noon we had the truck half empty and began to get the stairs made of pallets started. One pallet we emptied had been all of flour so I said to Cam that we had better start learning how to make bread as we were the only ones with an oven now. We had also found ten boxes of whole grain brown bread that had not gone stale which we put in the van so as to put in the freezer. Let's have lunch I said so we drove the van to the Rangers and parked by the freezers. I put four loafs in the fridge for tonight and filled the freezer with the rest. We had lunch from the leftovers in the fridge and then decided to go home for a snooze for our levels of fitness were not as good as we hoped. At 1.30 we were back at the hall unloading the truck again and by 2 Bruce and the girls returned. We all set to work in the truck and tried to finish the job by 4.30 when we planned to stop. By the time we stopped we only had three pallets left and the hall was beginning to look like a supermarket, but I was happy because the job was nearly done and we would easily be finished by tomorrow. We closed the hall and the truck and headed to the Rangers for dinner. At the Rangers we found David at work filleting about six fish and he had about eight crayfish. You did well I said, maybe you should go fishing every 3 or 4 days as we don't want to eat them all up straight away. I was thinking the same David said that food truck has brought us time so it would be a good idea to save our reserves. I found I was really looking forward to my fish and tartare sauce sandwich. I sat back and watched David work and saw Angela and Jodie walking along the fence line on their way here. When Angela arrived she saw all the fish and crayfish and said what a feast. David said I will do the fish first and after we have eaten that I will start on the crayfish. I was just starting my crayfish when the Rev and Allen turned up. David put half a crayfish each on a paper plate for the new arrivals. What have you two been up to said Angela you look very sweaty and grubby? We've been rounding up livestock said the Rev between mouthfuls. We kind of got it all sorted out today. David put on the last of the steaks, bacon and sausages along with heaps of onions. I'll get us a beer while you are eating and you can tell us your story when you are finished. When everyone had their drinks Allen began their story. We were thinking about what we could do as we didn't want to overstock the place as we only have one paddock at the moment even though we can turn the park area on the other side of the boat ramp into another paddock which we will do latter on we still can't run a lot of cattle but we do need them to keep the grass down or we will be in big trouble when the fire season comes. So what we've done is sorted out from all the local livestock four pregnant milk cows and one young male to get them pregnant again latter. With all the cattle in the area we have opened up the paddocks into each other so they can move freely and get to water, we will butcher these for our meat starting with the largest herds. We've found a good small livestock truck which we can use and have got it set up for loading the cows we mentioned tomorrow. One of the main reasons we picked the cows we did is that they are fairly tame but we need to tame them down further as I would like to use them as lawnmowers and move them where we need to keep the grass down so the tamer we can make them the more easier they will be to handle. How are you going with the horses I asked? We've seen a few of them and even have a 4wd diesel and float ready to use when we make up our minds we even found a horse buggy along with heaps of saddles and other gear. You've been busy I said. So have you said the Rev, I had a look in the hall on the way over here, that food truck must be nearly empty. Yeah only three pallets left and they will be gone in a few hours in the morning. I asked Bruce how he felt in doing another truck in seven days' time as the trucks should still be able to start easily but this time we would go the other way to the truck stop closer to town. The Kmart truck might be worth collecting as well Bruce said. Yes I have been thinking about that myself but not really looking forward to it. Alright I will see you the same time in seven days. With that settled it was time to call it a night as Cam and I were both fairly tired and the full tummy and the beer was making it worse.

Day 21

Woke up at 7.30 and it was a very cold morning which made it hard to get out of bed. Guess what I found yesterday I said to Cam. What? I went into the Rangers kitchen to wash my hands and turned on the hot water thinking It doesn't matter which tap I use now as hot water is a thing of the past then the water went hot, so I went outside and walked around the house and found some gas bottles which were screened off from the house so you couldn't see them from the road. There were two bottles hooked up and two spare ones. So that means we can have hot showers again and if we take all the stuff stacked on top of the oven we would find that its gas as well which means we can use it to make bread. So next time we go out truck hunting we have to go gas bottle hunting as well. Right I'm getting up and going to have a shower Cam said. I got up a bit latter and headed over to the Rangers to see what was in the fridge for breakfast. I had just finished a nice steak and bacon sandwich when a happy and clean Cam came out for breakfast. Oh God that feels better, I'm so happy that we have hot showers back for a while. I'm hoping that there is some black plastic pipe in the hardware truck, I thought I saw some coils of them on top of the pallet, if so I can coil them flat on the roof and make a solar hot water heater so we will be set when the gas runs out. So, what are we going to do today Cam asked. First we will finish the food truck as there is not much left of it and then we will start on the hardware trailer. We will leave the wood on the front and the wire on the back and just concentrate on the center pallets and see what in them. Bruce was up and searching the fridge so I asked him what time he was thinking of going? In about an hour's time when the girls are ready. I told him what we were going to do today and said when he sees us again in a week's time all the stock from the hardware truck would be laid out in the Hall so he would be able to see and choose from what we had got. Cam and I got up and headed over to the Hall, Bruce said I will see you there and load up some more food. We opened the truck, Hall and the van and were ready to work. The first pallet was made up of cans of fish, tuna, salmon, mussels, oysters and even prawns and a very high pallet it was to, it took nearly half an hour for the both of us to get it into the Hall. Just as we finished Bruce arrived with the girls, this is beginning to look like a supermarket he said about the Hall. What's in the last two pallets Bruce asked. I don't know I have been kind of saving it so each pallet is a kind of surprise, sort of something to look forward to. Well let's get surprised said Bruce. We all headed into the truck and Bruce started pulling off the plastic until I gave him my knife. He cut from the top to the bottom and gave me my knife back and pulled the wrap away. It was a pallet of all different kinds of spreads, all the jams, peanut butter, vegemite, cheese spreads and lots more. The girls were thrilled to see all their favorite spreads especially the jams. I used the knife to cut the wrap off the last pallet and found that it was two thirds full of vitamin and herb supplements with the rest being mostly batteries with a few different kinds of torches. You might as well help us with the spreads pallet I said to Bruce; from the look of the girls they will want lots off that pallet. With five people the pallet was soon gone with a fair bit of it going into Bruce's truck. By the time we had the spreads loaded in the Hall Bruce was ready to go and they all came to say goodbye. See ya in seven days' time I said, we will be round in the morning at about nine or ten. Right see you then. We started on the last pallet and took all the batteries off the top and put them in the hall and then came back and started on the supplements. The main packs in bulk were fish oil, evening primrose oil, Vitamin C, Calcium, Tea Tree Oil and Eucalyptus Oil. Everything else was in mixed cartons. We put most of the bulk items except for the Tea Tree Oil in the Hall and put the mixed boxes in the van so as to take them home. We dragged the last of the pallets out of the trailer and finished the stair case going into it. We might as well do a bit of shopping ourselves I said to Cam, so we went into the hall and loaded the van with all the spreads and cans of fish that we liked. We drove home and emptied the van in the kitchen, stacking up all the supplements against the kitchen wall to be sorted out latter. As it was only 11am we drove out to the hardware trailer to start work on that. We undid the tarp at the front of the trailer and I got on top and pulled the tarp up and walked backwards carefully over the load uncovering about half the trailer. On top of the wood packs at the front were four garden sheds, two big ones on the bottom with two smaller ones on the top. These are going to be heavy I said to Cam, I think we will drive the Rangers Ute alongside and slide them straight into the tray. Let's see what's in the pallets. The first three pallets looked to be mixed loads while the next two looked like bags of different fertilizers. I cut the wrap off the first pallet and said to Cam let's get this one out of the way then we can stand up on the trailer. By the time we had finished the contents of the pallet was spread around the van. We had a collection of hoses both garden and black plastic with all types of attachments, then there were seeds, secatuers, spades, forks, saws, plant boxes, seed trays, complete dripper system kits and much more. Soon we had the other three on the ground all spread out and to add to our haul we had lots of solar water pumps for fountains, hedge shears, small garden hand tools, liquid concentrate plant food as well as pellet form, weed killers and much more. I went up on the trailer and checked out the bags of fertilizer and found that they were a mixture of potting mixes and other products as well. What's in the next two pallets down Cam asked? I laid on top of the bags and started cutting open selected cartons at the top of the pallet and saw they all contained paint. I passed the knife down to Cam and told her to cut open the ones further down. These were also paint. We did the same to the other side and found paint again. Let's go get Angela so she can have a look at all the gardening stuff. We walked to the Rangers and took his Ute for the sheds and while there I checked out the sheds to see if I could make some room for our new stock. We decided to move the fire trailer out of the shed after we took the pump out. This left a fairly large area for storage. We dragged the trailer in front of the tractors shed door and left it there for the time being. Just as I was turning I noticed a half pallet of concrete blocks which gave me and idea. Let's go get Angela I said but first I want to put 6 of those concrete blocks in the Ute. What for Cam asked. It will be a lot easier to show you then tell you and I can show Angela at the same time. We picked up Angela and Jodie who sat in the back of the Ute while we drove to the trailer. Angela was very happy with her haul as everything fitted in with her plans and she could find a use for everything eventually. I showed her the 2 small garden sheds and told her that I could easily turn them into a Goose house and use the same concrete pavers we used for the chooks for the floor. Now the big question is where are you going to put it all. I watched her think and then told her we had removed the fire trailer so she had room in the shed and then I said I had another idea as well, I'll show you. I got the cutters I had put in the Ute and cut the straps on the wood pile at the front of the truck and took six batons off the top. I jumped down and went to the Ute and took out three blocks. I put a baton on the ground and put a block at each end and one in the center then put three batons on top of the blocks. Shelf one I said, then I put three blocks on top of the wood and directly over the other blocks and added the wood and said shelf two and we can go as high as you want. We can do this to the back wall of the shed where the trailer was and then do another at a right angle going out towards the door and then you have lots of shelves to sort out your new stock on. I like it said Angela and it still leaves us lots of space. I was thinking of putting some in the hall I said. Good thinking 99 Cam said. We loaded the van with most of the garden stock and put the rest in the Ute along with lots of batons then Angela took the van and Cam the Ute back to the Rangers shed. It was time for lunch and a rest so Cam and I went home for a while. After lunch we went back to the shed and unloaded the Ute for Angela and then headed back to the hardware trailer. Just as we were leaving I noticed that there were cows in the paddock so we went over for a closer look. We went to the fence but the cows would not come over to us regardless what we did. Oh well they probably have had a stressful day, it looks as if the Rev and Allen dropped them off and went back again. We drove back to the trailer and I got Cam to drive really close to it so we could drop the bags on the pallets straight in to the tray of the Ute. Half an hour later we were done and as we were about to go we decided to put the pallets on top of the load so Angela would have something to stack them on. We drove back to the Rangers and swapped the Ute for the van leaving Angela and Jodie their work for the day. Before leaving we loaded the vans floor with concrete blocks and headed to the Hall and unloaded them just inside the door and drove back to the trailer. Next to come off were the two pallets of paint. We emptied one pallet into the van and then I passed Cam down some batons to lie on top of the load then we headed off to the hall. We started making shelves with the blocks and batons going five high along the back left wall and then brought the paint in. We repeated the process with the next pallet and continued the shelves along the side of the wall. The paint was a very mixed load, it was more bits and pieces and we only had about thirty cartons of the same color and those were mostly small cans but we did have about twenty four large pales of white and brown fence coat which had been loaded on top of the pallets. Let's go see what the last two pallets are said Cam as they look strange. The pallets were loaded with large upright cartons, some about two meters high but only about a foot wide. I jumped up on to the trailer and used my knife to cut the wrap off so I could read any writing on the cartons. I read that they were Galvanized Metal Shelves in kit form. I told Cam and said I will pass you down two and we will take them to Angela and build them up for her that should make her happy. When Cam had them both in the Ute she said what about the sheds? That can be tomorrows job I said. We drove back to the Rangers and showed Angela the shelves and said we would build them up for her. The rest will be good for the Hall as it will make it easier to see what we have got. Cam and I started on a shelf each, we are usually competitive like that as for years in the chemist we both had to assemble the display stands that arrived with stock which were sometimes more like a demented jigsaw puzzle and we prided ourselves for being able to complete the other staffs failures. We finished both at about the same time with Jody enjoying the competition. For the last job of the day we helped Angela sort out the bags and reload them on pallets with mostly potting mix on one and fertilizer on the other. After that we called it a day. We both had the luxury of a hot shower and had a fairly decent meal from the frozen bread and a few selected cans. We had an early night as we were both fairly sore from the day's efforts but were happy with a job well done and knowing that tomorrow would be an easier day.

Day 22

Another cold morning, it was very hard to get out of bed. We were not used to such cold, coming from the sub tropics to the high country was a shock to the system. I got up and looked out of the window and saw there was fog so thick that you probably wouldn't see your hand in front of you. I jumped back into bed and told Cam who said that's good I want to go back to sleep. So back to sleep we went. Lots of fog is one of the joys you get from living next to a lake. We finally got up at 10am and had our breakfast. What are we going to do today cam asked? Today is Jodie day. We are going to get the CB radio and battery out of the truck after we show her how to use it and also get Johns old monitor going plus we have to get the radio logs set up for her. There are some school exercise books in the hall said Cam we can use them for the log. Good thinking, I will get the monitor and see what size batteries it takes and we will get them for her and some spares to. We walked to the Hall via the back of the Rangers place and the front of the lake. It was a cold morning and you could still see patches of fog over the lake. We got four books and the batteries for the monitor and walked back home. How are we going to lay out the book said Cam? We have got to have the date and time so we will put a calendar in the book for her. Next we need the frequency, AM, FM, long wave and short-wave etc then the message. We wrote Monitor on one book and set it up with Date, time, frequency and message. On the other book we wrote CB and set it up with date, time, channel and message. We turned on the monitor and checked it on all frequencies but no signal stood out. Looks as if we are on our own now I said to Cam. They can't all have gone there's got to be someone out there. Well that's for Jodie to find out I said to Cam. We eventually found Jodie in the Rangers shed where she was sorting out with her mum some of the hardware trucks load. We told Angela what we were doing and took Jodie with us to the prime mover truck so she could learn the CB radio before we took it out of the truck. I showed her how the radio worked and went through all the channels with her and listened for a while on each but no one was on the air. I explained to her that when there were storms or lots of low clouds around then that was a good time to put more effort into it as the radio waves would bounce off the clouds to the earth then up again and so on and this would give you extra-long range. After we took the radio, aerial and battery out of the truck we went back to see Angela. Angela said it would be better to set everything up in the Rangers kitchen as we will be here a lot of the time now especially since the showers here as well as a lot of our work. We set the CB and radio monitor up in a corner of the kitchen with the battery on the porch and the aerial and solar charger on the roof and then got Jodie to organize everything how she wanted. I told her not to stick to regular times at first but to listen randomly and see what happens and explained to her that the most important thing was to log and record everything she did especially in covering different frequencies at different times but save your first entry till you find something. It was lunch time now so we took a break and had a feed and discussed what we would do in the afternoon. We decided we would build all the shelves so we took the van to the hardware trailer and cleared out all the shelf kits and took them to the hall and started assembling them we had about 16 cartons of shelves from the pallet. We were getting good and by 3pm we had assembled them all. We took two shelves and delivered them to Angela who was still sorting out the gardening supplies and left the van there and picked up the Rangers

Ute so as to pick up two of the garden sheds. We drove the Ute close to the side of the trailer so as to slide the heavy cartons from the top of the wood pile straight into the Utes tray. This worked well and we were soon loaded. We drove back to Angela and with her we tried to decide where to build the new house for the geese. In the end we decided to build it against the small side of the Rangers main shed facing the lake as this would be in the shade all the year so the geese would stay cool in the summer. We spent the next hour figuring out how we were going to build it and finally decided to build a shed on each end and fence off the gap in the middle bringing it out so they would have a spacious run and build another door in the center of the fence. We would load up the sheds with nesting boxes and use the gap between for water and feeding, it would be a good lock up for them till they got used to their new home. We opened up one of the shed cartons and laid it out on the ground to see what we had. The walls were just slightly over head height so it was and ideal size for the geese and as we were using the Rangers shed wall I had to figure out how to join everything together. Eventually I decided the easiest way would be to put two batons together so as to make a 4 by 4 and bolt two of them to each end of the shed wall and build the sheds out from this. We decided to use the rest of the day transporting and laying the concrete pavers from Johns store that we had used for the floor of the chook house. By the end of the day we had two floors nearly complete and everything we needed to complete the job for tomorrow. It was still cold and cloudy and looked as if it was going to get worse so I suggested to Cam that it might be a good time to test our new oven and have a nice warm evening. We headed home and went in the kitchen. Well there's no point having a fridge and electric oven in here anymore let's get rid of them. Cam emptied what was left of the fridge while I went out and got the trolley. Soon we had them both out of the kitchen with the only problem left being the big mess on the floor especially behind the oven. Cam cleaned up while I got the new oven ready for its first fire. The fire box was very large so I had the room to build a decent fire. In about twenty minutes the fire was going well so I added to it a bit of coke and coal and closed the door. John had a really big pot maybe about ten liters in size so I filled it up with water and put it on the element with a lid on. I figured that if we wanted to boil water we could use a little sauce pan and take the water out of the big pot but at least while the oven was going we would have a constant supply of hot water. In about an hour our new oven had warmed the room so much that we had to take some clothes off to stop ourselves from sweating. It works well Cam said and I'm so glad we have the couch in here. We had a rest for a while and then made dinner. In the early evening the Rev came and paid us a visit. He was looking tired but happy. They had sorted out all the livestock that they wanted and had just transported 2 pregnant mares who were now in the paddock with the cows temporarily until they started fencing and setting up the stables. They also had a stallion that they were going to bring in latter, it was the one at the place where the horse buggy was and apparently it had been used for the buggy so there would not be much training needed. I got us all a bottle of beer made cold by being in a bucket of water under the house. The Rev was very impressed with our oven as he already had to take his coat and jumper off. So what are you and Allen going to do next Cam asked the Rev. We are going to put a fence between the last holiday house and the garage and turn the last holiday house into a stable. Then join up the fences to the first paddock. Then we are going to fence off from the back of the garage and my place including the big field area on the other side of the boat ramp by the hall so in the end we will have three separate paddocks. You're going to be busy especially turning the house into a stable and that's heaps of fencing you're talking about. What about when we have finished empting the trailer hooking it up to the truck and taking it into the back corner of the paddock on the other side of the boat ramp and reversing it into the lake, That way you don't have to do fencing in the water as the trailer would be twenty to thirty feet into the water which would stop most animals getting around it, you could use the legs of the trailer as the first straining post and start from there. That's a good idea the Rev said, it would save us a lot of work and I don't think you could get a better straining post then a semi-trailer, I'll tell Allen tomorrow. Jodie's got the battery from the truck powering the CB in the Rangers kitchen so we will have to put it back in the truck to start it. What are you up to tomorrow the Rev asked? We are building a house for the geese using the Rangers lake side shed wall as the back wall. We took two garden sheds off the truck and will use them by having a shed at each end joined by a fenced off enclosure. There are still two really big garden sheds left on the trailer. Also we had two pallets of galvanized steel shelving and have assembled some for Angela and also for the Hall. Well I'm off said the Rev, your beer did the trick of making me want to go to sleep; besides I am stiff and sore from the day's work. We said goodnight to the Rev and decided to sleep ourselves.

Day 23

Woke up to another very cold morning with fog so we slept in till about nine then got up and had coffee and breakfast. After breakfast we headed over to the Rangers to continue building the goose house. We decided to do the hard part first which was to bolt the four thick pieces of wood to the existing sheds wall so as to build out our new sheds from them. So the first job was a trip to the hardware trailer to get the wood then followed by a lot of cutting. I already had the bolts that I needed but the problem was going to be drilling the holes and there was no way to do that except with the electric generator. I found the drill and bits that I needed along with the extension lead and plugged into the generator which I had just started for the freezer so as to keep the last of our bread frozen. I had been running the generator for about 45 minutes every 4 hours during the day so as to keep the bread frozen. It took nearly an hour to get all four of the pieces of wood bolted to the wall of the shed with me on the outside and Cam on the inside putting the washers and nuts on the bolts. After that it was fairly straight forward and by lunch the two sheds were up. Each shed had a door on the front had a window on the side looking out away from where the caged area was going to be. After lunch we came back to finish our work and saw Angela there with Jodie looking at the sheds, she said don't worry about putting nesting boxes in as I will use the ones in the old chook house. I told Angela that tomorrow all the herbal tinctures we were making would be ready to be finished and it would be an all day job so she wouldn't have Jodie with her tomorrow as she would be finishing her lessons on how to make tinctures. She's been looking forward to that Angela said. In a few hours our work was complete, there was now a chicken wire fence running from shed to shed which extended out from the sheds and had another door in the middle. Cam and I decided to spend the rest of the afternoon sorting out the hall. Now that we had shelves we thought we would sort out all the hardware that had been mixed in with the food which was mainly batteries, cleaning products, bags of barbeque coke, a few cartons of cheap motor oil and all the stationary as this would make it a lot easier to find things in a hurry. Latter when we were finishing Cam said we are getting quite a lot of loot aren't we. There will be a lot more yet I said we might as well get all we need while it's still easy, remember our fuels only going to last for a year then that's it. Let's go for a walk and check out the new paddocks they want to make said Cam. The paddock went for a fair distance, about 150 meters along the lake with about 100 meters away from the lake to the bush line. There weren't any picnic tables in this area and they would save a lot of work by not having to fence the lake front and you wouldn't have to worry about water for the livestock. It was a nice walk along the waterline and there were lots of bird life especially ducks. As we started back we could see in the distance a boat coming in by the Rangers. Must be David coming in said Cam, yummy fish and crayfish for dinner, I can't wait. By the time we got to the Rangers David was already there. I thought it was time for another protein hit said David. What did you get asked Cam? Seven fish and seven crayfish David replied. Are you going to do them like last time she asked, as they were really yummy? Sure am David replied. Jodie came out of the shed to have a look at the fish and crayfish. Do you know where the Rev and Allen are I asked Jodie? Yes they are next to the first paddock putting up a fence along the bush line. Do you want to go over and tell them that dinner will be ready soon? Alright Jodie said and ran off. I might get half a dozen bottles and put them in the freezer I said to Cam. I'll come with you and help you carry them. We went home and put three bottles into two different bags so we could carry back a bag each and went back to the Rangers and put them in the freezer and buried them deep in the bread so as to cool them rapidly. Jodie told us the Rev and Allen was just finishing and were going to clean up and come over. David had everything prepared and ready to go. We had better get the tables and chair ready I said to Cam. Soon all was ready and David came out of the kitchen with a couple of loaves of bread which he had thawed out along with a tray full of different sauces, vinegar and salt. Next Jodie came out of the kitchen with a couple of big bags of chips and some peanuts and paper plates along with plastic knife and forks. The Rev and Allen arrived and on seeing them David started his cooking and Jodie went to find her mum. Soon we were all sitting and comfortable and Cam went to the freezer and got us a beer each and a cold can of lemonade for Jodie. Cam said to Angela why don't you give Jodie a small shandee. What's a shandee Angela asked? Half a glass of beer or smaller topped up with lemonade, that's what my parents used to give us on special occasions like this, mind you we only got one of them. Alright make her a shandee then. Cam got a glass and filled it half with beer and half with lemonade and gave it to Angela for a taste. I like it Angela said I might have one for myself she said giving the glass to Jodie. Jodie took a curious sip and said that's nice. We all had a battered fish sandwich on which I put on mine tartare sauce, that was followed by a crayfish each cut in half soaked in garlic butter with seafood sauce spread on top or in my case one half with tartare sauce. We were all happy and quiet as the freshness really added to the taste. My pretty seafood glutton Cam was in heaven. A pleasant night was had by all and time went by fast and it was soon time to call it a night as the temperature was dropping fast.

Day 24

Woke up to a very cold foggy morning, winter was really beginning to set in. I said to Cam we need more blankets, I think I will get one of those sleeping bags and open it up and use it as a quilt. That's a good idea Cam said can you do it now? Not really I replied but after a while I decided to get up anyway as I had a very busy day ahead of me as today all the tinctures that we had made were now ready to be shook for the last time and then double filtered and bottled. The filtering part takes a long time so I had better start early. I told Cam what I was going to do and got up. I'll get that that blanket for you now. I got dressed and went through the sleeping bags and found the thickest and unzipped it and opened it up turning it into a blanket and then put it on the bed. I made breakfast and had a coffee to wake up and decided to fire up the oven to make it warm as we would be spending most of the day in the kitchen. After the fire was made I decided I would make the tinctures of Echinacea and Licorice first for these were the main herbs and they were going to be in the largest quantities of tinctures to be made. Another reason was because Jodie already knew a lot about these herbs so I'll get them out of the way while she is not here. After that I will start on Andrographis because that one is my largest quantity and will take some time to filter and Jodie should arrive while I am doing that. Luckily John had lots of large measuring jugs which are what I normally use for filtering tinctures. I started with Echinacea and got two jugs and put a funnel in each and a coffee filter in each and shook the large jar of Echinacea for the last time. I then opened the jar and was careful not to let too much herb fall on the filter and block it which would lengthen the filtering time. Next I got my bottles and adhesive labels ready and put the biggest funnel into the mouth of the bottle along with the filter. The tincture would be filtered once going into the jug and a second time going into the bottle. In half an hour I was finished with the Echinacea and started with the Licorice. When the Licorice was finished I started on the Andrographis which would be the last of the large quantities to do and went out to get Jodie. I showed Jodie where we were up to and how much we had left to do. I will tell you about the herb we are filtering now as it's not a well-known herb but one of the good things about being a western herbalist is that we use anyone's herbs especially when they are really good. The actions of Andrographis are antiviral and bacterial along with being an immune stimulant. It has an anti-inflammatory action as well which is important especially in the strain of flu that we have now because it is the inflammation that kills you. The herbs mainly used in India and China and some people claim that it stopped the Spanish flu in India in 1919. Now this herb is a popular treatment for stopping or reducing colds and flu. So for this herb in fighting our flu the most important actions are anti-viral, immune booster and anti-inflammatory as we can combine them with lots of other herbs that share the same action thus adding to the strength of our formula and attacking the roots of our disease. The joy of talking is that it makes time go by faster and work more pleasant. Right, now that one is finished we shall start on Boneset next. We gave Boneset its last shake and started filtering it in our two jugs and found and labeled a bottle for it and set up a funnel and filter. Boneset is the specific for fevers but more of the nasty type of fevers where it feels as if you have been belted all over with a baseball bat and you hurt and ache all over especially in the limbs. The name comes from break bone fever and in our flu we use it for the mid to last stages as an immune stimulant, diaphoretic which means for reducing fevers and as an anti-inflammatory for reducing the pain. This was used in America during the Spanish Flu with good results. For your information the Spanish Flu was called the Spanish Flu because all the countries at war in WW1 were under censorship so it was not mentioned in their newspapers but as Spain was neutral and didn't have censorship they could write about it in their newspapers while all the countries at war tried to keep it a secret. The Spanish flu killed more people then WW1 did. My grandfather caught it while fighting in the trenches during that war and says the only reason he survived is because their sergeant forced them to eat. When we had finished with Boneset I told Jodie to bring over Pleurisy Root and give it a good shake. After we were set up and filtering I started to tell Jodie the story about Pleurisy Root. This is a bit like Boneset as you use it for fevers but with this it is usually fevers associated with the lungs. Its other actions are expectorant which help with coughing usually by letting you bring up all the mucous in your chest or by making it easier to. The other main action is as an antispasmodic which means it works on the nervous system. Spasms are like twitches or cramps and are usually painful. Sometimes when you cough and cannot stop that's a spasmodic cough. But in the lungs the scary spasms are when the little pipes called the bronchioles start spasming and you can't breathe this happens in asthma. This strain of flu is taking out all the asthmatics which make this herb very important. Pleurisy itself is a very nasty and painful disease, I have had it myself so I know. To give you an idea of how it works imagine the inside of your ribcage being a big plastic bag coated all over with oil. Now inside this plastic bag is the lungs, one on each side in their own plastic bag but this bag is covered in oil on the outside. When you breathe in and out your lungs go up and down and when this happens the bags are sliding freely against each other even when you are running and breathing fast. This is what it is like inside the body, imagine what it would be like without the lubricant with everything scraping against each other and jamming up. When something goes wrong and the oil is not produced which is usually during a very serious infection it feels as if the lungs are scraping against the ribs and it is extremely painful. Some people during this condition like me lie on the side that is sore usually with a pillow there and they try to crush it into the ribs as much as they can so as to reduce the pain, it can be common to see them lying on the floor crushing the pillow into the side of their chest and breathing as shallowly as they can. If you see someone doing this then you know what they have got. For our flu we would use this herb with Boneset in the middle to last stages of the flu depending on the individual's symptoms. When we had finished I decided to do Mullein next so I got Jodie to find it and give it a last shake. When we had it set up and filtering I started to tell Jodie about the herb. Remember the last herb we talked about it was more about pain especially about pleura pain, what other pains can you think of that happen with the lungs. Jodie thought for a while and said when you cough and your chest hurts and all your pipes feel sore. Yes that's a really good one I replied and coughs can also make you hoarse and give you a sore throat. I picked this herb because it's mostly about soothing pains in the chest and is an anti-inflammatory so it tries to reduce inflammation which in turn reduces pain but also it is a strong demulcent which means it can soothe and coat inflamed areas and make them less sensitive. And what other herb have we used recently that is an anti-inflammatory and demulcent. Licorice Jodie replied. I thought to myself this girls brighter than me. Very good, have you ever had lots of Licorice like maybe those Licorice straps that you can buy? I think so she replied. What did your tongue and throat look like when you were finished? They were all black. That's Licorices demulcent action at work it coats and soothes and whatever we coat we will also get the anti-inflammatory action as well. Mulleins specifics are bronchitis and hard coughs and like Licorice it is also an expectorant. I think we will stop for lunch now I said to Jodie as I don't want to overload your mind, have lunch then a rest and come back in a couple of hours say about 1.30. Jodie went on her way and I decided to carry on filtering and get most of the work out of the way and leave only three herbs to do for when she come back, these would be the most important of the herbs left. After setting up I stoked up the oven fire again and went to see what Cam was up to. I found her in the spare room working on the next brew and told her Jodie had gone home for a few hours and that we might as well have lunch now. After lunch I carried on with the filtering lying on the couch snoozing between top ups and thinking that we were very lucky to have such a big comfortable and warm kitchen. I was wondering how cold the winter would get here and thought I would ask Jodie when she returned. Soon it was 1.30 and Jodie was back. Could you get the Elderberry and give it a last shake I asked Jodie. I set up the jugs, funnels and filters then she came over and carefully filled up the funnels with tincture. This tincture is made from the flowers and the berries it has more flowers then berries. Elder is the main European herb for colds and flu's and has been used for this for hundreds of years. It works mainly in the upper respiratory area in the chest so it's good for colds and runny noses etc. For this flu we would combine it with Boneset which would add to Elder's work of fever and aches and pains. After Elder I got Jodie to get Elecampane. When Jodie was ready and had the tincture filtering I told her that this herb was very useful for children especially when used with Horehound which will be our next herb. Elecampane is used for irritating coughs especially in children and is used when there is lots of phlegm and mucous to help bring it up as it is also an expectorant and gets the rubbish moving. This herb is known to soothe the cough to but one of the main reasons I use it is because it is also an antibiotic and the other reason is that it is good for asthmatics so I chose this herb in case I have to deal with asthmatic children which this flu seems to pick on. I got the last herb Horehound to add to this one especially for anyone whose cough was getting bad or out of control. Horehound is the main herbal expectorant with its main problem being its bad taste as it is very bitter so it's usually mixed with sweet syrups. So Horehound is the main herb for coughs, it has a antispasmodic action as well so it's helpful in the nasty coughs such as whooping cough were sometimes you can't stop coughing to breathe. Well that's it I said to Jodie, don't worry Ill clear up the mess. She smiled and said see ya latter and was off. I went to find Cam and see what she was up to and found her in the spare room brewing. How's it going? Good she said when this batch is ready it will replace all that we have drunk already. That's good we are doing well, what are we going to have for dinner I asked? Haven't a clue Cam replied. Let's go for a walk to the hall when you are ready and we will figure it out. Let's go Cam said. We walked down the streets for a change and could see the Rev and Allen in the distance putting up the fence along the bush line. So what are we going to get, we are going to need some protein and we are not going to get much out of canned food except fish other than that I think the only other protein is those cans of Spam though beans have a small amount. We went into the hall and started looking round trying to make up our minds. After a while I said we will just have to experiment, how's this for a start. We will go for a sachet of flavored precooked rice which will give us our carbohydrates, take a couple of cans of vegetable soup for flavor and fiber and a can of Spam and dice it up for our protein. We might as well give it a try said Cam we have to start somewhere. I was thinking that in the past before fridges and electricity they had what was called eternal soup in other word a pot with everything in just left on the stove or fire all the time and just emptied and added to all the time with the heat keeping the bacteria away. I don't know said Cam it sounds a bit scary we will just have to see what happens. Maybe before we go to bed we stoke up the fire so it will be warm for breakfast. We got home and I decided to start cooking while it was still light. The first thing to figure out was which pot I should use as the eternal pot. I decided to use an old mid-size stainless steel one and soon had all the ingredients in leaving the Spam till last but I had it out of the tin all diced up. It wasn't long before it was ready. The meal was alright but a bit bland for our tastes. I'm missing meat already I said to Cam, even if Allen butchered something we haven't a fridge or freezer to preserve it and you had better be careful to as you need your iron, we had better start taking our multivitamins I miss butter the most Cam said and milk as well. We talked through the evening of all the things we needed, liked and missed the most and started to make plans to get them back. The fridge was important we would have to hunt down caravan LPG fridges or maybe if we were really lucky we could find a kerosene fridge. We should be able to get power back by finding a house with solar power and stripping it for what we need. We decided that a month from today we would go into town and get what we needed and stay for a few days to get it all done. Finally at 9 we called it a night and headed to bed.

Day 25

This is where the novel finishes as the small community has survived. Next year's strain will still most likely be a killer but isolation could save them though those who try to establish big communities could be in trouble.

Medical Terms

Adenopathy - Disease of the Lymphnodes.

Bradycardia - Is the resting heart rate of under 60 beats per minute although it is seldom symptomatic until the rate drops below 50 BPM. It sometimes results in fatigue, weakness, dizziness and at very low rates fainting. A waking heart rate below 40 BPM is considered absolute bradycardia.

Catarrh - Inflammation of the mucous membranes in one of the airways or cavities of the body. It is a symptom usually associated with the common cold and chesty coughs, but can also be found in patients with infections of the adenoids, middle ear, sinus or tonsils. The phlegm produced by catarrh may either discharge or cause a blockage which may become chronic.

Coryza - Is a word describing the symptoms of a "cold". It describes the inflammation of the mucous membranes lining the nasal cavity.

Cutaneous - The adjective cutaneous means of the skin.

Desquamation - Meaning "to scrape the scales off a fish, also called skin peeling, is the shedding of the outermost membrane or layer of a tissue, such as the skin.

Dysphagia - Medical term for difficulty in swallowing.

Dyspnea - Also dyspnoea; shortness of breath or air hunger, breathlessness.

Ecchymosis - Is the medical term for a subcutaneous purpura larger than 1 centimeter or a hematoma, commonly, but erroneously, called a bruise. That is, bruises are caused by trauma whereas ecchymoses, a type of purpura, are not caused by trauma. The term also applies to the subcutaneous discoloration resulting from seepage of blood within the contused tissue.

Epigastrium - Is the upper central region of the abdomen.

Erythema - Is redness of the skin, caused by hyperemia of the capillaries in the lower layers of the skin. It occurs with any skin injury, infection, or inflammation

Febrile - Means fever.

Hemoptysis - Is the expectoration (coughing up) of blood or of blood-stained sputum from the bronchi, larynx, trachea, or lungs (e.g., in tuberculosis or other respiratory infections or cardiovascular pathologies).

Macule – A macule is a change in surface color, without elevation or depression and, therefore, nonpalpable, well or ill-defined, variously sized, but generally considered less than either 5 or 10 mm in diameter at the widest point.

Malaise - Is a feeling of general discomfort or uneasiness, of being "out of sorts", often the first indication of an infection or other disease. Malaise is often defined in medical literature as a "general feeling of being unwell".

Myalgia - Means muscle pain and is a symptom of many diseases and disorders. The most common causes are the overuse or over-stretching of a muscle or group of muscles. Myalgia without a traumatic history is often due to viral infections.

Nares - Is one of the two channels of the nose, from the point where they bifurcate to the external opening.

Nephritis - Inflammation of the kidney.

Papule – A papule is a circumscribed, solid elevation of skin with no visible fluid, varying in size from a pinhead to less than either 5 or 10 mm in diameter at the widest point.

Paroxysmal - attacks or paroxysms are a sudden recurrence or intensification of symptoms, such as a spasm or seizure. Can be observed in various clinical conditions such as multiple sclerosis or pertussis, but they may also be observed in other disorders such as encephalitis, head trauma, stroke and asthma.
Paroxysm means "sudden attack, outburst.

Parotitis - Is an inflammation of one or both parotid glands, the major salivary glands located on either side of the face, in humans. The parotid gland is the salivary gland most commonly affected by inflammation.

Petechiae - Refers to one of the three major classes of purpuric skin conditions. Purpuric eruptions are classified by size into three broad categories. Petechiae is generally used to refer to the smallest of the three classes of purpuric skin eruptions, those that measure less than 3 mm.

Prodrome - Is an early symptom that might indicate the start of a disease before specific symptoms occur. For example fever, headache and lack of appetite frequently occur in the prodrome of many infective disorders.

Purpura - Is the appearance of red or purple discolorations on the skin that do not blanch on applying pressure. They are caused by bleeding underneath the skin usually secondary to vasculitis or dietary deficiency of vitamin C (scurvy). Purpura measure 0.3–1 cm (3–10 mm), whereas petechiae measure less than 3 mm, and ecchymoses greater than 1 cm.

Pyaemia - Is a type of septicaemia that leads to widespread abscesses of a metastatic nature. It is usually caused by the staphylococcus bacteria by pus-forming organisms in the blood. Apart from the distinctive abscesses, pyaemia exhibits the same symptoms as other forms of septicaemia. It was almost universally fatal before the introduction of antibiotics.

Rhinorrhea - Is a condition where the nasal cavity is filled with a significant amount of mucous fluid. The condition, commonly known as "runny nose", occurs relatively frequently. Rhinorrhea is a common symptom of allergies or certain diseases, such as the common cold or hay fever.

Stridor - Is a high-pitched wheezing sound from turbulent air flow in the upper airway. Produced by narrowed or obstructed airway path. It can be indicative of serious airway obstruction from severe conditions such as epiglottitis or foreign body lodged in the airway. Stridor is indicative of a potential medical emergency and should always command attention.

Vesication - Means blister.

www.ingramcontent.com/pod-product-compliance
Lightning Source LLC
Chambersburg PA
CBHW080233180526
45167CB00006B/2260